Humane Health Care for Prisoners

Humane Health Care for Prisoners

Ethical and Legal Challenges

KENNETH L. FAIVER

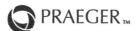

An Imprint of ABC-CLIO, LLC

Santa Barbara, California • Denver, Colorado

Library of Congress Cataloging-in-Publication Data

Names: Faiver, Kenneth L., author.
Title: Humane health care for prisoners : ethical and legal challenges / Kenneth L. Faiver.
Description: Santa Barbara, California : Praeger, [2017] | Includes bibliographical references and index.
Identifiers: LCCN 2016054652 (print) | LCCN 2016055723 (ebook) | ISBN 9781440855504 (hard copy : alk. paper) | ISBN 9781440855511 (ebook)
Subjects: | MESH: Prisoners | Prisons—organization & administration | Community Health Services—ethics | Community Health Services—legislation & jurisprudence | Holistic Health—ethics | United States
Classification: LCC HV8833 (print) | LCC HV8833 (ebook) | NLM WA 300 AA1 | DDC 365/.667—dc23
LC record available at https://lccn.loc.gov/2016054652

ISBN: 978-1-4408-5550-4
EISBN: 978-1-4408-5551-1

21 20 19 18 17   2 3 4 5

This book is also available as an eBook.

Praeger
An Imprint of ABC-CLIO, LLC

ABC-CLIO, LLC
130 Cremona Drive, P.O. Box 1911
Santa Barbara, California 93116-1911
www.abc-clio.com

This book is printed on acid-free paper ∞

Manufactured in the United States of America

Contents

Preface   xi

Acknowledgments   xv

Explanatory Notes   xix

Introduction   xxiii

1. **Ethics in the Context of Correctional Health**   1
    Common Mission   1
        Recognizing Differences   2
    A Brief Historical Perspective   2
    Ethics   6
        Definition of Ethics   6
        Ethics and the Law   7
        Dignity of the Human Person   8
        Professional Codes of Ethics   10
            Meaning of a Professional Code of Ethics   11
    Important Ethical Issues in Corrections   14
        Beneficence, Medical Neutrality, Medical Autonomy   14
        Privacy, Patient Autonomy, Confidentiality, Acceptability   14
        Informed Consent and Enforced Treatment   18
        Informed Refusal   22
        A Caring Approach   22
    Some Practical Ethical Issues in Corrections   27
        Transgender Issues   27
        Forensic Use of Medically Obtained Information   30
            General Principles   30

DNA Testing   32
Body Cavity Searches   33
Strip Searches   36
Evaluation of Competence   39
Concept of Predicted Dangerousness and Medical
    Parole Issues   40
Medical Restraint   41
Directly Observed Therapy   41
Crushing Medications   42
Organ Transplants   43
Treating or Diagnosing under Less-than-Satisfactory Conditions 43
Patient Assessment through a Closed Door   44
Drawing Blood through the Bars or through a Food Slot   45
Undue Noise   46
Unnecessary Risk to Safety of Health Care Staff   46
No Sink or Running Water   47
Defective or Inadequate Equipment   47
Methods of Preventing HIV Transmission   48
Food Loaf   49
Hunger Strikes   50
Conclusion   53

2. Areas of Significant Ethical Role Conflict   **55**
Ethical Role Conflict Situations   55
Medical Clearance for Punishment   56
Use of Mace   58
Writing Tickets   59
Use of Medication for Behavior Control   60
Shakedowns Performed by Health Professional Staff   61
Witnessing the Use of Force   61
Participation in Executions   62
Position of the American Pharmaceutical Association   68
Treatment to Render a Person Competent for Trial   70
Determination of Competence to Be Executed   72
Treatment to Render a Person Competent for Execution   74
Involvement with Acts of Torture   75
Reporting Abuses by Staff   79
A Note of Caution—Erosion and Burnout   81
Conclusion   84

3. Other Challenging Topics in Ethics   **87**
Ethical Reasoning   87
Biomedical Research and Experimentation   88
Working in the Context of a Blemished History   88
First Steps toward Regulation of Biomedical Research
    in U.S. Prisons   90

Institute of Medicine Recommendations and Some
  Critical Responses   98
Encouraging Appropriate Research   101
How Do We Bring It All Together?   102
Housing the Mentally Ill in Isolation or Supermax Settings   104
A Vicious Cycle   107
Extreme Segregation, Isolation, and Supermax Settings   109
Chemical Castration by Court Order   115
Is It Legal?   115
Is Physician Participation Ethical?   117
Retrospective Clues for a Current Ethical Imperative   120
Conclusion   121

4. **Legal Issues in Correctional Health Care**   **123**
What the Courts Have Done   123
Hands-off Policy   124
A Break in the Hands-off Era   125
Holt v. Sarver   127
Newman v. Alabama   128
Estelle v. Gamble   128
Tort Liability   130
Deliberate Indifference   131
Qualified Immunity   133
Farmer v. Brennan   134
Civil Rights of Institutionalized Persons Act   135
*Bivens v. Six Unknown Agents of the Federal Bureau
  of Narcotics*   136
Pulling in the Reins   136
Prison Litigation Reform Act of 1996   137
Urgent Need for Reform of the PLRA   140
Miscellaneous Legal Issues   143
Adequacy of Funding   143
Persons with Disabilities   143
Adequate Documentation   148
Health Insurance Portability and Accountability Act   149
Special Problems of Juveniles   149
Some Important Legal Cases   150
Cases Concerning Adults   151
Cases Concerning Juveniles   156
Strategies to Avoid Litigation   159
A Checklist of Risk-Prone Areas   159
Don't Fight the Courts   162
Impact of the Courts   163
A New Challenge—The Impact of Mass Incarceration   167
Conclusion: Looking Toward the Future   169

5. **How Much Health Care Is Appropriate and Necessary?**   **173**
    A Complex Issue   173
        Practitioner Guidelines   176
        Universal Principles   178
    Conceptual Framework for Decision Analysis   180
        International Implications   182
    A Spectrum of Care Model   183
        From Whose Perspective?   187
    Factors That Should Not Influence a Decision to Treat   189
        Gender, Race, Ethnicity, or Sexual Orientation   190
        Nature of Crime or Behavior in Prison   190
        Self-Harm or Contributory Behavior   190
        Celebrity Status, Notoriety, Social Class, or Profession   191
        Preexisting Conditions   191
    Factors That May Influence the Decision to Intervene   192
        Dimensions of Necessity   192
        Cost Factors   194
        Description of Factors to Be Considered in the Decision
            to Treat   195
            Improvement in Health, Improvement in Function,
                or Relief of Pain   196
            Probability of a Successful Outcome with Few Adverse
                Side Effects   196
            Urgency   197
            Availability of an Acceptable Alternative   197
            Patient's Desire for Treatment   197
            Expected Remaining Duration of Incarceration   197
            Chronicity of Care   198
            Cost of the Intervention   198
        Avoid Confounding the Variables   199
            History of Compliance with Treatment   199
            Comorbidity   199
            Treatment Delays   199
            Age and General Health of Patient   200
            Quality of Life   200
    Conclusion   200

6. **Conceptualizing Mental Illness as a Chronic Condition**   **203**
    Mental Illness Should Be Treated, Not Punished   203
    Society's Failure—Deinstitutionalization   205
        The Consequences   209
        Scope of the Problem—Prevalence   209
    Jail and Prison Environments Are Countertherapeutic   212
    Mental Illness: A Chronic Condition That Waxes and Wanes   215

Acute Stress Disorder versus PTSD   218
Closed Head Injury   218
Special Units for Housing Mentally Ill Patients   219
Typical Characteristics of Mentally Ill Patients by Level of Care   220
Practical Consequences of Failing to Recognize the Chronic Nature
of Mental Illness   221
Conclusion: An Ethical Imperative   224

7. **A Patient or a Prisoner?**   **227**
Why Call Them "Patients"?   228
Is It a Health Care Unit?   234
Where the Lines Get Crossed   235
Patient Advocacy   236
A Lesson from the Captain   237
Conclusion   238

8. **Organizing Correctional Health Care**   **241**
Common Mission with Differences   241
Responsible Health Authority   242
Medical Autonomy   243
Rationale for Designating a Responsible Health Authority   245
Role of Responsible Health Authority   246
Role of the Medical Director   247
Organizational Models   248
No Central Health Authority   248
Outside Public Health Authority   251
Need for Patient Advocacy   252
Risk of Excessive Fragmentation   253
Coordination by a Central Health Care Authority   254
Line Authority from a Central Office of Health Care   254
Conclusion   256

9. **Corrections and Health Care Working Together**   **259**
Corrections and Health Care   259
Recognizing Differences   260
Purpose   260
Means Employed   262
Coercive Measures   263
Punitive Sanctions   264
Primary Client Served   264
Style of Staff Training   265
System of Beliefs   266
Interdependence   268
How Health Care Depends on Custody and Institutional Services   268

    How Custody Depends on Health Care   269
  Working Together   270
    Strategies   270
    Dialogue and Respectful Deliberation   272
  Cooperating in Training   274
    Health Aspects of Officer Training   274
    Security and Institutional Aspects of Health Care Staff Training   277
  Some Tough Questions   279
  Two Examples of Productive Cooperation   280
    Rhabdomyolysis   280
    Emergency Vodka   281
  Selected Problems for Cooperative Resolution   282
    Ensuring Safety and Security within Clinic Areas   282
    What Should We Call "Them"?   283
    Security Housing Units and Other Forms of Severe Isolation   283
    Physician On-Call Arrangement   284
    On-Site Specialty Care   284
    Privacy of Clinic Encounters   284
    Health Classification   285
    Transporting Prisoners   286
    Security Constraints That Impair Cost-Effective Health Care   287
    Rehabilitation—Start with Respect for Dignity and Self-Worth   288
  Conclusion—Speaking Out Loyally   288

Epilogue   291
Notes   293
Bibliography   317
Index   335
Index of Legal Cases   361
About the Author   365

Preface

Fyodor Dostoyevsky wrote: "The degree of civilization in a society can be judged by entering its prisons."[1] Although this was not a new idea, it was aptly expressed. It might even be seen as a specific application of words from the Sermon on the Mount: "Whatever you do for one of these least of my brethren, you do unto Me" (Matthew 25).

Each of the many times that I entered the Unidad de Tratamiento Intensivo—a small, ancient, highly secure prison adjacent to the former Penitenciaría Estatal in San Juan, Puerto Rico, I paused to read the words engraved above its portal: "Odia el delito, pero compadesca al delinquente" ("Hate the crime, but be compassionate toward the doer of the crime").

My friend Perry M. Johnson, former director of corrections for the state of Michigan and past president of the American Correctional Association (1993–1994), used to say, "Prisons are places *of* punishment, but never places *for* punishment."

It is also wise to keep in mind the oft-quoted classical definition of health, as given by the World Health Organization. "Health is a state of complete physical, mental, and social well-being, and not merely the absence of disease." There can be no meritorious reason to curtail or delimit the applicability of this definition in the context of corrections. This is the standard of health for which honorable medical personnel of all disciplines the world over have pledged and committed their professional lives on behalf of their patients. It is, moreover, the strong and central message of this book that this is the vision of health that must inspire the efforts of all who work in the field of prison or jail or juvenile correctional health services.

Like a familiar and lingering melody, all of these wise words somehow emerge as a unifying thread from my own years of active involvement in the field of correctional health care. They draw together and give focus to certain themes that need to be expressed, and they have provided motivation, energy, and direction for the preparation of this book.

ORIGIN AND PURPOSE OF THIS BOOK

This volume began as an effort to prepare an updated second edition of my earlier book, *Health Management Issues in Corrections* (Lanham, MD: American Correctional Association, 1997). Several new chapters were written and some chapters were expanded so much that they required division into two or three separate chapters. Thus, rather than a simple updating, the work grew until, in consultation with the editor, a decision was made to regard this as a new book, not a second edition. Because of shifting priorities, the American Correctional Association (ACA) decided not to publish a revised volume. I knew, however, that the field had changed dramatically since I wrote the initial book and I wanted to offer some new guidance to readers who work in and are concerned with correctional health care. Through the encouragement of my wife Rosemary, several friends, and my original editor, Alice Heiserman, we were able to get these new ideas out through ABC-CLIO/Praeger Publishers, under the gentle and capable guiding hand of its acquisitions editor Jessica Gribble. I am deeply grateful to ACA for granting full release of rights to the earlier volume so that I was permitted to find a new publisher.

The lapse of several years required a new update, but this time a pragmatic view prevailed and it was decided to break the 1,300-page work into two or more volumes. The first theme to emerge was the one dealing with ethical and legal challenges—unquestionably the heart of the entire project—and this has become the current volume.

The next effort will entail combining and updating the remainder of the manuscript material to cover topics of delivery and management of health care services in correctional facilities. These will include chapters such as "Ensuring Access to Care"; "Dental Health Care in Corrections"; "Infectious Diseases in Corrections"; "Mental Health Care for Correctional Populations"; "Special Concerns of Juveniles in Corrections"; "Special Concerns of Women's Health Care in Corrections"; "Special Concerns of the Elderly in Corrections"; "End-of-Life Care in Prisons"; "Privatization of Correctional Health Care"; "Substance Abuse Rehabilitation Programs"; "Physical Exercise in Confinement"; "Design Considerations for Correctional Health Space"; and "Developing a Policy and Procedure Manual." Undoubtedly an ethical thread will run through all of them because the author's central concern is more on why we ought to do these things than precisely how we ought to do them.

I hope this current book will make some small but unique contribution to the growing wealth and diversity of literature appearing in the field of correctional health. In the mid-1990s, there were but few offerings. The landscape is notably different this time. Nearly two decades later, there is already a wealth of literature. Reading much of this material was an enjoyable part of preparing this volume. Where they appear to be helpful, references are cited and some important quotable material has been excerpted.

As with the earlier book, the primary target audience is the correctional administrator (commissioner, sheriff, director, warden, jail administrator, correctional officials, correctional program staff), legislative committee members and other responsible government agents, and parties to litigation including judges and attorneys for both defendants and plaintiffs. When I was first approached at the ACA Conference in Fort Worth, Texas in January 1995 by Alice Fins (now Heiserman), who was then the ACA's publications and research managing editor, she invited me to write a book on correctional health care issues, but she explained that there were already many fine manuals instructing health care professionals on how to practice their disciplines. What was needed was a book that would tell correctional administrators and officials what they need to know about health care. I accepted this as the mission then, and have tried to remain faithful to the same mission in this book as well.

During the past 18 years, several wardens and correctional administrators have credited the previous book for useful insights into why certain medical practices are important and for enabling them to be more supportive of medical and mental health issues. Likewise, physicians, nurses, and mental health professionals have said that they found it useful as both a guide on how care should be delivered in a correctional context and an aid in preparing for dialogue with correctional officials on these matters. Various health clinicians have used the book as a study resource in preparation for their certification as correctional health professionals, and it has served as an official textbook for nurses in preparation for the ACA certification as correctional nurses. Some auditors and surveyors of correctional facilities remarked that they found it helpful in performing the accreditation function, primarily because it often provided a detailed explanation of why the standards said what they did.

It was my aim to look at the practice of health care in corrections from the perspective of *what is right* or *what is ethical*. What light do the essence of our humanity and the valued norms of our society shine on these practices? This criterion is both informed and influenced by what is legal, what is clinically sound contemporary practice, what is the professional standard of care, and what is safe practice. As a basis for appreciating the ethical dimension and enabling a common ground for reference, I made an effort to consult important formulations of ethical principles from highly regarded and widely respected sources. As various practice issues were discussed, I tried to include the reasoning behind recommended directions to help readers reach their own conclusions.

It will be apparent that this book often draws authoritative support for recommended practices from the standards and pronouncements of the National Commission on Correctional Health Care (NCCHC) and the American Correctional Association (ACA). These esteemed national agencies and their accreditation programs are of immense importance in the effort to improve and maintain the quality of correctional health care. There are few noteworthy differences in the thrust and direction of their two sets of standards, partly because both had a common origin some 40 years ago in the American Medical Association (AMA) standards for jails and for prisons, partly because some of the same correctional health professionals have played an active role in the development of both sets of standards and, perhaps most of all, because there is little dispute over the basic elements of what should constitute acceptable practice in this arena among experts in correctional health care. Where a relevant variance does exist among the sets of standards concerning the topic under discussion, this book calls attention to the difference.

In addition to the manuals of standards published by the ACA and the NCCHC, several other sources are frequently mentioned, because they represent authoritative references in the field and may treat a given topic in greater detail. These are:

B. Jaye Anno, *Guidelines for the Management of an Adequate Delivery System*

Michael Puisis, ed., *Clinical Practice in Correctional Medicine*

Nancy Dubler, *APHA Standards for Correctional Health Care*, 2nd ed.

APHA Task Force, *APHA* Standards *for Correctional Health Care*, 3rd ed.

Likewise the ethical codes and pronouncements of the World Medical Association and World Psychiatric Association, including the *Declarations of Helsinki, Tokyo, Malta,* and *Madrid* and also various statements of the United Nations, the Council for International Organizations of Medical Sciences (CIOMS), and the World Health Organization have been inspirational and enlightening. None of these principles should ever be lightly dismissed.

Acknowledgments

I have been blessed along the way with meeting or having the opportunity to work alongside many highly dedicated, moral, committed, skilled, and enthusiastic individuals. From them I have learned important lessons and I respect all of them. The list is quite long, and I will only name a few.

Some are no longer with us, but they stood as giants in terms of their contribution to correctional health care. I thank B. Jaye Anno, PhD; Robert L. Brutsche, MD; R. Scott Chavez, PhD, MPA; Bernard P. Harrison, JD; Glenn G. Johnson, DO, MD; Joseph E. Paris, MD, PhD; Joseph R. Rowan, MSW; and Armand H. Start, MD, MPH. These good friends I count also among my heroes. Each exemplified a deep concern, caring, dedication, and steadfast commitment to the health and well-being of prisoners. I am deeply grateful to each of them and to the many others who are not named. *Requiescant in pace.* From each I have liberally borrowed thoughts, ideas, principles, solutions, and examples. I trust that they would basically agree with what is said in this book, though likely they could have said it better.

Of friends who are living and whose continuing contribution to the field of correctional health care I also hold in high regard, the list I drafted is again too long to include. I will mention only a few—those who have, in various ways, made a tangible contribution in terms of inspiration and encouragement, review of drafts, helpful information, or important insights. John H. Clark, MD, MPH; Nancy N. Dubler, LLB; Jay K. Harness, MD, FACS; Edward A. Harrison, MBA; Craig L. Hutchinson, MD; Lambert N. King, MD, PhD; Catherine M. Knox, RN, MN; Vincent M. Nathan, JD; Michael Puisis, DO; Dianne Rechtine, MD; Dean P. Rieger, MD, MPH; William J. Rold, JD; Jayne R. Russell, M.Ed; Lorry Schoenly, PhD, RN; and Jaime Shimkus, BA.

I earnestly and especially commend all of the persons responsible for the good work of the National Commission on Correctional Health Care (NCCHC), whose statements I have copiously referenced. They have for several decades served as a bright beacon of guidance and inspiration to correctional health professionals at all levels, and I wish the organization long and continuing success in charting the course and setting the tone. I hasten to put in a word also for the American Correctional Association (ACA). This agency serves a worthy and important cause, and there is ample evidence around the nation—and even in other countries—of its beneficial impact. It has contributed enormously to the professionalization of corrections.

In addition, the American Jail Association (AJA), American Correctional Health Services Association (ACHSA), American College of Correctional Physicians (ACCP), Academy of Correctional Health Professionals (ACHP), American Public Health Association (APHA), Joint Commission (JCAHO), American Medical Association (AMA), and like professional associations each fulfill a critically important purpose and have earned my appreciation and recognition.

I would be remiss were I to fail to acknowledge the essential contribution made behind the scenes by the current editor—Jessica Gribble—whose wise guidance and perspective have enabled this work to come to fruition, as well as the ongoing effort, encouragement, and calm judgment of its first editor—Alice Heiserman—who has continued to engage actively through every phase.

My family has been a bedrock of strength and encouragement. Above all, Rosemary, my wife, stood as a constant source of support and inspiration through this long process. She graciously offered to read and critique portions of the manuscript and suggested clearer wording or raised challenging and insightful questions. She has a way of sharing the same ideals and principles yet approaching subjects from surprisingly different perspectives—a fact that inevitably yields better results. Nor must I overlook the many times she quietly excused me from pulling my fair share of household chores over this period. Even these words fall short of the true measure of her contribution. Our children—Daniel, Michelle, Rebecca, Christa, and Maleika—were genuine sources of encouragement and inspiration, each in his or her own supportive way. And the grandchildren—Cameron, Marrianna, Savannah, Lauren, Caleb, Joshua, Galaxy, and Elia.—have been a joy and a delight to observe. Their urgent interruptions for "grandpa time" were always welcome opportunities to take a needed break and enter their world for a short while. Their presence also served as a reminder that the choices we make and the values we embrace will shape the world they inherit.

One daughter warrants particular mention. Christa rescued me a few years ago from the extremely slow progress that I had been making on the manuscript. Had it not been for her welcoming invitation to come and live in her suburban Washington, D.C., apartment for a few months, this book would have tarried much longer in the writing. There I was removed from distractions and competing responsibilities. In addition, her background in sports medicine and athletic training enabled her to contribute most of the content of a chapter on physical exercise in confinement that will appear in my next book. Thanks, Christa, for the love, companionship, support, and the space. You are truly wonderful.

Two very close friends and coworkers are both recently deceased. Richard M. Campau, MBA, CCHP, a perceptive observer of human nature and a pioneer in advancing the principles of good correctional health care, kindly agreed to read critically the draft of each chapter and provide helpful feedback—ranging from grammatical construction to interpretation of standards to "whether I really want to say it that way." Robert S. Ort, MD, PhD, a true gentleman and a caring professional, served as my mentor over a period of years in the area of correctional mental health. They are both very much missed, and I humbly dedicate this work in their memory.

Any mistakes in the book remain my own, but I gratefully acknowledge that its value and usefulness have notably benefited from the assistance of others. Some colleagues and friends have willingly reviewed one or more chapters of the book, and these are given credit in the introduction to those chapters. It was because I respect their expertise that I sought their input.

Explanatory Notes

TERMINOLOGY

Some of the terminology used in this book warrants comment or needs clarification.

For sake of brevity, the term *warden* is often used in the generic sense and refers to the institution head, whether called a *warden*, *superintendent*, *facility supervisor*, *jail administrator*, or *director*. No slight is intended.

A *facility* is a correctional institution (or camp) that houses prisoners, jail inmates, juvenile detainees, or immigration detainees. Unless otherwise explicitly stated or evident from the context, what is said here about prisons usually applies also to other types of facilities. Jails ordinarily are county facilities, although in a few states they are operated by the state correctional agency. Jails are predominantly short-term facilities, usually for a stay of less than one year. Unlike prisons, jails also house detainees—that is, persons who have been arrested and are being held pending arraignment, trial, or sentencing, as well as those found guilty of misdemeanors. Juvenile facilities hold some persons who have been adjudicated guilty of a crime, but for the most part this is not the case. Those for short-term confinement are often referred to as *detention centers*, whereas those for longer-term confinement are called *juvenile correctional facilities* or *schools*. The standards and ethical principles are equally applicable to privatized operations. In large part, these distinctions are not relevant to the matters discussed, because the principles apply equally, *mutatis mutandis*, to the populations of each type of facility.

The term *physician* or *nurse* usually means exactly what it says, but quite often what is said of them can be applied generically also to all health care professionals. The precise meaning should be evident from the context.

When a person is mentioned in the context of the health care system or as a recipient of health care, the term *patient* (or sometimes *client*) is used. Otherwise, when the same person is referenced as an occupant of a correctional facility, terms such as *inmate* or *prisoner* may be used. The terms *offender* and *delinquent* are intentionally avoided unless they appear in a direct quotation because these words unnecessarily imply guilt and wrongdoing, which is completely irrelevant to the rendering of health care services. The term *inmate* is more neutral than *prisoner* or *offender*. See further discussion on this topic in Chapter 7, "A Patient or a Prisoner?"

REFERENCES TO THE STANDARDS

Because the standards of the American Correctional Association (ACA), National Commission on Correctional Health Care (NCCHC), American Public Health Association (APHA), and American Medical Association (AMA), among others, are frequently cited, certain simplifying conventions have been adopted in this book. First, the acronyms are often used, except for the first time they appear in any chapter. The first citation of a manual of standards in each chapter is accorded a full reference in the endnote or bibliography. Subsequent references to that volume are abbreviated. A similar convention is adopted for other endnote references that may appear in multiple chapters, with the first usage of that resource in a chapter cited in full, and subsequent references in shortened form.

Second, specific ACA standards are referenced in a shorthand fashion to avoid cumbersome repetition. ACA *ACI* refers to prisons (adult correctional institutions), ACA *ALDF* to local jails (adult local detention facilities), and ACA *JCF* to youth facilities (juvenile correctional facilities). Updates or revisions in the 2014 *Standards Supplement* have been duly noted. Similarly, the NCCHC standards are abbreviated so that the letter *P*, *J*, or *Y* distinguishes whether it addresses a prison, jail, or youth facility.

Third, the position of ACA or of NCCHC with respect to a particular topic or principle may be illustrated by citing only the prison standard, omitting mention of the corresponding jail and juvenile standard unless there are relevant differences. The fundamental principles of these standards do not differ among adult prison, jail, and juvenile facilities, although there may be specific differences in their application.

Fourth, the relevant NCCHC and ACA standards are often both cited, even when they agree. Their solidarity tends to emphasize the importance of the requirement, and the somewhat different wording, examples, or commentary can serve to clarify its intent. In a very few instances, the two sets of standards are not in full agreement, and these cases are pointed out.

Fifth, for simplicity and by custom, we have adhered to the traditional usage of the term *standard*, even while recognizing the convention officially adopted in ACA's fourth editions where performance-based *expected practices* is the preferred terminology for what had been *standards* in earlier editions.

Sixth, the fact that a referenced standard is rated "mandatory" (by the ACA) or "essential" (by the NCCHC) is noted in the text or in the endnote. Omission of this designation implies a "non-mandatory" or "important" standard.

Seventh, if referenced material appears in the associated commentary rather than in the expected practice (standard) itself, this fact is noted. Neither agency regards its "comments" as binding, and only holds the surveyed facility to the wording of the standard itself and to its *compliance indicators*. Nevertheless, the comment can be instructive and carry considerable weight because it often defines terms used in the standard or clarifies its intent.

In addition, both the NCCHC and the ACA have issued multiple sets of standards. The author did not always attempt to compare the wording in such ACA publications as: *Standards for Adult Correctional Boot Camp Programs, Standards for Juvenile Community Residential Facilities, Standards for Juvenile Correctional Boot Camp Programs, Standards for Juvenile Detention Facilities, Standards for Small Jail Facilities,* or *Standards for Small Juvenile Detention Facilities* or in NCCHC publications such as *Standards for Mental Health Services in Correctional Facilities* and *Standards for Opioid Treatment Programs in Correctional Facilities*. However, it is likely that their admonitions do not differ in principle or intent from the standards of the manuals referenced, and the reasoning can be expected to be the same although the content may be more explicit for the specific application.

Eighth, because new editions of the standards are released every few years, future readers may find that the wording of a standard has changed, or that an important standard has become essential or mandatory. Although major departures in the direction of the various requirements are unlikely, there can be differences.

Finally, the author makes no claim whatsoever that the statements made in this book represent official or authorized interpretations of the ACA, NCCHC, or any other standards. For a current official and authoritative explanation of any standard, the accrediting body itself should be consulted.

MISCELLANEA

Sometimes a subject is broader than the chapter or section in which it is primarily discussed and topics may be mentioned in more than one location. Cross-references to other portions of the book are frequently provided to assist the interested reader. Readers will, it is hoped, forgive some repetition because few persons are likely to read this book from cover to cover, but many will consult it as a reference to explore particular areas of interest. The index will provide further help in locating topics quickly.

Having resided in Michigan for most of my life, having worked for many years as the statewide administrator in charge of health care services for the Michigan Department of Corrections, and being quite familiar with some of the large jails nearby, it is only natural that many examples and illustrations used in the book are drawn from this state. However, the author has experience in facilities across the country and the examples chosen should be widely applicable.

In addition, some of the examples cited relate to situations observed during audits, surveys, or other tours of correctional facilities. In deference to the confidentiality that is professionally owed and which was promised by the accrediting agencies to these facilities, no identifying information is provided and the facility will remain anonymous, even when, as is often the case, the revelation would be complimentary.

To facilitate use of this volume as a reference manual, both a table of contents and an alphabetical topic index have been included. Besides the topic index, a separate legal case index is provided to direct the reader to pages where various lawsuits are mentioned.

Introduction

THE CHALLENGE

The challenge of providing adequate health care services to incarcerated persons can be daunting. In all fundamental respects, it is no different from supplying health care services to people in the free world. This book attempts to show why this is so within the context of ethical and legal principles. Yet, it is clear that notable discrepancies do exist between the way health care services are delivered to prisoners and to those living in free society. Apart from understandable and acceptable circumstantial or logistical differences, it should not matter that one is a prisoner. This book will address situations in which ambiguity, role conflict, or dual loyalty can tend to compromise professional ethics in the correctional setting.

You and I have our doctors and dentists. We have access to hospitals and clinics. We have our health insurance. And when we get sick or injured, we know how to get help. We also have our mom, or spouse, or a good friend whom we can always call for advice and support and assistance when things go wrong. So we may take it all quite for granted.

But now imagine the man or woman who is in prison or jail, or the youth in a juvenile detention center. Yes, there is likely a doctor and a nurse available—but who chose them? The prisoner had no say at all in which health professionals are available to serve his or her needs. Are there any really trusted persons around to call on for advice and support? This situation can be vastly different—even supposing that the correctional facility does have an excellent health care program.

The health needs of the incarcerated are no less than our own. In fact, data show that, in general, prisoners are sicker than their age, race, and sex counterparts in free society. And they live confined to a small cell, often without companionship or distractions, left to think and ponder and worry about their situation and the way they feel.

Until fairly recently—the late 1970s at the earliest—arrangements for providing health care services to those in prisons and jails in our country were primitive and woefully inadequate. Owing largely to intervention by the courts, it became clear that failure to make adequate health services available to an incarcerated person could violate the U.S. Constitution—a form of "cruel and unusual punishment." Although conditions are vastly better as we approach the year 2020, they still fall short in far too many instances.

Substantial differences can be seen in the way health care programs are set up and operated and monitored when serving an incarcerated population. This book explores, in particular, the ethical and legal principles that must guide delivery of health care to the incarcerated. A companion book (expected in 2018) will deal with practical and operational realities of delivering health care to prisoners, looking at access to care; cost of care; issues related to privatization; design considerations for health care space; medical and mental health and dental care; services to women, to juveniles, and to the elderly; quality-control programs; substance-abuse rehabilitation programs; physical exercise in confinement; and other aspects of care.

TARGET AUDIENCE

There are six kinds of people in this world, in terms of their awareness and concern about the quality of health care services for the incarcerated:

1. Those who neither know nor care about prisoners, believing they deserve what they get.
2. Those who have no idea what it is like to be in prison or, especially, to be sick in prison.
3. Those with some idea because a parent, child, spouse, cousin, or friend is incarcerated.
4. Those with a very personal awareness because they are (or have been) imprisoned.
5. Those who know it well because they actually provide health services to prisoners.
6. Those who need to know, because they have responsibility or authority over prisons or jails.

To persons of the first type—hopefully they are few—I would try to influence you to change your mind. What if you, or a loved one, fell into that unfortunate circumstance? As human beings, apart from the circumstance of guilt or innocence, of stubborn impenitence or deep remorse—do you (or they) deserve to suffer needless pain and anxiety, in addition to the court-ordered loss of liberty?

To those of the second type—likely there are many—perhaps I can enlighten you somewhat about what it is like to dwell in a world that you have never experienced and hopefully never will.

To those of the third and fourth types, this book will try to offer a perspective on where we have been and how far we have come and also give some insight into how much more we still need to do and why we should do it. There are indeed many of you. The Bureau of Justice Statistics shows that currently more than 2 million people were incarcerated in 2014 (1,561,500 under jurisdiction of state or federal prisons and another 744,600 in local jails), and nearly 650,000 persons enter and leave prison each year and some 11 million pass through our jails each year. At the same time, there were almost 4 million on probation and 856,900 on parole—all of these directly involved in the criminal justice system one way or another.[1] And if each of these millions of people has an average of 10 or more family members or close friends in the free world, calculate how many there must be who have had close direct or indirect experience with prison or jail! (These figures do not count persons held in youth facilities.) Consider also that the 2.3 million state and federal prisoners and local jail inmates were being held in 1,719 state prisons, 102 federal prisons, 942 juvenile correctional facilities, 3,283 local jails, and 79 Indian Country jails.[2]

If you are in the fifth group, there is little new that I can tell you about how things really are because most of you know it as well or better than I. But this book may help refresh what you learned in school when you studied medicine or nursing or psychology or pharmacy or dentistry. You were taught the principles of ethics that must guide your behavior as a healing professional. Perhaps this book can accompany you through an examination of some of the challenges that confront you every day and some of the things we know can go wrong—precisely because they have gone so terribly wrong in the recent past. This book may suggest resources and provide an impetus to keep the compass pointed in the right direction.

Finally, to those in the sixth group—the governors, legislators, bureau chiefs, directors and commissioners of corrections, jail administrators and sheriffs, wardens, deputy wardens, correctional officials, relevant professional associations, and anyone else who has some say in determining the amount of resources, the priorities, the staffing complement, and the policies and standards of correctional health care, I hope that some of what is written will provide a helpful perspective and perhaps incline you to take a closer look at the consequences of your decisions.

No, not quite yet. Let me also suggest a seventh group that consists of the American voters, the news media, religious leaders, ethicists, attorneys, and judges. Each of you can also contribute to changing and improving the situation. Understanding the background of the correctional health care system is the first step; after that one can learn about the laws and regulations that surround this vital topic. Beyond this, one may even wish to visit these facilities and then serve as a volunteer to help make things better.

OVERVIEW OF THE CHAPTERS

The current volume is divided into nine chapters. The first three will describe the basic principles of ethics that must guide the choices we each make in our lives. They are derived from what is fundamental to humanity—to our better nature—and to society. They are common to all peoples, of all times, of every culture. The great philosophers and theologians, sages and healers through the ages have espoused them and shaped their formulation. If we explore deeply within our own being, we will discover strong support for these principles. Starting with a simple notion of "Do unto others as you would have them do unto you" can give us a great deal of insight into what is essentially right and wrong. Some may prefer to base their behavior on religious principles and teachings.

Regardless of which faith tradition you follow—be it Christianity, Islam, Judaism, Buddhism, Hinduism, or indigenous cultural beliefs—there will be strong support for fairness, justice, truth, beneficence, and the notion that a healer's first and inviolable duty is to his or her patient and to cause no harm. These three chapters will also explore some areas of ethical conflict that can face health care professionals (and others) working in the correctional arena. We will look at lessons from history and at tragic examples—even very recent instances—when health professionals violated these principles, whether motivated by a conflict of loyalty to one's country or to one's employer, or perhaps by personal malice or greed, or even from long-held and deeply seated bias and prejudice. Such examples include participation by health professionals in extreme isolation, capital punishment, exploitative biomedical research, and torture. We will look also at examples of less obvious unethical practices that contribute to the unfortunate plight of prisoners but that also tend to inure professionals to more serious breaches of the norms of decency.

Chapter 4 will touch on the role of law, as legislated or as interpreted by the courts in determining the conditions of confinement and the access of prisoners to quality health care services. Courts have played a highly significant role from the 1970s through the 1990s, but since 1996, a particularly noxious piece of legislation—the Prison Litigation Reform Act—has severely impeded legitimate access of prisoners to judicial oversight and relief. Why and how this should be corrected are discussed in some detail. The legal system can be a powerful force for the good, and this chapter outlines ways that correctional systems can protect themselves by maintaining a high-quality health care program that will render them much less vulnerable to being sued.

Chapter 5 describes a way of thinking about and determining how much heath care prisoners are entitled to receive—a subject that has never been defined with precision.

Chapter 6 explores some aspects of mental illness and explains how we got into a situation in which an extremely high percentage of prisoners suffers from mental illness—leading to the undeniable realization that our society is actually punishing mental illness rather than treating it appropriately. Some of the disastrous consequences of misperceiving the nature and course of mental illness and ignoring its significance will be discussed.

Chapter 7 explains why it matters what we call "them." The terms *prisoner*, *offender*, and *delinquent*, when used by doctors and nurses to refer to their patients, connote a meaning not overtly intended, but one that can have serious negative consequence to the attitude and behavior of both speaker and listener.

Chapter 8 points out a factor that significantly conditions whether and how effectively a correctional system can ensure ethical practice and high-quality medical services for its prisoners. Organizational structure can be critically important.

Chapter 9 wraps it all up by dealing with what should be obvious. Doctors and other health professionals in correctional settings need to think and work closely and cooperatively with corrections personnel—from wardens to line officers—to accomplish what needs to be done. This final chapter outlines specific areas of similarity and of difference between corrections and health care, and points to practical ways of mutual collaboration.

The author readily acknowledges that the vast majority of correctional health care professionals, correctional officers, and program staff are dedicated, ethical, competent, and decent human beings who should take justifiable pride in their efforts to serve the incarcerated population of our country in a humane and professional manner. Yet it is clear that fundamental areas of difference between the worlds of health care and corrections can easily impede implementation of components essential to a good health care program. As pointed out by B. Jaye Anno et al. in 2004, "[t]he tension between care and custody in prisons has not, until very recently, been part of the biomedical ethical discussion. . . . Medical care is delivered in the context of informed choices, selectivity, and securing of patient satisfaction. On the other hand, prisons are authoritarian institutions, organized as hierarchies that tend to focus on expedient, time-honored, standardized solutions to problems. Prisoners, furthermore, are defined by the imperatives of custody and control."[3] In view of this reality, the sobering issues discussed in this book are intended to promote mutual respect and productive dialogue among members of these two worlds and to foster inclusion in the biomedical ethical conversation. These topics are not presented in a tone of negativity or pessimism, but rather in the spirit of hope and optimism, believing that we need to look candidly at each other, learn from our past experiences, and then together both plan and build a better future for all concerned.

Chapter 1

Ethics in the Context of Correctional Health*

COMMON MISSION

After *public protection,* the most commonly cited mission of corrections is the *care and custody* of prisoners. This formulation clearly entrusts correctional officials with the *care* of inmates and not solely with their custody or confinement. Meeting their *health* needs is undeniably an essential aspect of their care.

From this mission, it thus follows that the policies and practices of a good correctional system must be consistent with the requirements of good health care. As a matter of principle, a properly managed correctional system, like a properly managed health care program, will assign a high priority to each of the following characteristics:

- adherence to ethical and professional standards
- prevention of harm
- safety and well-being of each person
- a safe and secure environment for staff and patients
- proper hygienic practices and sanitation
- confidentiality of private and sensitive information
- respect for inmates' dignity and basic human needs
- emergency preparedness

---

* Some of the content of this chapter and Chapters 2 and 3 has been excerpted and extensively revised and expanded by the author from Chapter 13, "Issues in Health Professional Ethics: Some Practical Considerations," in Kenneth L. Faiver, *Health Care Management Issues in Corrections* (Lanham, MD: American Correctional Association, 1997).

- due attention to maintaining and improving program quality
- orderly management of the institution
- conservation of scarce resources (avoidance of waste and inefficiency)

Each characteristic is critically important to the success of both correctional programs and health care programs. Neither system can properly achieve its mission in an unsafe or disorderly environment. Good hygienic practices and sanitation measures protect the health of staff, inmates, and visitors. To be successful, each discipline requires clear and consistent policies along with ongoing staff training and development that reflect due concern for human dignity and respect for fundamental human needs and rights. Each must have a quality-control program, a focus on patient safety and prevention of bad outcomes, a solid ethical and professional foundation, and an emphasis on efficiency. All priorities must be balanced and optimized with mutual cooperation and respect by both the custody and health care sectors.

Recognizing Differences

Even though the two systems share elements of a common mission, they have important and fundamental differences. Correctional and health care programs differ in their purpose, the means used to achieve that purpose, primary client served, use of coercive measures, type of employee training, and system of beliefs. Although they share similar priorities and goals, they will (or should) not choose to implement them in exactly the same manner. They have decidedly different functions.

A BRIEF HISTORICAL PERSPECTIVE

Before delving into the topic of correctional health care ethics we will briefly review the recent past so readers can gain insight into the stark realities of health care services in prisons and jails in the United States just five decades ago.

Prior to and into the 1970s, prisons and jails in the United States had almost no qualified medical staff or anything resembling properly equipped clinical areas. Inmates were widely used to deliver health services, impaired or unlicensed physicians were sometimes employed, proper equipment and supplies for diagnosis and treatment were often lacking, and inmates with serious medical needs were frequently denied access to care. Medical, mental health, and dental services were scarcely regarded as a "program" and garnered little of a facility's budget. When these appalling conditions finally reached the attention of courts and the public, the revolution in correctional health care practices of the 1970s and 1980s began, as will be described in Chapter 4, "Legal Issues in Correctional Health Care."

The highly unsatisfactory conditions that generally prevailed in prison health care have been documented inter alia by Brecher and Della Penna, by Faiver, by Anno, by several commissions, and by numerous court documents. The excerpts cited in the following may show newcomers to the field of correctional health care just how far we have come in a few short years—and into what depths we shall hopefully never return—provided we afford due deference to our ethical principles.

Doctors Edward M. Brecher and Richard D. Della Penna, on behalf of the Law Enforcement Assistance Administration of the U.S. Department of Justice, visited during 1974 and 1975 "a substantial number of state departments of correction and a broad range of individual institutions in all parts of the country," often joined by Dr. Kenneth Babcock, retired medical director of the Joint Commission on Accreditation of Hospitals. Their report provides little detail on findings, because it chiefly focuses on formulating an excellent set of recommendations to improve health services for prisoners. The following are some of the findings gleaned from their report, beginning with the observation that the medical care in correctional facilities consisted mainly of "sick call" in which inmates would line up in great numbers for a brief encounter with a physician. Their report made the following observations:

[At sick call] a little more than one minute of the physician's time per inmate attending sick call was available on the average, and many inmates received only a few seconds of time.

[Sick call took place in a small room typically called a "pharmacy."] A counter topped by a mesh screen which extended to the ceiling divided the pharmacy in two, and separated the doctor from the inmate. . . . At sick call, only sick-call records, and not medical records, were available to the doctor.

Continuity of care is conspicuous by its absence. . . . "Take an aspirin" becomes the common prescription.

Even a physician who takes a post in a correctional institution with a genuine concern for inmates, and with a determination to practice the same high-quality brand of medicine within its walls as he formerly practiced on the outside, soon "burns out." He may lose all empathy with the endless stream of inmates who parade through his office at three-minute intervals or less, openly voicing their disrespect for him and his medical skill, sullen and manipulative at best, hostile, and at times even threatening.

"Inmate nurses" are . . . not in fact nurses at all, and many have no nursing training whatever. Yet they may be found not only nursing the sick but also diagnosing illnesses, dispensing medicines, giving injections, suturing wounds, and otherwise practicing medicine in some institutions today. Untrained and inexperienced inmates may similarly be found operating X-ray equipment, performing laboratory tests, giving physical therapy treatments, and performing other duties for which they are wholly unqualified.[1]

Faiver found deplorable conditions in the Michigan prison system in 1974. His year-long comprehensive study involved a team of largely university-based physicians, nurses, psychiatrists and psychologists, dentists, pharmacists, and other health professionals. They documented serious problems that were far too numerous to recite here. Under the overall direction of a handful of licensed civilian health care professionals—approximately 28 for a population of 8,000 inmates housed in five institutions statewide—most of the health services were being provided by inmates who possessed few if any qualifications for the procedures they performed and who received woefully inadequate supervision. The following are a few excerpts from his two-volume report.

[T]he so called "nursing care" is provided by civilians, some with prior experience in the military services as hospital corpsmen and by attendants and inmate resident aides with varying degrees of training, experience, and abilities.

Records of sick call . . . are generally recorded in all the institutions on a 5" × 7" card which provides one line for each successive clinic visit, specifying "date," "medications," and "treatments." Nature or seriousness of the complaint or problem prompting the visit and specific diagnosis of condition are not ordinarily recorded and can only be surmised from the information given. Further, the forms do not call for an indication of the date of any scheduled follow-up visit.

The largest Michigan prison, with 4,226 inmates at the time, had one full-time equivalent physician, 0.1 psychiatrist, two registered nurses, three dentists, three psychologists, two registered pharmacists, an x-ray and laboratory technician, and a few former military medical corpsmen.

[One of the two registered nurses] also functions in two other roles (nurse-anesthetist for surgery performed in the prison hospital and responsibility for conducting a special shoe clinic). In addition, . . . there is a registered nurse supervising the psychiatric nursing care, and another part-time serving the outside clinics [in several correctional camps located within about 20 miles of the facility] and conducting training courses for civilian and resident aides.[2]

> Inmates were widely used to deliver health services, impaired or unlicensed physicians were sometimes employed, proper equipment and supplies for diagnosis and treatment were often lacking, and inmates with serious medical needs were frequently denied access to care.

In writing about this period, B. Jaye Anno said:

In contrast [to jails], most prisons tended to have some facilities for health care onsite and hence may have been more reluctant to send an inmate to the "free world" for care. The health staff in prisons, though, often consisted of unlicensed foreign medical graduates or physicians with institutional licenses, supplemented by unlicensed medical corpsmen and untrained inmate "nurses. As noted below, these and other factors scarcely meant that health care in prisons was adequate.[3]

In Ohio, a report issued by the state's advisory committee to the U.S. Commission on Civil Rights in 1976 included the following:

Medical decisions in Ohio prisons are sometimes made by non-medical personnel, probably unavoidably so in some cases since access to doctors or nurses must be granted by prison personnel. Procedures for getting medical attention in an emergency can be extensive. . . .

With fewer than 300 inmates in the Ohio Reformatory for Women, two official figures place the number of drug prescriptions in 1973 at between 800 and 10,000. The institution had no staff pharmacist at the time these figures were current. . . . [It was reported that] drugs are a main control device used by Ohio's prison administrators. . . .

[A physician, Amasa B. Ford, a professor of medicine at Case Western Reserve University School of Medicine, said:] I believe that there is a conflict between security and health priorities in any prison system, at all levels from the allocation of money at the State level down to whether a guard ignores or responds to a prisoner's request for medical assistance. . . . The final decision lies with the corrective [sic] authorities and not with health professionals.[4]

A team of physicians appointed by the Washington State Medical Association inspected three Washington prisons and made specific recommendations in 1976. Among their findings:

We must detach ourselves from the colonial mores of public reluctance to spend money and time on "bad people." The old idea of punish, isolate, and forget them must be substituted by a real effort and program and attitude for rehabilitation. . . .

[The criminally insane] are being simply isolated under security. . . . [We recommend that they] should be treated in a mental unit, with provision for maximum security, and that such treatment be intensified under qualified specialists and auxiliary trained personnel. . . .

At the present time, medical care is low on the list of priorities in the prison budget. In importance, it unfortunately follows the kitchen and laundry services. We feel that there needs to be a complete re-evaluation of our priorities if we are to affect the change necessary to rehabilitate the men in our state penal institutions.[5]

In his opinion in *Newman v. Alabama*, Judge Frank Johnson said:

Perhaps the most deplorable deprivation is that which is the product of the knowing and intentional mistreatment of sick and injured inmates. Inmates held in lockup at the M&DC (Medical and Diagnostic Center), sent there for the purpose of treatment, are arbitrarily denied by correctional staff the right even to attend sick call. At the M&DC and elsewhere, correctional personnel, well knowing that an inmate has been prescribed medicine which he is entitled to receive, deliberately refuse it.[6]

In addition, numerous federal court cases documented the woefully inadequate conditions of medical services in prisons and jails in the 1970s and 1980s, finding their medical care programs to be constitutionally deficient. The ruling in *Battle v. Anderson* said this of the Oklahoma system:

For many years, the penitentiary system has, for all practical purposes, been without any professionally trained medical support personnel whatsoever. Due to shortages in staff, defendants have continuously relied on unlicensed, untrained, and unqualified correctional officers and other penitentiary employees, as well as inmate personnel, to perform clinical and related medical services [that] should be performed solely by licensed and qualified professionals. Such services performed by unqualified inmate and civilian personnel include, for example, screening medical complaints to determine which inmates on sick call will actually get to see a doctor, as well as providing actual treatment and nursing care.[7]

ETHICS

Definition of Ethics

Ethics is a branch of philosophy that addresses morality—whether a course of action is morally right or wrong. A subtle but important distinction is made between what is legal and what is right. Our legislatures and courts define for us what is legal and illegal. Under most circumstances, we hold it as right to obey the law and wrong to disobey it. The exception would be for laws that are intrinsically and patently evil. Nazi Germany's laws to exterminate Jews, Poles, gypsies, and the disabled clearly fall into this category and should never have been obeyed.

Some actions can be wrong even though they may not be illegal. They are wrong in and of themselves regardless of whether prohibited by a legislature and whether anyone else knows about them. Thus, murder would be wrong even if no law prohibits it. Wanton disregard of another person's dignity and feelings, although not illegal, would also be wrong. So also is any participation by a health care professional in the legal process of capital punishment. Some behavior can be ethical and moral, even though illegal. An act of civil disobedience such as trespassing or disobeying a lawful order in protest of a societal injustice would be an example. Thus, the domains of ethics and law are not coextensive.

In expressing judgment about what constitutes ethical or unethical behavior, the author is well aware that good and wise persons may at times hold differing opinions. Nevertheless, the explicit reasoning and examples presented here can provide a model for thinking about these difficult situations. Also, slight variations in the circumstances of each individual case could lead to differing assessments. The study of ethics offers a framework for defining what behavior is right and what behavior is wrong in a given set of circumstances.

> "But we must consider this more carefully. For we are discussing no trivial matter, but rather the very direction our lives must follow."
> —Socrates

Prisoners are the only persons in United States society with a constitutionally guaranteed right to health care. Not all free citizens in America enjoy adequate access to health care. Consequently, some people—including corrections personnel, health care staff, and legislators—resent the fact that prisoners may be receiving better health care than they or their families can afford or that is not available to many disadvantaged persons in society. The result can be pushback that tends to challenge or undermine the ethical concerns and standards affecting the delivery of health care to prisoners.

People in a free society rightly expect their physicians will care for them, carefully diagnose their illnesses, prescribe proper treatments, and serve as their advocates—always looking selflessly after their best interests. They trust their doctors and want to feel their doctors respect them and that health professionals will do them no harm. Prisoners, too, should have the same expectations. The big difference is that people living freely in the community are able to choose their own medical care providers. In prisons, jails, and juvenile correctional facilities, this choice is not available.

Most prison doctors and other health professionals are skillful as well as caring, careful, and attentive to their patients—but some clearly are not. A few health care providers actively or subconsciously dislike prisoners and are antagonistic to them. These persons should not be working in correctional settings. Others are incompetent or impaired and also should not be allowed to work in such environments.

The ethical principles and values that guide physicians and other health professionals in the community apply equally in the correctional setting and should not be abandoned or disregarded. All correctional physicians should ask themselves whether they are practicing health care that consistently adheres to the principles they adopted when undertaking their practice.

In this book, we are attempting to apply the principles of medical ethics to the correctional context. Given the major differences between the arenas of corrections and health care, it is not surprising that we encounter difficult and controversial topics. As Socrates said 2,400 years ago, "But we must consider this more carefully. For we are discussing no trivial matter, but rather the very direction our lives must follow."[8]

Ethics and the Law

Considerable interplay can occur between ethics and the law. Ethics seeks to define what is "good" or "right" behavior. Ethical insight may be found in the deliberative reasoning of courts that strive to balance competing entitlements by applying the principle of "rightness," although this reasoning can be nearly obscured amid the maze of finely honed distinctions, appeals to precedent, and arcane procedure.

Court decisions and laws can be said to reflect, albeit imperfectly, the current values and norms held dear by society. They may also reflect the basic and fundamental human values and societal norms that undergird and inform our moral and ethical principles. Hence, there are similarities. Much of ethics is based on the golden rule. We hate being lied to or ridiculed, so it is unethical and wrong to lie to or ridicule others. Ethics does not derive from the law but does often parallel it. Ethics and law are not coterminous and sometimes sharply diverge.

Although law addresses what one is required to do, ethics deals with what one *ought* to do. A court ruling or a statute is binding and must be followed or there can be civil or criminal consequences if one is charged and duly convicted. On the other hand, an ethical precept (unless also codified into law) is generally unenforceable, although it can serve as a significant moral or professional guideline for behavior.

Unethical behavior is often punished by what the wrongdoer sees in the mirror. Some might term this a *guilty conscience*. Little happens in the way of retribution or punishment for unethical behavior except a loss of self-respect and good reputation and possibly the retaliatory behavior of a wronged party. Failure to comply with a code of professional ethical conduct may result in penalties, even including expulsion from the profession.

Both ethics and the law are dynamic and constantly evolving in response to challenges, including new technology, scientific discoveries, and society's perception and appreciation of the standards of decency. Sometimes the moral conscience of society is a precursor to legal rules.

This book occasionally cites significant court rulings when they cogently express an ethical principle or when they afford insight into the thoughtful rationale applied in resolving difficult and contested matters, especially those that affect the behaviors of health professionals. To an extent, professional codes of ethics may derive some of their precepts from legal precedent.

Courts often defer to the tenets of medical ethics, although some courts have not done so when rendering decisions in death penalty cases.[9]

Dignity of the Human Person

We begin with the concept that prisoners are human beings and that their basic human rights are not abbreviated, except to the extent necessary to carry out their sentences. Their intrinsic worth or dignity as human beings is not diminished, and all people—regardless of gender, sexual preference, race, age, ethnicity, nationality, history, politics, or present circumstance—share in the same humanity.

From where does the ethical obligation to provide medical care to prisoners derive? Medical ethicist Felicia Cohn gives an excellent summary of the ethical rationale and foundation for prisoner entitlement to the same basic rights as other human beings. She ascribes the ethical basis of the rights prisoners enjoy to:

- their inherent human value as persons,
- the social contract theory,
- the definition of justice,
- the notion of just deserts, and
- a utilitarian calculus of societal benefits and burdens.[10]

Value of Persons—People matter as ends in and of themselves and not solely in relation to their ability to benefit or harm society. Respect for each individual person is fundamental and central to most religious belief systems—certainly to

Christianity, Judaism, and Islam. We recognize socially approved norms of human conduct as forming a common morality that embodies basic human rights and corresponding obligations, which have been summed up as "doing unto others as we would have them do unto us." To impose suffering or inflict harm on another when that suffering or harm can be avoided is to devalue that person as a human being.

See the further discussion on the value of each human person in Chapter 5, "How Much Health Care Is Appropriate and Necessary," under "Cost Factors." There the "social value theory" is rejected because it would allocate scarce resources such as organ transplants on a priority basis to persons deemed of greater worth to society.

Social Contract Theory—Within a free society, justice is commonly believed to be based on fairness. We can theorize[11] that people, under an original veil of ignorance with respect to their own unique characteristics in society—that is, not knowing who is rich or poor, majority or minority, male or female, prisoner or free—would be unable to tailor the social principles of the larger group to favor their own particular circumstances. Each person who operates in that world and is motivated by self-interest would necessarily seek to design principles as advantageous as possible to whatever position each ultimately will be in when the veil of ignorance is lifted. Thus, it is postulated that fair principles would arise from this process. Reason can tell us that we would all prefer to live in a society in which being in jail does not threaten our lives but also one in which heinous crime is maximally discouraged. Society then would create principles allowing for the fair and equitable treatment of inmates without rewarding criminal behavior. Seriously ill prisoners should receive appropriate care because the original self-interested parties had to allow for the possibility that they themselves might turn out to be prisoners afflicted with serious illness. The same theory would accord as much liberty as possible to all persons—even to prisoners. Criminals have breached the social contract, impinged on the liberty of others, and are sanctioned with a loss of freedom as a result. However, this loss of liberty is not comprehensive or absolute, and some measure of liberty is retained according to the security classification ascribed for the particular offense and offender—that is, prisoners maintain as much freedom as possible under the system of sanctions developed and accepted by society.[12]

Despite their limited liberty, certain interests of prisoners are constitutionally protected. When the state incarcerates people and thereby interferes with their freedom and ability to provide for all of their basic needs, the state itself assumes the obligation to provide for those needs. "Prisoners, as a consequence of their status, cannot independently secure medical services; they must rely on the system and the practitioners within it."[13]

"The degree of civilization in a society can be judged by entering its prisons."
—Fyodor Dostoevsky

Justice Defined—Justice can be defined in the *distributive* sense as rendering to each person what is his or her due. It can also be construed in the *corrective* sense—that is, the righting of a wrong. It is in this latter sense that we find the principles applicable to our system of criminal punishment. Victims of crime experience injustice from the perpetrators, and consequently society attempts to right this wrong by imposing punishment on the perpetrators—typically by enforcing limits on their freedom.

Perhaps because retribution and restraint have become the prominent functions of the criminal justice system, other important goals of justice—specifically *rehabilitation*—are too often obscured or downgraded in priority, especially under conditions of limited resources. Thus, programs such as education, job training, counseling, substance abuse treatment, and social skills development should also be seen as central to the purpose of correctional systems. The development of such programs, Cohn points out, "may not only fulfill the requirements of justice in terms of giving each his due, but it also may provide the opportunities for rehabilitation that justice also evokes.[13]

Just Deserts—Some theorists hold that inmates deserve an unpleasant life and a miserable death. But criminals are incarcerated *as* punishment, not *for* punishment. Sentences do not mandate additional punishments once confined. Consequently, their basic human needs are to be met while incarcerated. "To suggest that inmates deserve to suffer when they become seriously ill and approach death is to use prison unjustly as a forum for additional retribution," says Cohn.[14]

Utilitarian Calculus—What type of society do we wish to be? Society's ethical imperative to provide proper health care to prisoners arises from its fundamental commitment to care for its members. But who is responsible for the inadequate conditions that now obtain for so many inmates? There are choices to be made regarding our moral identity and values: we can be the type of society that allows fellow human beings to live and die in deplorable conditions, including unnecessary pain and suffering, or we can be the type of society that chooses to care. The insightful statement of Dostoevsky echoes this point: "The degree of civilization in a society can be judged by entering its prisons."[15]

Cohn concludes:

Ethical arguments can be useful in making a case for valuing prisoners as human beings, fulfilling our social contract with them, recognizing the need for just policies, and allowing for social utility. What remains is action on those philosophical arguments. . . . If we can learn to care for what is arguably one of the least valued populations in our society, then we certainly can provide care for other population groups. Our society should not have to rely on the courts, as it has in the past, to serve as its moral conscience.[16]

Professional Codes of Ethics

Virtually every learned profession develops and publishes a set of ethical standards. Though worded and arranged differently, each bespeaks the thoughtful commitment of leadership within that profession to adhere to high standards of integrity and, for medical practitioners, a dedication to the health and well-being of the patient or client.

People have a right to expect that a police officer will help rather than harm them, that a priest will not betray their confidence or abuse them, that a teacher will not knowingly mislead them, that a doctor or nurse will not intentionally cause injury, and that a correctional official will not abuse the power and opportunities that she or he possesses over them.

Meaning of a Professional Code of Ethics

Codes of ethics formulated by professional societies tend to be distillations of the accumulated philosophy, tradition, and moral precepts of dedicated members of that profession over the years that have been handed down to current practitioners of that profession as a concise set of fundamental principles to guide their conduct and relationships. Thus it serves to inform both its members and the general society of the ethical standards that the profession itself requires and expects its members to follow.

All health professionals are ethically bound, for example, to protect the confidentiality of private matters entrusted to them by their clients or patients. Even if not covered in law or regulation, professional persons have a duty in this regard. Ethical codes are compiled and promulgated by professional associations that can and do revoke membership for flagrant violations.

Becoming familiar with the principles of the professional disciplines and their practical significance is an integral part of the acculturation and socialization that occurs during formal academic preparation for the professions. A lawyer, doctor, priest, psychologist, or nurse learns not only the cognitive and technical skills of the respective profession but also the moral and behavioral expectations, obligations, and boundaries of its practice. Sanctions for deviating from these norms are intended to protect society and preserve the integrity of the profession.

Not every conceivable situation can be explicitly covered in a code of ethics. Application of ethical principles to individual situations is an ongoing, daily task. Choosing from apparently conflicting obligations in a specific circumstance can be difficult. The correct solution is not always obvious. Good and intelligent people may sometimes legitimately disagree on an interpretation or application of these principles. What might first appear to be a minor or scarcely relevant circumstance could affect the analysis significantly.

The health professions and the criminal justice professions have different starting points, objectives, philosophies, policies, methods, and standards as discussed in greater detail in Chapter 9, "Corrections and Health Care Working Together," under "Recognizing Differences." Some policies and practices of a correctional institution may place health care professionals in situations that conflict with the principles of medical ethics. The doctor, nurse, or psychologist may then question the procedure or decline to follow it. This can be troublesome for a correctional supervisor in systems that are tightly managed by detailed policy manuals that all employees are expected to observe.

Stanley Brodsky wrote,

While psychologists come from backgrounds of scientific discipline and helping concerns, correctional administrators are a part of the justice process. . . . The law, from the courts through corrections, holds to the principle that truth arises from the adversary presentation of opposing views. Psychology and other helping professions assume that cooperation and collaboration are the essence of finding truth, through research endeavors and therapeutic procedures. Psychology tends to value trust; corrections values control. . . . [17]

People have a right to expect that a police officer will help rather than harm them, that a priest will not betray their confidence or abuse them, that a teacher will not knowingly mislead them, that a doctor will not intentionally cause injury, and that a correctional official will not abuse the power and opportunities that she or he possesses over them.

In most cases, health professionals who question an established or proposed correctional policy on ethical grounds are not troublemakers or unruly persons and should not be viewed as such. They are conscientious employees facing a real dilemma. Perhaps it can be resolved by a simple clarification. At other times, a policy may need to be changed. A highly principled, honest employee who thoughtfully and respectfully challenges a system to rethink some policies and practices should be viewed as an asset to the agency, and he or she is far better in the long run than a "go along to get along" employee who just obeys the rules. The following pages illustrate this with examples and attempts to explore some boundaries of these ethical principles.

Correctional professionals regard as a sacred trust their duty to safeguard the public through confinement of legally detained inmates. They also subscribe to maintaining the good order of the institution and the humane and safe management of prisoners.

Physicians are bound by a fundamental principle to render service to a patient only when this intervention is deemed to be in the patient's best interest and not for any other purpose. The physician is taught *primum non nocere*—that is, "above all, inflict no harm." The Hippocratic oath states: "I will use treatment to help the sick according to my ability and judgment, but I will never use it to injure or wrong them."[18] The World Medical Association holds out the following pledge: "A physician shall respect a patient's right to confidentiality. It is ethical to disclose confidential information when the patient consents to it or when there is a real and imminent threat of harm to the patient or to others and this threat can be only removed by a breach of confidentiality."[19] Other health professionals subscribe to similar principles.

In recent years, economic realities have required recognition of legitimate interests outside of what had for a long time been widely regarded as a dyadic relationship[20] between physician and patient. The growth of medical insurance since the 1950s created a disconnect between *payment* for services and *receipt* of services. The rise of health maintenance organizations and managed care since the 1980s focused attention on costs and broke away from the traditional notion that cost should not limit needed medical care. As a result, third-party payers (insurers, governments, and employers) now have an active voice in doctor–patient decisions to prevent unreasonable escalation of costs. In some circumstances the need for access to a particular treatment by other patients must also be considered in allocating scarce resources. The physician's obligations to the patient must now balance the patient's interests against the legitimate competing claims of other patients, payers, and society as a whole.[21] Through all of this, however, it must remain clear that the physician's primary client is the patient, that the patient's well-being is preeminent, and that the physician must always be the patient's advocate.

Most of the time the issue will not reflect clear all-or-nothing or black-and-white dilemmas in which the medical professional or correctional professional must choose between two conflicting or opposing principles. Usually, concerns of both sides require open and candid recognition and discussion so that decisions can be made that acknowledge important nuances and attempt to balance the legitimate demands of both parties in a reasonable manner.

> It must remain clear that the physician's primary client is the patient, that the patient's well-being is preeminent, and that the physician must always be the patient's advocate.

Decision makers should not hesitate to seek the advice of thoughtful persons from outside the agency who may bring a greater objectivity and fresh insight to deliberations concerning sensitive and complex ethical issues. For a while during the late 1980s, the Michigan Department of Corrections added a medical ethicist[22] from the community to its health care advisory board. The Florida Department of Corrections established a bioethics committee in 1993 with a majority of its members being ethicists from outside the field of corrections. This bioethics committee held regular meetings to consider ethical problems within the correctional system, consult on individual cases, and propose positions and policies. There are similar examples elsewhere, but unfortunately the practice is not yet widespread. Examples of topics that can benefit from multidisciplinary bioethics review include organ transplantation, end-of-life decisions, informed-consent issues, religious objections to health care interventions, and management of transgender patients.

Thomas and Thomas[23] have proposed a national bioethics forum for corrections that is modeled after hospital bioethics committees and comprises a panel of recognized experts. Cases could be presented for consideration, and the results would be advisory in nature. Deliberations could be kept confidential, but the generalized findings would be publicly available so that a body of knowledge could be compiled on ethical matters in corrections. How such an effort would be funded and how members would be appointed are important questions to be resolved, but a central resource of this nature would be of value so long as full independence from outside pressure is ensured.

The situations demanding a careful application of sound ethical principles are numerous and frequent in correctional settings. A thoughtful guide for setting up a bioethics program in a correctional system is described by Reams et al.[24]

IMPORTANT ETHICAL ISSUES IN CORRECTIONS

Beneficence, Medical Neutrality, Medical Autonomy

The fundamental ethical principles of beneficence and autonomy are explained in Chapter 5, "How Much Health Care Is Appropriate and Necessary," under "Universal Principles." Briefly, the principle of *beneficence* requires that no intervention be undertaken unless it is expected to result in a net benefit for the patient. Some theorists also identify the principle of *nonmaleficence*, which is the mirror image of beneficence—"Do no harm"—and logically precedes it.

Medical neutrality dictates that the health professional treat patients regardless of their background, race, gender, ethnicity, nationality, status, affiliations, or position. Thus, a doctor in wartime must treat all wounded, whether co-patriots or enemy, and medical decision-making should not be affected or influenced by loyalty to either side.

Medical autonomy requires that health care providers are not directed by non-medical authorities in making clinical judgments and decisions affecting their patients. Providers are free to make clinical judgments based on clinical reasons, and without interference.

Privacy, Patient Autonomy, Confidentiality, Acceptability

In *Olmstead v. U.S.* (277 U.S. 438 [1928]), Justice Louis Brandeis defined *privacy* as "the right to be left alone—the most comprehensive of rights, and the right most valued by a free people." It embraces the right to confidentiality of medical information. It is also the foundation for the principle of *patient autonomy*.

The principle of patient autonomy requires that treatment not be enforced on an unwilling patient. The right of the individual for self-determination is important and can only be overridden when exercise of that freedom results in harm to another. This "harm principle" was clearly expressed by 19th-century philosopher John Stuart Mill (1806–1873) as follows:

The only purpose for which power can rightfully be exercised over any member of a civilized community, against his will, is to prevent harm to others. His own good, either physical or moral, is not sufficient warrant. He cannot rightfully be compelled to do or forbear because it will be better for him to do so, because it will make him happier, because, in the opinions of others, to do so would be wise, or even right. These are good reasons for remonstrating with him, or reasoning with him, or persuading him, or entreating him, but not for compelling him.[25]

A related principle is that of *least restrictive alternative* so that the treatment selected is the one that best balances the benefits and risks. In a similar vein, the U.S. Supreme Court in *Shelton v. Tucker* (364 U.S. 479) declared in 1960 that "even though the governmental purpose be legitimate and substantial, that purpose cannot be pursued by means that broadly stifle fundamental personal liberties when the end can be more narrowly achieved."

Confidentiality relates to the promise made by health professionals to their clients that their private and personal information will be safeguarded as "privileged." It is this promise, along with the pledge to hold patients' well-being above all other considerations, that enables and encourages patients to place trust in their health care providers. Physician–patient confidentiality is fundamentally an ethical obligation that is derived from the essential trust that a patient must have in the health care professional. This duty to maintain confidentiality may also be codified in statute.

People rightly expect the doctor–patient privilege to safeguard in strict confidence whatever the health professionals have learned about them in the process of rendering health care. They do not want their personal secrets revealed at a cocktail party or over the back fence. This is analogous to the attorney–client privilege or the inviolable confidence between priest and penitent. The expectation that this confidence will be respected is essential to the trust required in any of these relationships. Codes of correctional health care standards of the National Commission on Correctional Health Care (NCCHC),[26] American Public Health Association (APHA),[27] and American Correctional Association (ACA)[28] require that medical records of patients be kept separate from the institutional records and that their contents be held in strict confidence and only be available to those persons with a legitimate need to access the information.

Health care personnel go to considerable lengths to protect patient confidentiality. Medical and mental health encounters with patients should take place in relative privacy and as appropriate to the situation. Health record files should be kept locked and inaccessible to officers and inmates.

In addition to the obligation to accord patients due privacy and confidentiality, *patient acceptability* is another concern that ought not to be lightly dismissed. Certain types of medical and psychiatric examinations and procedures are inherently embarrassing to many people. Patients become uncomfortable when they feel their privacy is being invaded. As a result, some patients may not seek needed care, or they may give the provider incomplete or inaccurate information. Great sensitivity and empathy on the part of care providers is needed to detect this concern and gently assist patients in managing it. Sensitivity to issues of gender, ethnicity, culture, and age are highly important.

It is easy to imagine areas of potential conflict, even in a well-managed correctional system. Secrecy and privacy are problematic in the correctional setting. Patients known to be dangerous should not be left alone with a health provider. Correctional officers do need to know what is going on with inmates. Suppose a maximum-security institution has a policy that all inmates living in certain housing areas will have an officer present in the examining room during each medical encounter because the warden or other appropriate authority has determined this to be necessary for safety and security. Here, careful examination of the intent and the content of both conflicting requirements can lead to a satisfactory resolution. Medical ethics do not intend to create unsafe conditions for the practice of medicine, and the health care professional may be less likely than the correctional officer to assess accurately the current security risks. Neither does the correctional concern for security intentionally seek to breach the doctor–patient privilege. Perhaps the officer could stand just outside the door and observe the doctor and patient through a window. If the patient does not behave appropriately, the doctor should be instructed to terminate the encounter at once. On the other hand, this may not always be adequate, and sometimes good judgment may require the officer to remain physically close during the encounter.

Such decisions are best reached on a case-by-case basis rather than be dictated as a general routine practice. If the policy directs that an officer be present whenever either the officer or the health service provider has reason to believe that a particular patient is likely to present a security risk on a specific occasion, then the intrusion into privacy rests on a judgment regarding individual circumstances and not merely on the fact that the person belongs to a particular class.

At a minimum, each correctional agency must have a policy that indicates that any officer who observes or overhears confidential or privileged information derived from the process of rendering health care to an inmate is obliged to respect that confidence and is strictly prohibited from discussing or revealing this information to any other person. This is not a matter to be taken lightly but it also should not present an insoluble dilemma. It must, however, be incorporated into officer training and supervision as well as into formal policy.

Confidentiality and privacy have limits, and neither is absolute. When they conflict with other societal goods such as safety or the common welfare, there is a need to achieve balance among the values. In recognition of a greater good, laws require that free world doctors report gunshot wounds or signs of child abuse to the proper authorities, even when this information is obtained while giving medical care to the patient. Most states also require that certain infectious diseases be reported to the health department. These provisions are justifiable because they are intended to prevent greater harm to the larger community. When a patient reveals an intent to harm a third party and the mental health professional determines that disclosure of client information is necessary to protect the third party from a clear, imminent risk of serious injury or death, there arises an obligation to warn the potential victim. Under such circumstances, health professionals are protected from liability in most states if they breach a client's confidence.[29] Correctional officials have a need to know certain information to facilitate provision of care, for example, to escort a patient to a specific type of provider or to permit certain medications or devices to be in a patient's possession. Also, when appropriate, they need to know the specific disease-prevention practices to be observed. This does not suggest, however, that HIV-positive individuals should be identified for the protection of officers. The concept of *universal precautions* for blood-borne pathogens, if correctly understood and applied, offers far greater protection to the officers because those known to be infected represent only a fraction of all persons who may be infected. Whenever there is potential exposure to blood and body fluids, the only safe course is to regard *all* persons as if they were infected. Using "extra care" with known infected persons implies use of "lesser caution" with the others—thereby incurring additional risk.

Each correctional agency must have a policy that indicates that any officer who observes or overhears confidential or privileged information derived from the process of rendering health care to an inmate is obliged to respect that confidence and is strictly prohibited from discussing or revealing this information to any other person.

Any information that indicates a danger to self or others must be shared with institutional authorities, including suicidal intent, possession of a weapon, or a plan for escape, as required by the APHA standards.[30] The clinician should let the patient know in advance just how much the patient can reveal before the therapist will be obliged to inform custody staff.

Good facility design considerations can assist greatly with meeting the requirements to provide care in a *safe* as well as *confidential* manner. For example, doors to examination and treatment rooms should have windows that are large enough to permit an officer to ascertain that all is secure. Some health care staff unwisely attempt to cover windows with paper or curtains and thereby defeat their important purpose. This practice should not be allowed. Another solution is the use of a partition that does not reach to the ceiling, thus allowing loud cries or sounds to be heard easily. Generally, for mental health situations, privacy of sound is more important than privacy of sight. For certain medical procedures, the opposite may be true.

Above all, the patient ought to be informed about any limits to the confidentiality she or he otherwise has a right to expect. These limits should be explained by mental health professionals when interviewing a new patient and at other times when relevant.[31]

Informed Consent and Enforced Treatment

Medical and mental health practitioners are justifiably concerned with ensuring that patients give their informed consent for all therapeutic interventions. Ultimately, it is the patient alone who must determine what happens to his or her own body. This is an important application of the right to *privacy* and the principle of *autonomy*. Informed consent requires communicating, in language understood by the patient, the relevant risks and the benefits of a test or treatment in a way that allows the patient to decide whether to authorize the intervention. The practitioner who obtains the patient's informed consent generally will place a note to this effect in the patient's health record. For minor procedures, verbal consent or even implied consent usually is sufficient. When working with juveniles, there is an additional obligation to obtain parental consent for all significant procedures. State law and community practice are relevant here, both as to age of majority and who may be designated as a surrogate for the parents. Generally, it is good practice to make a reasonable effort to contact a parent or guardian directly.

For invasive, intrusive, or risky procedures, a more formal process is required. An explanation is given to the patient concerning the advantages and disadvantages of the procedure, as well as the availability, benefits, and risks of alternative therapies or of no treatment at all, followed by a signed consent to treatment. Failure to obtain consent for treatment exposes the provider to tort liability for "unwanted touching." In other words, the patient can sue the doctor for assault and battery and may prevail if consent was not granted. It matters not whether the touching harms the patient or if the intent (and result) of the touching is to provide benefit to the patient.[32] APHA requires that "[c]onsent should be witnessed by health care staff and documented in the record prior to performing invasive procedures."[33]

The use of preauthorization forms has become a common practice in many prisons and jails. Each new arrival is presented with a generic consent form applicable to all health services provided while an individual is in custody at that facility. This approach has little value and does not obviate the need for all health care professionals to obtain informed consent from patients for each procedure, formal or informal, as appropriate. A court would give scant heed to this generic consent if the matter were to arise in litigation.

An early judicial statement of the right of competent adults to refuse treatment is that of Judge (and later Associate Justice) Benjamin Cardozo: "Every human being of adult years and sound mind has a right to determine what shall be done with his own body; and a surgeon who performs an operation without his patient's consent commits an assault for which he is liable in damages. This is true except in cases of emergency where the patient is unconscious and where it is necessary to operate before consent can be obtained" (*Schloendorff v. Society of New York Hospital*).[34]

An unconscious or incompetent person can be treated in an emergency under the presumption that the patient would give consent if able to do so. When time permits, surrogate consent is advised. Family members are often appropriate for this purpose, as also may be the institution head or designee. This procedure involves explaining both the risks and advantages of the intervention to the patient's representative so that an informed decision can be made reflecting, as far as possible, the patient's own preferences and best interests.

The concept of informed consent can be thought of as a "meeting of the minds"—a *consensus ad idem,* to use the old legal term, meaning a "mutual understanding of the same thing." A person who is told the benefits of a procedure but is not told about its risks or alternatives has not been fully informed and there has been no meeting of the minds. In law, the parties to a contract are assumed to know what they are getting into. When one of the parties has been misled and is not fully informed of all the risks, then there has been no true meeting of the minds and the contract is not enforceable.

Attorney William Isele explained a subsequent development of law concerning the right to privacy:

A second basis for this right is grounded in the long-recognized constitutional right of privacy. There is no specific statement of this right in the U.S. Constitution or any of its amendments. Nevertheless, in *Roe v. Wade,* the Supreme Court said: "In a line of decisions, however, going back to . . . 1891 . . . the court has recognized that a right of personal privacy, or a guarantee of certain areas or zones of privacy, does exist under the constitution." The essence of this right, as the Supreme Court has defined it, is autonomy over matters of personal integrity, including control over one's body.[35]

In 1990, the Supreme Court upheld the legal standard that competent persons are able to exercise the right to refuse medical treatment under the *due process* clause (*Cruzan v. Missouri Department of Health,* 497 U.S. 261 [1990]). For prisoners, sometimes legitimate state interests are superior to the individual's constitutional right to refuse. Each case is fact specific, and the patient's medical condition and prognosis, the benefits and burdens of treatment, and the impact of the refusal on other persons are all factors that weigh on this issue. The state's interests include protecting and preserving life, preventing suicide, protecting the interests of the parties, and maintaining prison security, order, and discipline.[36]

Psychiatric treatment sometimes is administered involuntarily. The principles and guidelines that apply in a correctional setting are generally the same as for a patient in the free world under similar circumstances. In the community, commitment to a mental hospital is a process involving strict legal safeguards for the patient, partly because involuntary hospitalization deprives an otherwise free citizen of liberty. Some have argued that, because this liberty already has been taken away from prisoners by a court of law, it is within the authority of the institution head to assign the patient to a mental health unit even when the patient does not wish to go, as long as no involuntary treatment is administered in the psychiatric unit. However, the U.S. Supreme Court in *Vitek v. Jones*[37] would disallow this interpretation on grounds that the stigma attached to psychiatric commitment and the possibility of involuntary subjection to psychiatric treatment constitutes a deprivation of liberty requiring due process. This principle of *Vitek* was found applicable, even if the mental hospital is part of the correctional department (*Baugh v. Woodard* and *Witzke v. Johnson*).[38]

Although the exact language may differ, in most jurisdictions the decision to enforce psychiatric treatment rests on a triple finding that the patient:

1. is mentally ill;
2. as a consequence of the mental illness, is imminently dangerous to self or to others, or is unable to care for his or her own bodily needs essential to the preservation of life, or whose judgment is so impaired that she or he is unable to understand the need for treatment and whose continued behavior as a result of this mental illness can reasonably be expected, on the basis of competent medical opinion, to result in significant physical harm to self or others, and;
3. that no less invasive or less restrictive alternative will suffice.

In most states, a psychiatrist who makes such a determination may treat only in an emergency and may continue the treatment for a period not to exceed 48 hours. When prolonged involuntary treatment is determined to be necessary, a court order should be obtained or other due process followed, according to the established procedures in the jurisdiction. At this point also, the patient probably belongs in a hospital.

In view of the shift of patients with serious mental illness from long-term institutional care to community settings, some mental health professionals such as Munetz, Galon, and Frese have advocated expanding this concept to include mandatory outpatient treatment, under strict conditions and well-defined circumstances, for free world patients with serious mental disorders (such as schizophrenia spectrum and bipolar and major depressive disorders) who do not voluntarily adhere to treatment regimens and who appear unable to live successfully in the community without coercive interventions. Their reasoning is that many such persons are incompetent because they lack insight into their illness or their need for treatment and therefore suffer from a persistent lack of decision-making capacity:

A strong argument can be made that there are patients with schizophrenia who meet the description of the revolving-door patient who cannot make an autonomous refusal. Their brain disorders prevent them from making an informed decision. In such cases, rights-based arguments [against treating unwilling patients] appear to give way to the notion of *beneficence,* using the *parens patriae* powers of the state to make decisions on behalf of individuals who are unable to make informed decisions for themselves. [39]

Without such imposed treatment, it is argued, a patient would be allowed to be a victim of his or her own illness. Munetz et al. acknowledge that this reasoning has been criticized for defining "lack of insight into one's illness" to mean "disagreeing with one's doctor." Although their argument relies on the contested theory that rational decision-making capacity in these mentally ill patients is prevented by a brain disorder, overall the authors make a strong utilitarian case that the benefits to society and these individuals themselves can be maximized by mandatory outpatient treatment under carefully defined limitations and circumstances. They also point out a "slippery slope" concern, "especially if we are not careful with the criteria used for such interventions" and caution against expanding these criteria to include other populations such as substance abusers and sex offenders.

In *Washington v. Harper* (494 U.S. 210 [1990]), the Supreme Court ruled that, although prison inmates have a liberty interest in resisting unwanted psychotropic medications, due process can be satisfied by a competent physician deciding to protect the inmate or others as long as this decision can be challenged in an administrative proceeding. The treating physician may not be included in this proceeding.[40]

Policies in some correctional systems have inappropriately condoned enforced medical treatment. Such a policy might state, in effect, that any treatment prescribed by the doctor must be taken by the patient as directed or the patient will be ticketed and be subject to punishment. The reasoning (of at least one prison system several years ago) was that each able-bodied prisoner was required to work in the fields every day. Remaining sick longer than necessary was not tolerated. Hence, the institution regarded compliance with prescribed treatment as an issue of good order and discipline. Whether legitimate penological concern or state interest justifies enforced treatment under these circumstances is a matter that ultimately a court could decide. However, it seem clear that the ethical concern for a patient's fundamental right to privacy should take precedence.

Similarly, some states require by policy that inmates submit to tuberculosis (TB) testing and faithfully take all TB medications prescribed by the doctor. Failure to do so results in a disciplinary infraction and segregation until the prisoner agrees to comply. The rationale is to prevent spread of disease, but the means used is punitive. A better alternative is to use the public health authority of the physician to place a person in quarantine until such time as it can be determined that he or she is no longer contagious. The quarantine might be achieved in a segregation cell, but the prisoner should understand that this is not a disciplinary proceeding or punishment and is a public health measure to protect others from disease, and care should be taken to ensure that undue loss of privilege does not accompany this restricted housing. The only justification for employing this strategy is a determination by the medical authority that the health of the population cannot otherwise be adequately safeguarded.

In *Sell v. United States*, the state sought to administer antipsychotic medications forcibly as the only viable hope of rendering the defendant competent to stand trial. The court agreed that involuntary treatment was "necessary to serve the government's compelling interest in obtaining an adjudication of defendant's guilt or innocence of numerous and serious charges." The court of appeals found that even though Sell was not a danger to himself or others in the institution, the governmental interest in bringing him to trial was itself sufficient to justify the administration of medications that would render him competent. However, the Supreme Court stated that administration of antipsychotic drugs against an inmate's will is constitutionally permissible, "but only if the treatment is medically appropriate, is substantially unlikely to have side effects that may undermine the fairness of the trial, and, taking account of less intrusive alternatives, is necessary significantly to further important governmental trial-related interests." [41] In other words, there would have to be an essential or overriding state interest.

Some patients especially dislike injectable medications. However, it may be possible to persuade a disturbed mentally ill patient to consent to open his or her mouth to take oral medication in order to calm down and feel better. If the patient agrees to do so, the newer orally disintegrating tablet or "wafer" form of medication can be placed on the patient's tongue where it will dissolve within a few seconds. This is vastly preferable to going through the ordeal of a forcible injection. Zyprexa and Klonopin are medications available in wafer form that may be suitable, depending on the patient's condition.[42]

Informed Refusal

Prisoners must be allowed to refuse treatment. Most facilities provide a form for signing an "informed refusal" to follow medical advice. This gives some protection to the provider and the facility from liability should the patient subsequently suffer adverse consequences. Care must be taken, however, to ensure that the patient is duly aware of the nature of the service being refused. When, for example, the patient signs a refusal slip because his tooth is feeling better, this is not an informed refusal if the callout was, instead, for a comprehensive dental examination or for follow-up on a different problem such as gingivitis. A patient who had put in a sick call request because of cold or flu symptoms might refuse a callout appointment on grounds that she or he is feeling better, being unaware that the callout appointment was, instead, for follow-up of some other medical problem or for an intake physical examination or a blood pressure check. The best solution is to require that refusals take place in the presence of the nurse rather than an officer so that any ambiguity or misunderstanding can be cleared up.

Some institutions will not allow an inmate on a special diet to take both a diet tray and a regular tray for the same meal. This is acceptable. Other institutions inform the physician each time an inmate with a special diet order elects instead to take the regular meal. Should this occur frequently, the doctor is justified in advising the patient that the special diet order will be discontinued. However, the patient should later be able to ask for reinstatement of a medically necessary diet on condition of promised compliance—as long as the medical need still exists and when there is some expectation that the promise will be kept.

A Caring Approach

"Caring" is a matter of central import for the health care professional. Other qualities are also critically important and essential—especially diagnostic and treatment skills—but caring is a *sine qua non*. Clinical skills can be and have been grossly misused by noncaring persons. Some seasoned, experienced correctional health care professionals and supervisors, out of concern with preventing problems with boundary issues and helping new staff avoid being naïve and vulnerable in their contacts with prisoners, stress the need to "toughen up," put on a stiff and hard exterior, demand that prisoners always address them formally, and refrain from giving any sign of caring, concern, or trust. While it is true that boundary issues require careful attention, it is neither required nor appropriate that health care staff present themselves in a harsh, noncaring manner.

Some experienced health care providers have become jaundiced and pessimistic about the potential of prisoners to succeed. This tendency is not limited to their beliefs as to whether prisoners will ever amend their life and avoid future crime. It extends even to nurses, doctors, and mental health professionals who believe that their patients will not cooperate with treatment, as well as substance abuse professionals who do not believe their clients can ever succeed in overcoming addiction. Sex offenders and violent offenders may be assessed in the same way. Often the belief derives from a preconceived notion or from prior experiences and is not based on an individual patient assessment. Senior or supervisory staff who have these beliefs may discourage new treatment staff from exerting extra effort to elicit a therapeutic alliance with a patient or from "going an extra mile" in the hope of achieving a better response. They warn staff about wasting their time, allowing themselves to be manipulated by the attention-seeking behavior of patients, and blurring the boundaries they must maintain.

This is self-defeating in two ways. First, such expectations can be self-fulfilling prophecies. Treatment providers who do not believe in the efficacy of their efforts will not succeed. Second, if the message explicitly or even implicitly conveyed to the patient is that the therapist has given up, that "You'll never make anything out of yourself," or that "You're just a loser," the patient may be discouraged from actively cooperating with treatment. The therapist should always communicate that she or he believes in the patient and expects the patient to be successful. Many prisoners grew up at home and school rarely hearing words of encouragement and constantly being judged as failures who would never amount to anything. As important as this advice is for all prisoners, it is even more so with juveniles. It is critically important for their therapists and caretakers to say that they believe in their clients.

Much the same can be said regarding patients with personality or behavioral (formerly called Axis II) disorders that are so common among prisoners. Starting with the pervasive belief of many that these conditions are not treatable, often little effort is devoted to treatment. Yet there are documented claims of successful interventions for these disorders, including sound evidence that psychotherapy, especially cognitive behavioral therapy (CBT) and dialectical behavioral treatment (DBT) interventions are often successful when other therapeutic approaches have failed. Using insights and knowledge gained in therapy, patients learn healthy ways to manage their symptoms. Recognizing the extreme financial burden shouldered by society and prison systems from the negative behaviors of persons with sociopathic personality disorders, it seems reasonable to take a fresh look at the potential benefit from spending resources to treat these disorders with the expectation that the lives of at least some of these patients will be improved.

The principles of quality listed by the Institute of Medicine[43] require that care be *patient centered* and *equitable.* Patient-centered care is respectful of and responsive to individual patient preferences, needs, and values, and it must ensure that patient well-being guides all clinical decisions. It is important to treat each patient as a *person,* not as a diagnosis or a medical condition. Moreover, equitable care does not vary in quality because of personal characteristics such as gender, ethnicity, geographic location, or socioeconomic status. We add that quality of care must not vary because of the fact of incarceration.

Nurses, doctors, and other health professionals have been taught to care about their patients. Work in a correctional environment has been known to have a corrosive effect on this caring approach. Examples are sometimes noticed in reviewing documents of a lawsuit brought against a correctional system alleging a wrongful death or injury. Too often, a disturbing pattern emerges as one reads through the medical record entries, looks at kites and grievances and their responses, examines notations made in logs, and reviews other related documentation. Something bad has clearly happened, but no one appears to have done anything really wrong. It is hard to assign blame or to point to the one thing that led to the unhappy event. None of the actors appears to be malicious or to have evil intent. But a general sense emerges that no one really cared. Nurses and medical service providers seem to comply with the rules and policies—but just barely. They do what is necessary, but nothing extra. Perhaps they are short staffed. Money is tight. There are many patients to see and a lot of kites to look at. There are grievances to answer, rounds to make, chronic patients to see, reports to write, and medications to pass. The ball simply gets passed from one person to another, each trying to dodge responsibility.

To illustrate from just one case known to the author, a patient submitted a kite saying that her keep-on-person medications would be gone in three days and she needed a refill. She was sent a form to complete for renewal of the medications (even though she had already made it clear in her kite which medications were in need of refill). She completed the form. But a week later she wrote another kite saying she still did not have her prescribed pain medications. After a few days she received another blank form for medication renewal. A couple of weeks later, she wrote a fifth kite, explaining in detail that she had now filled out four reorder forms but was still without her medications. Then she filed a grievance, indicating the date of the accident that caused her knee injury as the date the problem began. (Clearly this was a misunderstanding. She should have cited the failure to supply her medications as the date the problem began.) The grievance responder determined that the grievance was untimely since it must be filed within 10 days of the event that precipitated the grievance—completely omitting any reference to the substantive issue that was grieved. A responsible grievance responder should have investigated why the nurse did not simply phone the pharmacy on the first or second occasion and inquire whether the refill form had been received. Actually, this would have saved everyone time in the long run. The patient would have had her medications sooner. Why was the grievance responder so quick to find an irrelevant technicality as an excuse for dismissing the grievance rather than look at its substance and recognize a serious problem that needed to be addressed?

The same patient wrote a kite explaining that the orthopedic surgeon had wanted to see her in a month and that it was now five weeks and, as far as she knew, no appointment had yet been set up for her. The kite was answered: "Referral to PA next Monday." Now the patient had to wait for nearly another week to see the physician assistant who would look at her chart and discover that no appointment had been made for her. Why could not the nurse herself have checked the chart or made a phone call? She wrote another kite asking for some calcium, indicating that the orthopedic surgeon suggested that a calcium supplement would be helpful for her bone tissue and noting that it was not available in the commissary. The nurse replied that an appointment would be scheduled with the physician assistant in two weeks.

Over and over again in reviewing this chart it became apparent that staff routinely took a minimalist approach. No one ever went the "extra mile" or took that additional step to attempt to resolve the problem and reassure the patient. What had happened? These health care professionals seem to have forgotten about *caring* for their patients. Instead, they "did their job" and followed procedures each day to supply health services to the prisoners. At times it appeared that their primary concern was to see that patients did not take advantage of staff.

In another case, also known to the author, a diabetic patient in his late teens was lost to follow-up for some months. When he complained of eye problems, it was discovered that his routine blood sugar checks and his insulin treatment had been inadvertently omitted. A close review of the record showed there had been inadequate care. The physicians at this large jail were medical residents who rotated through the assignment, and there was little continuity and no supervision. The staff did their jobs but did not appear to follow up on important details. The boy became blind.

Among the ways that the corrosive or punishing effect of working in a corrections environment can begin to manifest itself is when a patient fails to show up for an appointment and the nurse decides to reschedule at the bottom of the appointment calendar in order to "teach him a lesson." Never mind that failure to keep the appointment may have been unavoidable.

Without question, a little extra care can go a long way to reduce costs and avoid problems. Take the extra minute or two with each patient to see if there are any unaddressed concerns or issues. Make the extra effort to look up the answer or make the phone call so that it is not put off for another appointment. Let patients feel that they have been examined, listened to, and cared for—and not walk away from the clinical encounter feeling confused, dissatisfied, and worried. Take grievances seriously and look past their technical deficiencies to see if you can identify the substance of the matter. If you cannot, then give the grievant a hearing. There are important lessons to be learned here from private practice settings where doctors and nurses know that their patients have other choices and could decide to change doctors. Patient satisfaction should be important in any clinic. There is likely a problem with the way the grievance system is being managed when the percentage of health care grievances found in favor of the inmate is extremely low.

"Any profession that loses its values loses also its soul and heart and sense of worth. Caring should take place every time a nurse-to-patient contact is made," [44] declares Mary Muse. It is the duty of clinical professionals to offer hope and commitment, honesty, sensibility, listening, and comfort. They need to be supportive and protective. Appropriate touching and calling the patient by name can sometimes be the key to breaking through barriers, depression, and defenses. If an inmate's wife, parent, or child just died, it may be reasonable for a nurse or social worker to put a hand briefly on the shoulder or touch the hand and say, "I understand how hard this is for you."

The following wise advice given by Mary Muse, RN, MS, correctional nurse leader for the Wisconsin Department of Corrections, is relevant and helpful:

- Care needs to be delivered in a professional caring manner. "I'm just here to give medication" is the response of an overworked medication pass nurse to patients who attempt to express complaints and symptoms.
- If we hope to change their behavior, we cannot do it punitively. Engaging the patient can help inspire accountability rather than anger over being written up.
- Some nurses just do not like the population they serve. They should get another job.
- Many think that nurses are "guests" in the correctional setting. But when do we stop being guests? We are partners.
- Caring means letting patients know that their welfare is important.
- We have opportunities to help inmates turn their lives around, minimize disparities that exist for our patients, and improve the quality of care.
- It is okay to be frustrated. But we have ethical boundaries. We need baseline measures for caring and ethics, and we should include them in performance appraisals.
- Caring can occur without curing, but curing cannot occur without caring.[45]
- When nurses' actions violate personal beliefs, they experience moral distress. When one knows the right thing to do but institutional constraints make it difficult, the nurses' moral values conflict with the reality of the workplace.
- Some staff cope with conflict by manifesting frustration, anger, backbiting, confusion, helplessness, cynicism, bickering, withdrawal, and bad relationship with security. Some also become punitive toward their patients.
- Recommended remedies: Acknowledge that moral distress exists. Enhance the knowledge of clinical team members about it. Develop a system to identify nurses experiencing it. Set up an ethics committee. [46]

Lorry Schoenly, PhD, RN, an experienced correctional nurse educator, points out that caring is the essence of professional nursing practice, but that some persons have questioned whether correctional nurses can care for their inmate patients. In fact, "nurses must continually negotiate boundaries between the values of custody and the values of caring; continually guarding against co-opting security values in practice. [47] Caring can be difficult in an antitherapeutic environment." [48] Schoenly then identifies some unique boundaries that exist in the nurse–patient relationship in corrections:

The real and potential danger to physical and psychological well-being when working closely with the inmate population threatens the ability to genuinely care for the patient over time. The manipulative nature of some patients in this setting encourages the development of cynicism and erodes the essential nurse-patient relationship.[49] Finally, the heinous crimes committed by some patients can make it difficult for nurses to overcome repugnance for what the patient has done to see the inherent humanity of who the patient is. Caring in nursing practice is challenging in the corrections environment.[50]

After cautioning that "constraints made necessary by the security environment limit the more intimate qualities of the care relationship," Schoenly then provides a useful operational definition of caring by presenting selected concepts adapted from Jean Watson as follow:

- Care is provided in a transpersonal relationship in which there is a moral commitment to protect and enhance human dignity.
- Caring is the intention of doing for another and being with another who is in need.
- Care is authentic presence where the nurse honors the patient's dignity and vulnerability. [51]

"Any profession that loses its values loses also its soul and heart and sense of worth. Caring should take place every time a nurse-to-patient contact is made."
—Mary Muse, RN

Certainly, caring is the essence of nursing. Nursing practice in corrections also takes on some special characteristics. Nurses tend to work with greater autonomy than many of those in the community. A balance needs to be achieved so that nurses fully use their skills yet do not exceed the boundaries of their legal scope of practice. They need to be highly skilled in making assessments. And they must be able to develop therapeutic relationships with patients that do not violate professional boundaries or legitimate security concerns.[52] Needless to say, virtually all that has been said about nurses in this section applies equally, *mutatis mutandis*, to all other health professionals who care for patients in a correctional setting.

SOME PRACTICAL ETHICAL ISSUES IN CORRECTIONS

Transgender Issues

Gender dysphoria is distress caused by discontent with a person's biological sex. Persons experiencing significant gender dysphoria may have the diagnosis of gender identity disorder. This is a medical problem that leads to emotional suffering if untreated. It needs to be addressed. Too many correctional jurisdictions have tried to ignore it or sweep it under the rug, oblivious to the pain this condition may cause. Policies in many correctional systems do not provide adequate protection and add unnecessarily to the patient's suffering. Gender identity disorder is a serious medical condition with a well-defined community standard of care.[53]

One issue of concern has to do with correctional classification of these persons. Housing can be a difficult decision, but each case needs to be considered individually on its merits. Whether the person will be housed among male or female inmates should give due regard to the individual's own views, preferences, and safety. The transsexual prisoner is highly vulnerable, and too frequently is subjected to deliberate humiliation and indignity by other prisoners and even by staff. Their safety is a preeminent concern. By the same token, they should not be isolated from reasonable social contact. They should be housed in general population whenever feasible, and due privacy for personal hygiene must be accommodated. A single cell is usually preferable.[54] Recent court decisions suggest that it may be ruled an act of discrimination to house transgender inmates in facilities that are not consistent with their gender identity.

Another issue has to do with continuing the process of gender change after it has begun in the community. Some prisons have a policy that no transgender treatment will be given. Others will place such a person on a gradual withdrawal from hormonal therapy. Still others will continue what was started in the community, especially hormone therapy, but not surgical procedures. The first two policies are essentially a "freeze-frame" approach with the second being only slightly more humane than the first in that abrupt cessation of hormones causes suffering. It is unreasonable to freeze a gender transition to what it was at date of entry into the prison. Such practice is not in keeping with modern standards of medicine. This is simply not the way other medical conditions are treated.[55] Hormone therapy should be maintained as closely as possible to previous levels in the community. This will prevent the side effects of withdrawal and prevent loss of changes that have already occurred.

Ceasing or denying treatment because of the personal bias of the physician would be unethical. It is important to remain nonjudgmental. These patients deserve to be treated humanely and equitably. A thorough medical history should be taken, and a release should be obtained permitting consultation with providers of prior care in the community.

Should transgender treatment be started in a prison? Such a decision should be made on a case-by-case basis after careful review of the relevant facts, including a thorough medical and behavioral assessment. In the community, gender reassignment is customarily initiated after a reasonable period of observing the person endeavoring to live as the sex she or he wishes to become. There should be no a priori policy decision that transgender treatment will never be initiated in the prison. It is reasonable to regard treatment of gender dysphoria in the same way as treatment of other serious medical conditions, and consequently there is a duty to treat when it is determined to be medically necessary for this patient.

This approach is supported by the NCCHC's position statement:

12. Transgender patients who received hormone therapy with or without a prescription prior to incarceration should have that therapy continued without interruption pending evaluation by a specialist, absent urgent medical reasons to the contrary. Hormone therapy should not be discontinued precipitously as this will likely cause depression and anxiety.

13. Gender dysphoric patients who have not received hormone therapy prior to incarceration should be evaluated by a health care provider qualified in the area of gender-related health care to determine their treatment needs.

14. When determined to be medically necessary for a particular patient, hormone therapy should be initiated and regular laboratory monitoring should be conducted according to community medical standards.

15. Sex reassignment surgery should be considered on a case-by-case basis and provided when determined to be medically necessary for a patient.[56]

These people present a unique set of issues making them highly vulnerable to abuse, assault, and self-injurious behavior. Serious and potentially lethal consequences of untreated gender identity disorders include autocastration or autopenectomy—which are performed as acts of self-treatment—as may be the self-mutilative actions of persons with certain personality disorders or psychotic disorders. Brown and McDuffie point out that they can quickly bleed to death because they are unable to stop the bleeding. "Few individuals who autocastrate appreciate the elasticity of the testicular arteries that can quickly retract into the peritoneum, making self-hemostasis of the wound nearly impossible."[57] Their survey in 2008 found that only 20 percent of states had any formal policies addressing transgender health care and housing, while another 20 percent reported having "informal policies." They also found that "issues related to their medical care and housing are substantial and out of proportion to their small numbers in institutions" and that they "present a unique set of issues generally not seen in other inmates that could increase the probability of assault and self-injurious behavior."

> There should be no a priori policy decision that transgender treatment will never be initiated in the prison. It is reasonable to regard treatment of gender dysphoria in the same way as treatment of other serious medical conditions, and consequently, there is a duty to treat when it is determined to be medically necessary for this patient.

In view of these findings, it is indefensible for a state law such as that enacted in Wisconsin to prohibit spending of any state dollars to treat a transgender inmate with hormonal therapy or sex-reassignment surgery.[58] Failure to treat diagnosed gender dysphoria could be a constitutional issue. In fact, the federal court for the Eastern District of Wisconsin struck down the Wisconsin law in March 2010 as unconstitutional and a violation of the Eighth and Fourteenth Amendments (*Fields v. Smith*).[59] This decision was upheld by the U.S. Court of Appeals for the Seventh Circuit on August 5, 2011.[60] The appellate court wrote: "Surely, had the Wisconsin legislature passed a law that inmates with cancer must be treated only with therapy and pain killers, this court would have no trouble concluding that the law was unconstitutional. Refusing to provide effective treatment for a serious medical condition serves no valid penological purpose and amounts to torture."

In *Phillips v. Michigan Department of Corrections*,[61] the federal court ordered hormonal treatment for a patient with gender identity disorder, finding denial of continuation hormone therapy to be deliberate indifference and cruel and unusual punishment. She had been taking estrogen for 17 years prior to incarceration and experienced severe symptoms of withdrawal when denied the treatment.

In one prison visited by the author in 2011, the only co-payment fee charged for prescribed medications was for estrogen therapy given to transsexual prisoners. This clearly discriminatory practice appeared to reflect a predetermined judgment that these treatments were not medically necessary.

In the opening words of his majority opinion on same-sex marriage in June 2015 (*Obergefell v. Hodges*), Justice Anthony Kennedy declared: "The Constitution promises liberty to all within its reach, a liberty that includes certain specific rights that allow persons, within a lawful realm, to define and express their identity."[62] Especially after *Obergefell* and other recent court decisions, the issue of lesbian, gay, bisexual, and transgender equality status in the community—derived from the U.S. Constitution and the Civil Rights Act of 1964—is becoming increasingly clear. Consequently, there should be no room for transgender discrimination or harassment in corrections.

Rodney Fry offers seven tips for dealing with transgendered inmates:

1. Treat the person humanely.
2. Provide a safe environment to avoid rape or physical abuse.
3. Supply appropriate clothing (brassieres when necessary).
4. Provide privacy for hygiene needs when possible.
5. Assign classification and housing placement appropriately.
6. Provide appropriate medical care, including hormonal therapy.
7. Provide behavioral health support when the need is identified.[63]

Forensic Use of Medically Obtained Information

General Principles

The ethical standards of health care professionals forbid their participation in obtaining tissue specimens or performing unconsented tests to obtain information for use in prosecuting or punishing inmates. This is an area related to (1) *benefi-cence* (and *nonmaleficence*), (2) *confidentiality* and *privacy*, (3) *informed consent*, and (4) *therapeutic relationship*. It derives especially from the medical principle that—above all else—a doctor must not inflict harm on a patient. Examples of forensic tests include blood, urine, or tissue samples for DNA or to establish paternity or the presence of alcohol or drugs; body cavity searches for contraband; evalua-tion of competence to submit to punishment; and evaluations for parole board decisions.

Suppose a prosecutor needs a blood or tissue sample from a prisoner to assist in convicting or clearing the prisoner of a crime. This action is not directed toward the delivery of health care services to the prisoner. It even may do some harm, although perhaps the "harm" is itself lawful and might even have a noble purpose. The patient likely did not freely consent to the procedure. The concept of informed consent also requires that the true reason for the test be explained in advance. Deceit or trickery should never be countenanced.

In a case that the author encountered while surveying a prison, the medical labo-ratory technician had been requested by the internal affairs investigator to draw blood from an inmate but was not told the purpose of the test. Consequently, he was unable to inform the inmate of its purpose. It would, of course, be a violation of pro-fessional ethics to draw the blood without informing the inmate of the intended use of the specimen, and consent would be obtained deceitfully if the inmate were led to believe that this were just a routine medical procedure. This concern could be remedied by a court order requiring the inmate to supply the specimen. The court order also could override conflict with confidentiality and the doctor–patient privilege. However, another principle still may stand in the way. Regular health care staff at the facility must be regarded by patients as persons who can always be counted on to act in their patients' best interest. A trusting relationship arises between clinician and patient, one that is termed a *therapeutic alliance*. Effective medical and mental health care for patients requires this continued trust. A patient who does not trust his or her doctor is likely to withhold relevant symptoms and history or may fail to comply with prescribed treatment. Confidence in one's doc-tor has been shown to be important to the healing process itself.

Participation in the unconsented collection of blood or tissue specimens for the purpose of prosecution and eventual punishment of the prisoner is inconsistent with the role of a trusted healer, particularly in a correctional setting in which the patient is given no opportunity to choose his or her providers. Thus arises the recommen-dation of the National Commission on Correctional Health Care[64] that tissue spec-imens for forensic uses be obtained by an outside health professional. Although this is somewhat more costly, the reasons underlying this precaution are important and should be respected. Because these cases should only occur rarely, the cost would not be prohibitive. Hair samples for DNA or substance-use testing and urine tests for drugs or alcohol do not require the skilled intervention of health care staff and thus are not an issue if they are obtained by officers at a location apart from the clinic setting.

It is important to distinguish among the following situations where the inmate:

1. freely consents to (and perhaps even desires) the testing or the procedure,
2. does not give free consent but acquiesces and does not actively resist, and
3. not only withholds consent but actively resists the procedure.

Situation 1 does not generally present any problem. Here the informed inmate perceives the test as beneficial or at least not harmful. Consequently, the correctional health provider is not placed in a position antagonistic to the well-being of a patient. Such might be the case of a prisoner who desires the test to prove his or her own innocence.

In situation 2, the health professional who bears a provider–patient relationship to the inmate should not participate in obtaining specimens for forensic purposes against the patient's will. However, as previously indicated, when legally required it may be performed by a qualified health professional who does not bear a provider–patient relationship.

Situation 3 poses serious problems and ought to be performed only in cases of the greatest necessity, preferably with a court order, and by a qualified provider who does not have a patient–provider relationship. The risk of causing physical injury to the actively resisting patient needs to be carefully assessed and may weigh heavily against performing all but the most urgently required procedures. It would be wrong for correctional officials to misrepresent the facts or exaggerate the urgency of retrieving the secreted contents from a body cavity in order to elicit the willingness of the physician to perform the procedure.

DNA Testing

As with all interventions conducted for forensic purposes, DNA testing generally should not be carried out by correctional health care staff. This practice confuses the role of the health care provider who should be seen and respected as a caregiver acting completely on behalf of and in the best interests of the patient. The health care provider should not be expected to use medical skills to perform procedures that can lead to prosecution or punishment of a patient.

In cases where acquisition of the DNA specimen must be accomplished by a health professional, it is best carried out by one from the outside who does not have and is unlikely to have a provider–patient relationship with the inmate.

An increasing number of state laws are requiring DNA testing of all inmates (or of a subset of inmates such as sex offenders or those convicted of violent crimes). Under these circumstances, the cost of arranging for separate staff to obtain the specimens could be excessive. A reasonable case can be made for allowing a portion of the blood routinely drawn for intake medical screening of new inmates to be used for legislatively mandated DNA testing, provided that a state law indeed requires the testing and that the inmates are duly informed that a portion of the blood supplied will be used for this purpose. Failure to disclose this information carries the risk that health care providers will not be seen as trustworthy by their patients. The rationale enabling this strategy is that the specimen is obtained routinely for all or most inmates, does not involve a separate invasive procedure, and the possibility of an eventual forensic use of this information is remote from the act of collecting the specimen. This situation is readily distinguished from drawing a specimen from a particular inmate for a legitimate medical purpose but also with the express intention of using the specimen to derive data for use in a current prosecutorial application.

Some state laws specify that the DNA testing shall be performed by an institution's health care staff. Even this need not be interpreted as requiring that the regular medical staff, with established or potential provider–patient relationships, conduct the testing procedures. The institution might contract with outside providers on a part-time basis for this sole purpose. On the other hand, these special arrangements can be quite costly. When unavoidably faced with this situation, medical staff should take care to protect the therapeutic relationship by appropriately informing the inmate in advance as to the purpose and the reason for the procedure, clearly distinguishing this from a medical procedure undertaken for the prisoner's health. Staff also should be alert to occasions when this process appears in any way to undermine or compromise patient confidence in the health care staff. An important proviso in the NCCHC standard[65] is that health services staff may be involved in the collection of forensic information when complying with state laws that require blood samples, as long as the inmate has given consent and health care staff are not involved in any punitive action taken in cases where the inmate refuses consent.

The principle discussed at the beginning of this chapter is applicable here: an act may be legal but unethical and therefore would be wrong. State correctional leaders are cautioned not to suggest or lobby legislators to enact such a provision because they will find it more problematic in the long run. There are sound and convincing reasons to promote and protect the trust and confidence that patients have in their physicians and other health care providers, and these reasons ought not to be lightly dismissed.

Many of the issues just described could easily be avoided by simply not involving health care staff in the process of gathering or processing specimens. It may be that buccal swabs or hair samples, for example, which can be collected by nonmedical law enforcement personnel, would provide acceptable DNA evidence for the legitimate intended purpose.

Body Cavity Searches

A sure way to engender a lively discussion in some jurisdictions is to raise the subject of body cavity searches in the mixed company of corrections officers and medical staff. (Of course, this intensity of feeling usually is lacking in those settings in which medical staff have already acquiesced to performing these procedures or where the incidence of requiring a body cavity search is so rare as almost to be a nonissue.) The standards of both the NCCHC and the APHA reflect strong ethical concerns when they so clearly prohibit the conducting of body cavity searches by health care staff who are routinely assigned to provide medical care at the facility. The ACA standard fails to acknowledge the ethical issue but does address the concern to avoid injury to the person being searched. ACA standards for juveniles specify that "when there is reason to conduct a manual or instrument inspection of a body cavity based on risk to the security of the facility, the juvenile is referred to a health care practitioner. Any inspection is completed in private."[66] For adults, ACA allows the alternative of using correctional personnel trained by health care staff.[67] The discussion to the NCCHC standard says it presents an ethical conflict for health services staff and that such acts undermine the credibility of these professionals with their patients.[68] The standards issued by the APHA include "Participation in this purely custodial function [strip and body cavity searches] compromises the ability of the health provider to relate to the health needs of the inmate population" (1986)[69] and "Correctional health providers' clinical skills should not be applied to non-clinical situations such as strip and cavity searches, forced transfers, health certification for punishment, or evidence gathering" (2003).[70]

The ethical concern is twofold. First, because body orifice searches are invasive procedures, they would require informed consent if performed for medical reasons. If consent is freely given (as may be the case with an inmate anxious to demonstrate his or her innocence), the nurse or doctor ethically may proceed unless it were judged that doing so would impair the doctor–patient relationship. Often, consent can be obtained if the health care worker approaches the patient with a proper attitude and gives a careful explanation.

The second concern is that the health care professional is not acting in the patient's best interest when conducting a search for concealed evidence that could lead to punishment. This procedure makes health care staff appear to be "police." Nurses and physicians work hard to achieve and maintain a therapeutic alliance with their patients. An unconsented invasive search for contraband is clearly a breach of this trust. A special situation exists if the prisoner explicitly requests that the body cavity exploration be performed by a health care provider.

Some experts[71] have suggested that body cavity searches be performed by corrections officers who have received training by health care staff on how to explore body cavities with a gloved finger. Although this may appear reasonable, at best it is a highly unsatisfactory compromise. No single officer is likely to perform the procedure frequently enough to maintain the skills necessary to avoid causing injury or infection. An additional concern is the appearance of impropriety when health care staff train officers how to perform a procedure that, by definition and intent, is contrary to the well-being of their patients. The procedure can also be a frightfully traumatic experience, especially for those who have been sexually abused in their childhood because of the memories and images that it can evoke. In view of such considerations, the National Commission on Correctional Health Care omitted this recommendation from its 1997 and subsequent editions of health care standards, as did the American Public Health Association in its third edition.

As already indicated, some experts advise the employment of health care professionals who are not associated with the provision of health care at the institution for this type of function. This can be quite costly and inconvenient. Also, the patient may not comprehend the subtle distinction of the nature of the health profession-al's employment contract, so that it still may appear that the procedure is being "inflicted" on him or her by a member of the institution's medical staff. More-over, the safe exploration of bodily orifices of an inmate who is not only unwill-ing but also actively and aggressively resisting can be extremely difficult. In this situation, the trained correctional officer is at great risk of inflicting injury, while the highly skilled health professional simply may refuse to proceed under such circumstances.

Legislation that explicitly permits nurses and doctors to perform body cavity searches has been sought in some states. While such legislation would make the procedure legal, it would remain unethical and therefore is not a solution. Any facility or system that seeks to attract and retain good staff and respects the profes-sional integrity of its medical personnel will never ask them to compromise their ethi-cal principles. What remedies, then, remain?

Each agency should honestly and carefully review its policy and practice regarding body cavity searches and explore relevant questions such as the following. How necessary are the searches that are currently being performed? In what percentage of searches is contraband actually found? Are the searches being ordered only when probable cause exists and when other less invasive or potentially harmful methods have been exhausted? Is each order signed by a high-level authority such as a warden or a jail administrator? (ACA requires authorization by the warden or designee.)[72] Are all body cavity searches carefully documented and periodically reported to a higher authority such as the director of corrections or sheriff for ret-rospective review and monitoring to prevent abuse and overuse? If all of these safeguards are in place, then the actual use of body cavity searches may become so rare that the few truly justified and necessary procedures can easily be handled by outside medical personnel without a major cost burden.[73]

To reduce the need for body cavity searches, some correctional agencies place an inmate suspected of having inserted contraband into the rectum in a dry cell with only a "potty" bucket—that is, no sink, no toilet, no drain—under observation until any contraband is excreted naturally. Others make use of advanced imaging technology.

Protection of the inmate from risk of serious harm in the event that a balloon filled with drugs were to burst within the body cavity is generally not sufficient jus-tification for an unconsented body cavity search. Instead, medical staff should advise the inmate of the serious consequences of a ruptured balloon and encourage its voluntary removal. In the meantime, she or he may be transferred to a medical bed and closely monitored by nursing staff.

The necessity of body cavity searches should be called into question in any location where they occur frequently but produce few results. Strict standards and careful monitoring can minimize abuse. There should be probable cause in every case, and each search should require written authorization of the warden or jail adminis-trator. (If the actual warden is not available, then the author recommends that the authorization come from the acting warden rather than a "designee.") Further, a report of each instance, its rationale, the alternatives considered, the names of all persons involved, and the outcome should be made to the higher level of authority on a regular basis for retrospective monitoring on at least a quarterly basis.

Documentation of the outcome (specifically, what was found during the search) is important because a retrospective review can draw useful inferences. A high percentage of positive findings might suggest that security procedures are too lax and contacts with visitors need to be more carefully monitored. On the other hand, a close to zero percentage of positive findings could indicate unnecessary and unjustified body cavity searches.

Body cavity searches should be ordered only when there is good reason to believe that contraband is there and when no satisfactory alternative can be found. For sentenced prisoners, a court order is not required as long as there is an order signed by the appropriate authority, but in cases of determined and aggressive resistance and when the procedures must be done by force, a court order is advisable. This ensures that the special circumstances, rationale, and alternatives all have been considered and weighed by a disinterested party. The World Medical Association recommends that,

to the extent feasible without compromising public security, alternate methods be used for routine screening of prisoners, and [that] body cavity searches be used only as a last resort. If a body cavity search must be conducted, the responsible public official must ensure that the search is conducted by personnel with sufficient medical knowledge and skills to safely perform the search. The same responsible authority [shall] ensure that the individual's privacy and dignity be guaranteed.[74]

Strip Searches

Strictly speaking, this section on strip searches does not belong in this chapter because it is not a function that health care professionals are likely to be called on to perform and it does not involve the forensic use of medically obtained information. The author has chosen to place it here, however, in part because it is cognate to the preceding section, "Body Cavity Searches." Of greater importance, because this practice can adversely affect the health of prisoners, health care professionals are duty bound to raise the issue should it become excessive or abusive.

The traditional ritual of strip searching prisoners on a routine basis may be inappropriate and largely unnecessary, and it can have implications for mental health. As practiced in many facilities, inmates are required to disrobe and present themselves for inspection each time they enter or reenter the facility or after they have had a contact visitation. Even though the strip searches are conducted by security staff rather than medical personnel, doctors and other health professionals have an ethical responsibility to speak out when they become aware of practices that may be harmful to prisoners' health.

Correctional facilities have legitimate reasons to prevent drugs, weapons, and contraband from entering the system. From a legal perspective, it is recognized that a balance must be struck that protects both the individual's constitutional rights (in the context of the Fourth Amendment right to be free from unreasonable search and seizure, the Eighth Amendment right to be free from cruel and unusual punishment, and the Fourteenth Amendment right to due process) as well as the legitimate security and penological interests of the institution. This balancing requires an even stronger justification when dealing with pretrial and juvenile detainees than with convicted offenders.

The courts have recognized the extreme invasiveness of these body searches. One court referred to strip searches as "demeaning, dehumanizing, undignified, humiliating, terrifying, unpleasant, embarrassing, repulsive, signifying degradation and submission" (*Mary Beth G. v. City of Chicago*).[75] Another said that "the experience of disrobing and exposing one's self for visual inspection by a stranger clothed with the uniform and authority of the state, in an enclosed room inside a jail, can only be seen as thoroughly degrading and frightening. Moreover, the imposition of such a search upon an individual detained for a lesser offense is quite likely to take that person by surprise, thereby exacerbating the terrifying quality of the event" (*John Does 1–100 v. Boyd*).[76] Yet another court stated, "A strip search, regardless of how professionally and courteously conducted, is an embarrassing and humiliating experience" (*Justice v. City of Peachtree City*).[77] Though these court pronouncements may not have widely applicable binding force, they do give clear testimony to the view that searches of this kind are deeply offensive to human dignity and can brutalize not only the victims but also the officials who perform them.

In *Jordan v. Gardner* [986 F. 2d 1521, 9th Cir. en banc (1993)], the court found that random, suspicionless cross-gender clothed body searches of female prisoners by male officers violate the Eighth Amendment's prohibition of cruel and unusual punishment and amount to deliberate indifference to the unnecessary and wanton infliction of severe mental pain and psychological injury, including exacerbation of symptoms of posttraumatic stress syndrome.

Although it is outside the competence of health professionals to judge the necessity of this practice, it is well within their right—if not also their duty—to raise thoughtful questions about its usefulness, necessity, and universality. It is an inherently debasing and humiliating intrusion into the privacy of a person with serious health implications. It is an assault on the human dignity of that person and must be balanced with a weighty rationale and justification. A body of court decisions [especially *Bell v. Wolfish*, 441 U.S. 520 (1979)] that provide guidance on balancing the rights of the prisoner and the interests of the state may not yet be the final word. Societal standards of decency continue to evolve (*Trop v. Dulles*).[78] Imaging technologies and detection methods have vastly improved over what they were two and three decades ago, as is abundantly apparent in the scanning procedures used at airports by the Transportation Security Administration. The societal awareness and opposition to interpersonal violence—especially violence against women and youth—are more clearly defined. We continue to gain insight and understanding into the nature of posttraumatic stress disorder. Consequently, it may now be the time to revisit these practices and policies in view of their implications for the mental health and well-being of incarcerated persons. It may be found that suspicionless and routine strip searches are neither necessary nor sufficient to maintain security and therefore can no longer be justified based on an institution's legitimate security interests.

Peter Williams and Joan Hirsch Holtzman support this position and offer the following commentary:

In fact, it is possible to show that the strip search rule is neither necessary nor sufficient to maintain security. That it is not necessary has already been argued . . . where several alternatives were proposed. Insofar as those alternatives afford the same, or better, protection, and are also more humane, they must be preferred. That the strip search rule is not sufficient can be seen from the fact that contraband continues to find its way into and out of prisons. It can also be seen from the possibility that someone bent on smuggling could resort to inserting the forbidden article beyond the anal sphincter or swallowing it.[79]

Many prisoners—especially women and girls—have suffered physical and sexual abuse before they were incarcerated and, to the shame of correctional systems, even while incarcerated at the hands of other inmates and staff. Each time these people are subjected to strip searches and asked to publicly expose their private parts, they are invariably and uncontrollably reminded of the horrors they previously experienced. Unwanted evocation of these powerful images can be debilitating, disorienting, and extremely painful.

Wardens of facilities that still engage in this practice are urged to sit down face to face with a psychiatrist or psychologist who can explain the notion of posttraumatic stress disorder and similar manifestations that are applicable to the impact of strip searches on vulnerable persons. Add to this the knowledge that some of the staff enforcing this procedure will further contribute to the intense humiliation of their prisoners by their looks, guffaws, gestures, and remarks. Any lewd, depraved, or mocking attitude is truly dehumanizing to the victims as well as to the perpetrators themselves and to the officers who stand by and condone this behavior. Suffice it to say that these behaviors will not easily be extinguished by the stroke of a policy writer's pen. The warden, in contemplating this issue, should consider whether it might be decided any differently if it were his or her own spouse or son or daughter who was being subjected to these procedures. It is relevant to point out the fact that the warden, more than any other person, sets the tone for the behavior of his or her staff and subordinates.

It may now be the time to revisit these practices and policies in view of their implications for the mental health and well-being of incarcerated persons. It may be found that suspicionless and routine strip searches are neither necessary nor sufficient to maintain security and therefore can no longer be justified based on an institution's legitimate security interests.

Without question, there are situations and circumstances in which the security and good order of a correctional facility require that inmates be subjected to a body search. Modern technology offers many devices to detect concealed items without requiring a prisoner to disrobe. Their use is appropriate whenever feasible.

Perhaps a good rule to follow would be something like the following. When deemed necessary in situations of specific and probable cause with no effective available alternative strategy, and with the explicit approval of the agency head in each case, the procedure may be performed—but only in private and by a person of the same gender as the inmate being searched. The author believes that few such procedures would actually be found necessary if this were the institutional policy.

Much the same could be said about the excessive use of pat-down searches. They should not be done without clear necessity, and any required touching near the private areas should be limited to officers of the same gender and without any spectators.

Dr. Pamela Dole, a gynecologist who worked at Bayview Correctional Facility in New York City, has considerable experience working with sexually traumatized women. She says that as many as 60 percent of incarcerated women have a history of sexual abuse. She describes how difficult it can be for many of these women to submit to a pelvic examination. She suggests not attempting the pelvic exam until the second or possibly third clinic visit so that the patient has a chance to become acquainted with the physician and discuss any fears, hesitations, or past experiences. Women often feel vulnerable and embarrassed. It is important to give the patient a sense that she retains control over her own body. It is important to avoid revictimizing the patient by a rushed or rough or insensitive examination.[80] If this concern is so evident in the private and caring performance of a medical procedure, how much more invasive and victimizing would be a strip or body cavity search performed by custody staff in a prison, jail, or juvenile facility?

Evaluation of Competence

Three important steps in the judicial process often raise a question about the sanity of a defendant. One step is meant to determine whether a defendant was mentally competent when the crime was committed. Another is to determine whether the defendant is currently competent to stand trial.

A psychologist or psychiatrist who is responsible for the treatment of mentally ill inmates should not be consulted or assigned to make either of these determinations, nor should the record of treatment for mental illness be reviewed or employed in reaching such a determination. There needs to be a clear and evident separation between the process of treating mentally ill patients and that of rendering evaluations that may result in adverse legal consequences to these patients.

The third and extreme case of determining competence for execution will be discussed in Chapter 2, "Areas of Significant Ethical Role Conflict," under "Determination of Competence to Be Executed."

Concept of Predicted Dangerousness and Medical Parole Issues

No satisfactory or reliable test has been developed for predicting whether a person will become dangerous, especially over the long term. Psychiatrists and psychologists are not experts at foretelling future events.[81] Past behavior of an individual may be the best available predictor of future actions, but it is far from reliable. Despite this, parole boards, judges, and others continue to call on psychiatrists or psychologists to advise whether an inmate is or will become dangerous or will harm someone if released. They are really asking behavioral experts to make an "educated guess" about the credibility of a person's stated intent and the relevance of past behavior to the likelihood of some future event. Although their best guess may be "better than nothing," it is not a prediction and should not be regarded as such.

From an ethical perspective, a psychiatrist or psychologist who has been treating a patient and subsequently uses the clinical insight obtained through the process of treatment to prepare a prediction of dangerousness may be violating patient confidentiality and privacy. Moreover, if the opinion or recommendation of the health professional could result in harm to the patient such as failure to grant parole, this can be seen as an unethical gathering and use of forensic information by a health care provider. Treating physicians and mental health professionals should have no role in length-of-stay decisions unless the question is limited to the area of medical appropriateness.[82]

When a "prediction of dangerousness" is needed, it should always be sought from a source not engaged in providing treatment to the patient. Often, this is done at a center for forensic psychiatry. An independent expert (psychologist, psychiatrist) also may be called in for this purpose. The forensic (legal) purpose of the evaluation must be made clear to the inmate at the beginning of the interview.

This situation, however, is not the same as when the treating health professional is being asked to advise on the type of treatment that the patient would require under a different set of circumstances. For instance, would this person, if paroled, require long- or short-term care for an acute or chronic physical or mental condition? Would she or he require hospitalization? Outpatient treatment? Assistance with activities of daily living? To provide advice about the needs of the patient is an appropriate application of the principle of continuity of care and does not present an ethical concern as long as there is at least presumed patient consent and as long as the health professional is not led into predicting dangerousness or recommending for or against release.

Joel Dvoskin, an experienced correctional psychologist, points out that the odds of future violent behavior are dynamic, not static, and that reasonable interventions have been shown to reduce the risk of violence, such as providing support systems for medication compliance or for maintaining sobriety or by granting increased freedom and reduced control in small increments to allow the patient to demonstrate trustworthiness and adapt to new situations.[83] Dvoskin has also aptly suggested that perhaps the best way to find out if individuals are planning to become violent or to injure anyone is simply to ask them.

Medical Restraint

When ordered for medical or mental health reasons, physical restraint should always be carried out in a medical setting with adequate nursing supervision. A segregation cell is unsuitable.

A facility without an acute psychiatric inpatient unit or at least a medical infirmary under full-time nursing direction should not attempt to employ medically ordered physical restraints or enforced psychotropic medication. Instead, these patients should be transferred to a hospital or other suitable medical setting where the procedures can be performed and monitored safely. In some cases, however, it may be reasonable to restrain or medicate as part of the process of transferring a patient to a suitable medical setting.

Soft leather or plastic restraints are preferred to metal restraints when used in a medical context. They should be ordered only when it is explicitly documented in the health record that less restrictive measures have been determined inadequate, and they should be employed for no longer than necessary. The order for application of restraints should state the condition for which the restraint is deemed necessary as well as the behavior or condition of the patient that will warrant removal of the device. Restraints should be ordered only by a psychiatrist, physician, or psychologist as consistent with the state mental health code. Likewise, an order for restraints should not be valid for longer than four hours or consistent with the state mental health regulations. When possible, ambulatory restraints should be considered in preference to restraining the patient to a bed. These principles apply as well to the use of a so-called restraining chair, which may be thought of as something between four-point restraint and ambulatory restraints.

> When ordered for medical or mental health reasons, physical restraint should always be carried out in a medical setting with adequate nursing supervision. A segregation cell is unsuitable.

The mental health statutes of various states contain regulations governing use of restraint, seclusion, and forced medication. These often are found in the section that deals with recipient rights. If there is no formal mental health code in a particular state, an acceptable guide may be found in the policy directive of a state or private mental hospital. Adherence to these local requirements can provide evidence that the correctional facility is following the accepted community standard of practice.

Directly Observed Therapy

Directly observed therapy (DOT) is the recommended mode of medication distribution for treatment and chemoprophylaxis (medical prevention) of tuberculosis and treatment of AIDS and hepatitis C. This is because intermittent taking or premature discontinuance of these medications can result in selecting strains of bacteria or virus that are resistant to treatment. These organisms can infect other persons and cause illness that is extremely difficult to treat.

DOT is not to be confused with forced treatment. A patient who previously had given informed consent but is now refusing to take TB medication should be counseled by medical staff, asked the reason for the refusal, reminded of the risks of intermittent or interrupted compliance, and told that the treatment will be stopped if refusal continues.

Patients may be required to ingest other medications in the presence of a nurse (or officer) who gives them a drink of water, orange juice, or Kool-Aid and watches them swallow. This is an acceptable practice, its purpose being to prevent the accumulation of quantities of medication, either for sale in the yard or for later ingestion of a large and possibly harmful or fatal dose. A clinical purpose may be verification of ingestion so as to determine if failure to achieve the expected results of treatment is caused by faulty compliance or inadequate dosage.

Some places also require a patient to open his or her mouth and roll the tongue around to show the medications have not been "cheeked." This is somewhat of an indignity and takes the officer's or nurse's time, but it is not wrong in principle. In fact, this practice is recommended if abuse of medication is known to be a problem with a particular patient.

On the other hand, the manner in which directly observed therapy is carried out can have unintended and undesirable effects. If patients are required to wait in line to have their medications administered by a nurse, there may be an opportunity for officers and possibly other inmates to learn what type of medications are being given. For HIV patients and for mentally ill persons, fear of "being discovered" may be a deterrent to taking the medication.

When the goal of DOT is to achieve a high rate of compliance with the prescribed medication regimen, the actual result may be quite different. Patients who have been properly educated and would responsibly take their medications faithfully if they had them in their own possession may find it overly burdensome to stand in long pill lines one or more times each day. If compliance is periodically checked by measuring viral load or blood levels, evidence of high compliance can be rewarded by allowing the patient to continue on the keep-on-person arrangement.

For these reasons, it is important to consider all sides of the issue rather than adopt a DOT program just because other prisons are doing so. A sincere attempt to discover and monitor the real impact of this practice on patients is essential. Failure to do so is unethical.

Crushing Medications

A few correctional institutions require all medications to be crushed before they are administered to patients. The stated reason is to ensure that the medications are ingested rather than saved for later overdose or for sale to other inmates. Despite legitimate interest in preventing these abuses, this might not be the appropriate method. Particularly with enteric coated, slow-release, and sublingual forms of medication, crushing of medications is ill advised. The manufacturer may have coated or specially formulated a product for any of several reasons, including protecting components from atmospheric degradation, preventing contact with a compound that is an irritant, separating reactive ingredients, protecting the patient's teeth, controlling the site of medication release, delaying absorption of the medication, or masking an unpleasant taste.[84]

Good medical practice encourages patients to comply with their prescribed treatment program. "A spoonful of sugar helps the medicine go down," as Mary Poppins sang in the familiar musical. Many people find taking medicine unpleasant. Requiring the ingestion of crushed medications exaggerates this association of unpleasantness with taking medicine. This is especially problematic for psychiatric patients, for whom faithful compliance with their treatment regimen is necessary to prevent decompensation and aggravation of their illness.

Although there may be legitimate security interests to suggest crushing medications, the important medical contraindications must be duly considered. Medical authorities need to advocate clearly and insistently with the custody authorities so that crushing all medications is not adopted as a generalized practice. There may be isolated instances where crushing is required, but other alternatives should first be evaluated. Although somewhat more costly to purchase and more burdensome to administer and store, the use of liquid forms of medication, if available, is preferable to crushing tablets when there is a problem of abuse and when compliance must be ensured.

Organ Transplants

The rules for selecting organ transplant recipients should be limited to medical criteria such as medical need and expected outcome. The fact that the potential recipient is a prisoner should have no bearing on the selection decision. In the words of medical ethicist Felicia Cohn, "Health care is to be provided according to assessments of medical benefit and likelihood of survival. When rationing decisions must be made, queuing usually ensues and resources are provided on a first-come, first-served basis, or according to triage criteria (that is, an account of medical need, probability of benefit, and likelihood of success)."[85]

This topic is discussed in greater detail in Chapter 5, "How Much Health Care Is Appropriate and Necessary," under "Cost Factors."

Treating or Diagnosing under Less-than-Satisfactory Conditions

Some circumstances and environmental arrangements are simply unacceptable for medical or mental health evaluation or treatment. In emergencies, doctors and nurses may have to work under less-than-satisfactory conditions. To do so routinely or when it is avoidable, however, cannot be justified and could represent a breach of professional ethics or even malpractice if it continues. Unfortunately, this concern is sometimes overlooked in correctional settings, where certain practices are rationalized under the rubric of "security" and may be tolerated or accepted without question by the medical staff. The following examples are posed for discussion, keeping in mind the premise that there should be no real contradiction between a legitimate security requirement and a legitimate medical need.

Patient Assessment through a Closed Door

In some facilities, nursing or mental health rounds of segregated or maximum-security prisoners are conducted by shouting to the patient through a closed cell door that has a tiny Plexiglas window. In others, both patient and staff must crouch down to talk through a waist-high food slot in the door. (This is often a small rectangular slot in a steel door near waist level through which food trays may be passed. They are also sometimes used by officers to apply or remove handcuffs while the inmate is securely inside the cell.) Shouting out one's medical or psychiatric symptoms for the world to hear and having the health care professional's questions and advice similarly broadcast are inexcusable breaches of privacy and confidentiality. Miscommunication in these circumstances is also a real possibility given the difficulties posed by the muffled and distorted voice and by background noises. This is not the way information is exchanged in a physician's office. We would all be outraged if our own private physician were ever to confer with us in that fashion.

Observing a patient, noting his or her skin color and texture, tremors, eye movement, and nonverbal body language often communicates more to a skilled medical or mental health professional than do the patient's words. This type of observation is not possible through a small security window or a food slot in a steel door. It is also uncomfortable and undignified for patient and staff to try to communicate in a crouched position through the food slot. Lighting is usually inadequate for proper clinical observation, even if the patient can be seen. Taking vital signs (pulse, temperature, and blood pressure), listening to the chest, and looking at the throat are not possible under these conditions, and injuries, wounds, and signs of trauma cannot be observed and evaluated. Should an adverse reaction to treatment ensue, there is no means of physically stabilizing the patient to prevent a fall. Besides, the patient does not feel as if she or he has been properly evaluated and may feel the need to send a kite or stop the next nurse who passes by to tell the same story all over again.

For these reasons, no health professional should attempt to diagnose and treat patients through a closed door. The level of assessment that typically occurs during segregation rounds is closer to a triage function in which the nurse attempts to learn the nature and urgency of the medical complaint and whether a face-to-face evaluation is needed.

A different door design is one possible solution and should be a consideration for any new facility or major renovation. At the very least, medical staff should never hesitate to insist that the door be opened or that the patient be taken to a different area whenever this is deemed necessary to resolve doubt about the patient's condition. When this is done, additional security staff may have to be summoned to ensure that it can be accomplished safely. Unfortunately, this extra burden on custody and health care staff time introduces pressure on health care professionals to "make do" with a less-than-satisfactory evaluation of a patient. Eventually, a serious problem will occur, and any ensuing lawsuit may hold the health care professional and the correctional system liable for their failures to evaluate the patient properly.

Observing a patient, noting his or her skin color and texture, tremors, eye movement, and nonverbal body language often communicates more to a skilled medical or mental health professional than the patient's words. This type of observation is not possible through a small security window or a food slot in a steel door.

ACA requires that segregated inmates receive daily visits from a qualified health care official[86] and that a qualified mental health professional personally interview and prepare a written report on any inmate remaining in segregation for more than 30 days.[87] Neither ACA nor NCCHC distinguish between administrative or disciplinary segregation in this regard. NCCHC requires that inmates in extreme isolation (defined as persons who have little or no contact with other individuals) be monitored by medical staff daily and at least weekly by mental health staff. Segregated inmates who have limited contact with staff or other inmates must be monitored three days a week by medical or mental health staff, and those who are allowed periods of recreation or other routine social contact among themselves while being segregated from the general population must be checked weekly by medical or mental health staff. The accompanying discussion explains that these "evaluations by health staff include notation of bruises or other trauma markings, comments regarding the inmate's attitude and outlook (particularly as they might relate to suicide ideation), and any health complaints."[88]

Drawing Blood through the Bars or through a Food Slot

The same remarks about the ill-advised practice of conducting patient assessments through a prison cell's closed door also apply to drawing blood, giving injections, and performing similar treatment procedures through the bars of a cell or through the slot in a closed cell door. Medical staff should clearly articulate to correctional administrators their serious concerns about the risks and dangers of such practices.

> The manner in which a medical procedure is carried out must always be a medical decision, not a custody decision. This is in keeping with the principle of medical autonomy.

First, venipuncture or similar procedures—drawing blood, performing a finger-stick blood test, or administering a skin test for TB—could occasion a fainting spell for the patient and result in serious injury from a fall. Second, there is risk of contamination and infection from nearby surfaces or if skin cleansing and antiseptic procedures are not properly followed. Third, the awkward or uncomfortable position for patient and provider, as well as the impaired visibility from inadequate lighting and view angle, can preclude a successful procedure, which is often seen in the process of finding a suitable vein, or could occasion a needle-stick injury. It is also dehumanizing to subject people to medical treatment under such conditions.

The manner in which a medical procedure is carried out must always be a medical decision, not a custody decision. This is in keeping with the principle of medical autonomy.

Undue Noise

Busy corridors can be extremely noisy. Following a decision to subdivide a large prison into separate areas with fencing, a satellite clinic was created to serve one of the new subdivisions and thus reduce patient traffic to the main clinic. Soon after its opening, it was apparent that the numerous wagons of food, laundry, waste, and supplies pulled by inmate porters through the corridor alongside the new clinic made such a racket that medical staff had difficulty listening to heartbeats and lung sounds with their stethoscopes. After some discussion and problem solving, someone suggested that pneumatic tires replace the steel-rimmed wheels on the wagons. This accomplished, the problem disappeared. Not to have taken effective action to solve this problem would have resulted in unacceptable quality of care.

Unnecessary Risk to Safety of Health Care Staff

Safety is an important concern for all health care staff, female and male. The inherent characteristics of the job duties of staff can affect the degree of risk involved.

The clinic of a minimum-security correctional camp was in a structure located at considerable distance from the administration building and was not routinely staffed by officers. Although there were no unfortunate incidents, nursing staff were uncomfortable—especially when only one health care provider was present in the clinic. There was a recognized potential for physical abuse or hostage taking. At first these concerns were dismissed by the superintendent on grounds that it was a minimum-security camp and officers are often alone with prisoners in this setting. It was pointed out that medical staff are not able to remain fully attentive to security concerns because the very nature of their work (e.g., listening to a chest, examining a patient, reading a medical chart, viewing an x-ray or laboratory test result) temporarily distracts the clinicians from the requisite security alertness and renders them vulnerable to any prisoner who would wish to take advantage. The result was a decision by the superintendent to assign an officer to be in the clinic whenever only one health care employee was present. Staff also were given personal alarm devices and required to wear them whenever on duty in the clinic.

No Sink or Running Water

From time to time, even in some relatively new correctional buildings, a medical or dental clinic or examination room can be found that is without a sink and running water. In those cases, the dentist, physician, or nurse must (1) rely on moist antiseptic towelettes or a waterless alcohol-based antimicrobial hand wash to cleanse hands between patients, (2) walk a considerable distance to a bathroom and thus lose valuable time between each patient (also unsatisfactory if there are one or more doors en route that must be opened by hand), or (3) attend patients without washing hands. None of these solutions is satisfactory, although option 1 is an acceptable temporary solution. A sink with running water, paper towels, soap dispensers, and adequate lighting is essential for any medical or dental clinic area. Suitable plumbing and fixtures should be installed, or the clinic should be relocated. Wrist-, foot-, or motion-activated faucets are preferable in order to prevent contamination.

Defective or Inadequate Equipment

Timely replacement or repair of defective medical equipment should be a priority if the responsible health authority presents this as a critically needed item. In a clinic without a properly functioning autoclave (sterilizer) for medical instruments and supplies, certain medical procedures and most dental procedures cannot be performed safely. Each dental clinic should have enough hand instruments so there are adequate supplies of presterilized packets for each day. Defective x-ray equipment can leak dangerous radiation, exposing patients and especially staff to the risk of cancer. It can also produce misleading results.

It is important that staff promptly report defective or malfunctioning equipment and arrange for its repair or replacement. A preventive maintenance program can avoid costly repairs and downtime. With expensive and highly complex equipment, it is wise to negotiate a maintenance contract with the vendor or other appropriate source, specifying an acceptable time frame for repair and including the loan of equipment while repairs are being performed.

One large county jail had constructed a new addition. Overlooking every two housing units was an officer station fitted with large unbreakable windows. Shortly after opening the unit, at the suggestion of officers, amber-colored reflective transparent plastic film was affixed to the interior of the windows in the officers' stations. As long as lighting was of higher intensity in the housing unit than inside the officer station, the window served as a one-way mirror that allowed officers to see the inmates but not vice versa. There were small-slotted openings through which a voice could be heard and small items could be passed (such as pieces of paper). Problems arose because three times each day the nurse would wheel a cart into the officers' station to conduct sick call and distribute medication. The patient could not see the nurse. Both nurse and patient had to shout to be heard, with the result that officers and other inmates were privy to the conversation. The colored plastic and the poor lighting made it difficult for the nurse to see clearly enough to evaluate a patient's appearance. If the nurse insisted, although with considerable inconvenience and delay, officers would admit a patient to a small anteroom (sally port) adjacent to the housing unit where the nurse could take a patient's temperature, pulse, and blood pressure. Even here, the lighting was not adequate and was so inconvenient for the officers that nurses only rarely requested to use this expedient.

Physicians and nurses are justified in insisting on adequate lighting. Not to do so is an unacceptable and unethical breach of the requisite standard of care.

Methods of Preventing HIV Transmission

Over the past few years, many prisons and jails have taken bold steps to reduce the transmission of HIV and other blood-borne pathogens. In addition to educational efforts, some facilities have provided (or permitted inmates to purchase) condoms. Although homosexual contact was prohibited in their institutions, the authorities decided to enable safer sex practices for those activities that would occur despite efforts to enforce the rules. At one large metropolitan jail, a bowl of condoms was located on the physician's desk, and patients were permitted to help themselves to a few. The facility established a policy that an inmate would not be charged with possession of contraband if he had three or fewer condoms at any one time. For similar reasons, a few facilities also have made small quantities of diluted household bleach or powdered bleach available to inmates so they could disinfect their intravenous drug equipment. These harm-reduction approaches recognize the seriousness of HIV as well as the reality of behaviors that can occur in these settings, so they were adopted as public health measures.

> Failure to employ known methods of reducing risk of fatal disease has serious ethical as well as public health implications.

Undoubtedly, more facilities will follow suit over the next few years. Policies such as these, however, are highly responsive to political pressures. No department head or elected official wants to see his or her agency's policy ridiculed in the headlines. Consequently, decision makers are afraid of conveying the impression that illegal or immoral behavior is condoned. The voices of medical professionals thus need to be raised in support of these practices, following the lead of Dr. Robert Greifinger: "We must advocate for programs that would be good for public health, such as providing condoms to prevent transmission of sexually transmitted infections and providing substitution therapy for opiate addiction. These are part of our ethical obligations and professional responsibilities."[89]

In the author's view, failure to employ known methods of reducing risk of fatal disease has serious ethical as well as public health implications.

Food Loaf

Some correctional institutions have adopted a creative approach to managing inmates who throw their food at officers in the segregation unit. The regular portion of food and drink normally served to inmates on that day is blended together and baked into a loaf to be eaten with the fingers and without table utensils. Although the food loaf may be as nutritious as the regular menu, it is decidedly less tasty and palatable.

Many correctional administrators consider the food loaf a humane and practical way to feed the type of prisoner it was originally designed for—an inmate in segregation who habitually throws (or threatens to throw) his or her food out through the bars or food slot at anyone who passes by. However, some jurisdictions have broadened its usage to all inmates in disciplinary segregation, or to a food thrower for a specified period such as thirty days, and not merely until he or she makes a credible contract not to repeat the misuse of food. Deprivation of palatable nourishment is not an appropriate punishment. Over a prolonged period, poor nutrition can adversely affect health.

ACA's standards prohibit the use of food in a punitive way: "Written policy precludes the use of food as a disciplinary measure." As its commentary explains, "Food should not be withheld, or the standard menu varied, as a disciplinary sanction for an individual inmate."[90] Thus a distinction is made that does not prohibit the use of food loaf to prevent misuse of food or food utensils. But it may not be imposed as a punishment or sanction, as would be the case if food loaf were made a routine part of the disciplinary segregation experience or were imposed as a sentence for a defined period of time. In addition, the ACA's standards explicitly address the fool loaf situation:

[A]lternative meal service may be provided to an inmate in segregation who uses food or food service equipment in a manner that is hazardous to self, staff, or other inmates. Alternative meal service is on an individual basis, is based on health or safety considerations only, meets basic nutritional requirements, and occurs with the written approval of the warden/superintendent, or designee and responsible health authority or designee. The substitution period shall not exceed seven days. [91]

The author recalls visiting a facility that attempted to circumvent this standard by serving food loaf to all persons in disciplinary segregation and offering regular meals only on Sundays. The audit team found this practice to be punitive and noncompliant.

Doctors should not certify that a patient is healthy enough to eat food loaf because this could suggest doctors are participating in the imposition of punishment.

Hunger Strikes

Hunger strikes pose extremely difficult situations for facility administrators and health care staff. They can quickly become media events with major political ramifications. A hunger strike may be an attempt to attract attention or for prisoners to get their way. It may be a protest against real or perceived wrongs. Hunger strikers are likely to be mentally competent persons acting in a purposeful and reasoned manner, perhaps even for a high and worthy cause. Outside of the correctional scene, the hunger strike tactic has been employed by such respected persons as Mohandas Gandhi and César Chávez as a nonviolent but effective means of inspiring support for the worthy causes in which they deeply believed. Less often, the hunger striker may be psychotic and acting on the command of hallucinatory voices.

Several alternative policy decisions are possible in these situations, assuming that a competent inmate's claims have some validity. First of all, the correctional authority should consider granting some or all of the hunger striker's demands if they are not unreasonable and this is likely to be a successful solution. An objective assessment should be made in each case. Reasonable demands should not be rejected out of a misguided belief that one should never "give in" to an inmate. Attempts also may be made to persuade the hunger striker to redirect his or her protest tactics to a more acceptable mode. In any case, it is prudent for the correctional authority to listen to the concerns and engage in constructive dialogue with the striker or strikers. When such efforts have failed and the competent inmate appears determined to continue the hunger strike, basically two courses of action are available, depending on the agency policy.

1. Advise the patient that the agency's no-rescue policy will be strictly followed. In this case, use all reasonable means to encourage the patient to eat. Do not rescue. Be willing and prepared to allow the hunger striker to die if refusal continues.
2. Intervene with forced feeding. It is best to seek a court order for this intervention to prevent such use of force on a competent person later being judged an assault. Without a court order, the author recommends that health care staff should refrain from participating in the forced feeding because it is unethical to force treatment on a competent unwilling patient. The fear of adverse publicity that may result from the death of a hunger striker is not a justification for enforced feeding.

On occasion, large numbers of inmates have participated in hunger strikes to give voice to their felt concerns. Witness the mass hunger strikes at Pelican Bay

State Prison in California (later joined by supportive hunger strikes at 13 other state prisons in that state) in 2011 and 2012, mass hunger strikes at the Red Onion State Prison in Virginia in May 2012, and the mass hunger strike of Ohio State Penitentiary prisoners in April and May 2012—all voicing protest over conditions in the security housing units (SHU) and solitary confinement.

> "Where a prisoner refuses nourishment and is considered by the physician as capable of forming an unimpaired and rational judgment concerning the consequences of such a voluntary refusal of nourishment, he or she shall not be fed artificially."
> —World Medical Association

Some court decisions have authorized the forced feeding of hunger strikers, as did Washington state's supreme court in 2008, affirming a 2005 lower court decision that the state was justified in force-feeding Charles R. McNabb, who had refused food for an extended period.[92] Although the facts specific to this case are relevant, the court distinguished between the case of otherwise healthy McNabb and cases in which a terminally ill patient declines treatment. The court concluded that the state's interests "in orderly administration within the prison system, the preservation of life, the protection of innocent third parties, the prevention of suicide, and the maintenance of the ethical integrity of the medical profession outweighed McNabb's limited right" to refuse artificial nutrition.[93]

However, to date there has been no U.S. Supreme Court ruling on the matter, and court precedents differ among jurisdictions. A Florida case (*Singletary v. Costello*) ruled that the state's interest in the preservation of an inmate's life "cannot overcome the fundamental nature of" the prisoner's privacy right but cautioned that this was not a universal holding that a prison inmate has the right to starve to death.[94] In *Thor v. Superior Court,*[95] California's supreme court ruled that Andrews, a prisoner who was quadriplegic, had a right to refuse feeding and medication, even if this meant death, and that the right to refuse treatment and food does not depend on the prisoner having a terminal condition.

In *Singletary v. Costello*, the court notably rejected the claim that the state was preventing suicide: "In the instant case, however, Costello testified that he did not want to die. Costello commenced his hunger strike as a form of protest, with the resolution of his complaints as the desired end. Thus, the purpose of the hunger strike was to bring about change, not death. Therefore, the state interest in the prevention of suicide is not implicated in the instant case."

The World Medical Association, through the *Declaration of Tokyo*, recommends:

Where a prisoner refuses nourishment and is considered by the physician as capable of forming an unimpaired and rational judgment concerning the consequences of such a voluntary refusal of nourishment, he or she shall not be fed artificially. The decision as to the capacity of the prisoner to form such a judgment should be confirmed by at least one other independent physician. The consequences of the refusal of nourishment shall be explained by the physician to the prisoner.[96]

The *Declaration of Malta* describes the ethical responsibility of a physician treating a hunger striker, pointing out the need to balance the principle of beneficence (to prevent harm to the striker) and that of nonmaleficence and autonomy (to respect the right to refuse treatment). Emphasis is placed on the fact that, especially in collective strikes or situations in which peer pressure may be a factor, it is critically important to ascertain the individual's true intention. Among the important points explicitly made by the *Declaration of Malta* are:

2. Respect for autonomy. Physicians should respect individuals' autonomy. This can involve difficult assessments as hunger strikers' true wishes may not be as clear as they appear. Any decisions lack moral force if made involuntarily by use of threats, peer pressure or coercion. Hunger strikers should not be forcibly given treatment they refuse. Forced feeding contrary to an informed and voluntary refusal is unjustifiable. . . .

3. "Benefit" and "harm.". . . . "Benefit" includes respecting individuals' wishes as well as promoting their welfare. Avoiding "harm" means not only minimising damage to health but also not forcing treatment upon competent people nor coercing them to stop fasting. Beneficence does not necessarily involve prolonging life at all costs, irrespective of other values.

4. Balancing dual loyalties. Physicians attending hunger strikers can experience a conflict between their loyalty to the employing authority (such as prison management) and their loyalty to patients. Physicians with dual loyalties are bound by the same ethical principles as other physicians, that is to say that their primary obligation is to the individual patient.[97]

If forced feeding is the choice, then it should be done at a relatively early stage rather than waiting until the patient has become unconscious or is too weak to offer resistance. Intervention should take place before permanent or irreparable organ damage occurs. Should serious and irreversible damage occur, costly and ongoing medical care expenses and permanent physical impairment will be the likely result.

In summary, the author recommends the following strategies in the event of a hunger strike:

1. Ascertain the nature of the complaint and the stated purpose and voluntariness of the protest. Have talk(s) with the patient—perhaps more than one.

2. If the stated claims and demands of the patient appear valid and legitimate, adopt a conciliatory stance and offer to make genuine efforts to assist in resolving the issues. If it becomes possible to grant the hunger striker's legitimate and reasonable demands, consider doing so as early as possible. Negotiate in good faith.

3. Arrange for a competency examination by a psychiatrist or psychologist. If the patient is deranged, incompetent, or mentally ill, consider seeking a court order for enforced nutrition.

4. Monitor all materials brought into a hunger striker's cell.

5. Monitor all food and liquid intake and output if the hunger strike continues beyond a few days. Accurate monitoring requires a cooperative subject, but some information is better than none.

6. Transfer the hunger striker to a medical area—such as an infirmary bed to facilitate close observation—when the patient becomes debilitated or exhibits medical need.

7. If it be determined that the hunger striker is competent and appears to be making a reasoned and purposeful choice, advise him or her that the facility has a "no rescue" policy. This means that if he or she becomes unconscious or comatose or too weak to resist, lifesaving emergency procedures will not be instituted to force-feed. Ask the patient to sign a release stating that he or she has been advised of the consequences of continuing the fast, understands there is a no-rescue policy, and does not want last-minute desperate rescue efforts.

8. Make every effort to determine whether the hunger striker's decision is being made without coercion or peer pressure from others. During a prolonged hunger strike, the physician should ascertain on a daily basis whether the individual wishes to continue the hunger strike and what she or he wants to be done when no longer able to communicate meaningfully. These findings must be duly recorded.

9. Continue to serve three appetizing meals a day. Estimate intake and output of fluids and solids. Keep up the contact by concerned visitors. Inform the hunger striker of the results and meaning of the medical tests being conducted.

10. Encourage liquids and vitamins even if food is being refused because this will delay the onset of serious or irreversible health problems. Remind the hunger striker of the no-rescue policy.

11. If the patient has access to commissary items (or other food sources) and presumably eats them while ignoring the food that is served, then perhaps the incident should be classified as something other than a hunger strike.

12. Arrange visits to the hunger striker by a physician, psychiatrist, psychologist, social worker, nurse, chaplain, and family members. The physician should advise both the hunger striker and the visitors clearly and truthfully about the short- and long-range health consequences from dehydration or prolonged malnutrition.

13. In a prolonged situation, hold a conference with the physician, psychiatrist, psychologist, nurse, warden, custody officer, central office representative, attorney, chaplain, and family member, as appropriate, to review what has taken place and discuss alternatives.

14. If it is determined that the patient is incompetent, advise him or her that a court order will be sought for involuntary nutrition. If this is the decision, it should be implemented as early as possible and before the patient becomes weakened or comatose.

CONCLUSION

The basic principles for guiding ethical decisions in correctional health care are chiefly those of beneficence, nonmaleficence, privacy, confidentiality, patient autonomy, and respect for dignity of the human person.

In many instances, the application of these principles can be obvious and easy with few dissenters. Other situations, however, can be more controversial and require more nuanced decisions, depending on the specific facts and a careful balancing of priorities. The actors always need to give due weight to ethical considerations in making decisions so as not to compromise their own principles or those of their professions.

This chapter has explored several frequently encountered ethical challenges. Much of the remainder of this book, and especially the following two chapters, will continue to present additional topics of ethical concern that may arise when providing health services in correctional settings. In so doing, the discussion will consider the ethical principles and reasoning involved, make reference to applicable codes and standards that have been promulgated, and also look at the positions of those who hold an opposing point of view and their supporting rationale when appropriate.

Chapter 2

Areas of Significant Ethical Role Conflict

ETHICAL ROLE CONFLICT SITUATIONS

From time to time, people who work in corrections can find themselves in situations of ethical role conflict. Job expectations may be discordant with their personal understanding of what is right or humane or ethical. Peer pressure can make them uncomfortable. Inappropriate behaviors are sometimes adopted because it is what policy or training requires or at least is believed to require. Other behaviors may arise out of ignorance, fear, or confusion. We will explore situations that can and do occur. To achieve immediate and unquestioned compliance, correctional systems often tend to prefer simple, black-and-white policies and directions that omit nuances and fine distinctions. However, failure to evaluate the nuances and specific details of given situations can have unintended consequences.

As will be evident from the situations discussed in the first three chapters of this book, role conflicts can range from relatively minor ethical dissonance (such as health care staff writing disciplinary tickets) to instances of obvious and overwhelming ethical conflict (such as participation in executions or acts of torture). Thus, there are degrees to which the ethical code can be violated. None are acceptable, but some are unthinkable. Habitual involvement in less atrocious forms of unethical behavior tend to condition a health professional so that more serious violations become easier. It is only by watchful and constant adherence to the spirit as well as the letter of our ethical principles that we avoid behaviors that will compromise our role as a member of the healing professions.

This chapter presents the following examples of role conflict for health professionals:

- Medical clearance for punishment
- Use of mace

- Writing tickets
- Use of medication for behavior control
- Shakedowns performed by health care staff
- Witnessing use of force
- Participation in executions
- Use of torture
- Staff abuse of prisoners

Additional examples of ethical issues in correctional health care are discussed in Chapters 1 and 3.

Medical Clearance for Punishment

To question the ethical propriety of seeking medical clearance for disciplinary segregation may at first appear puzzling. Is not the intent of this practice the avoidance of harm to a debilitated or sick inmate? Yet, disciplinary segregation is punishment, perceived as undesirable by the patient. The health professional must be guided by the principle, "above all, do no harm." The practice of medicine and the fundamental role of healer are always inconsistent with approving or enabling the imposition of punishment.

Still, even enlightened correctional systems have policies that require formal clearance or input from health care professionals in classification decisions that affect housing and work assignments. For all newly arrived inmates, the American Correctional Association (ACA) requires health professionals to develop and implement a "treatment plan, including recommendations concerning housing, job assignment, and program participation."[1] The ACA also requires that health care personnel be informed as soon as a person is transferred to segregation so that an appropriate screening and review can take place.[2] The National Commission on Correctional Health Care (NCCHC) requires communication between correctional officials and health care staff before any disciplinary measures are taken with patients who are diagnosed with significant medical or mental illness or disability to ensure these problems are considered and the prisoner's health and safety are protected. The rationale behind these carefully worded standards is to protect against unintended harm to persons whose medical or psychiatric condition would contraindicate such an assignment while avoiding any suggestion that the medical professional is condoning or approving the punishment.

NCCHC Standard P-A-08 reads:

Communication occurs between the facility administration and treating health care professionals regarding inmates' significant health needs that must be considered in classification decisions in order to preserve the health and safety of that inmate, other inmates, or staff. . . . Correctional staff are advised of inmates' special health needs that may affect housing, work, and program assignments; disciplinary measures; and admissions to and transfers from institutions. Such communication is documented.[3]

The accompanying discussion says, "This standard intends to ensure that correctional staff are aware of the special needs and any restrictions they are to accommodate in making classification decisions."

Medical *clearance* for classification that affects housing or work assignments is appropriate so long as the assignment is not punitive in nature or cannot reasonably be perceived as punishment by the inmate. There is a problem, however, with medical clearance for segregation or for movement from lesser security to higher security with consequent restriction of activity and privileges. Health care professionals certainly should be asked to *review and comment* before such assignments are initiated, and every such communication should be documented, but it is misleading to regard or label this process as "medical clearance" or "approval."

This is not a trivial distinction. The doctor (or other health professional) in these instances is not being asked for and is not granting *approval* for punishment. Whether the doctor personally regards the assignment to disciplinary segregation to be appropriate is not at all relevant. In fact, the doctor is not even involved in that decision process, and it should not be made to appear as if she or he were involved. Instead, the doctor is simply being asked to advise whether this inmate is known to have a medical or mental health condition that will require specific safeguards, precautions, or treatments or that makes him or her particularly susceptible to potentially adverse consequences (for example, in the segregation setting or from mace). Having so advised, it is up to the corrections officials to decide whether to make special arrangements and accommodations to ensure provision of all prescribed treatments and other medical precautions, to find another method for dealing with the behaviors and needs of this inmate, or to accept the risk and responsibility after being duly warned about likely adverse consequences.

For example, assume that a patient, whose psychotropic medications increase sensitivity to heat, is to be placed in a segregation unit where ambient temperatures are known to be often excessive. The doctor has done all that is required by asserting (1) this patient's vulnerability to excessive heat, (2) the likely consequences to the individual of prolonged heat exposure, and (3) the need for air conditioning or increased ventilation. At no time does the doctor "approve" or "disapprove" the punishment or "clear (or refuse to clear) the inmate for segregation." The doctor simply has evaluated the patient and the circumstances of confinement and accurately described to correctional officials the probable outcomes on a need-to-know basis and for the welfare of the patient. The doctor should document the date and content of all such recommendations.

To carry this theme to its extreme, it applies also to the question of determining whether or not a person on death row is well enough (physically or mentally) to be executed. Such a judgment should never be made by any health care professional because it is too closely linked with enabling the act of execution, as will be discussed in a later section of this chapter.

Certainly, prisoners on death row have the same right to health care as other prisoners. These patients also have the right to grant or withhold informed consent for diagnostic and treatment measures. If the patient is in a hospital, then discharge should not occur until it has been deemed medically appropriate.[4]

A key point is that the health professional is not charged with determining or evaluating the necessity, legality, or rationale for the use of force or punishment. If the forcible action is harmful to the health or well-being of the individual, the health professional does not approve or disapprove it, condone it, enable it, facilitate it, or participate in its implementation. On the other hand, if the forcible action is obviously illegal or inhumane or abusive, then the health professional has an affirmative duty to object or report such behavior to proper authorities.

Use of Mace

The use of mace presents a similar situation. Mace, pepper spray, tear gas, and other toxic sprays may be especially harmful to a person with chronic obstructive pulmonary disease (COPD), including asthma, or with heart problems or certain skin conditions. In fact, the potentially harmful effects of respiratory irritants are not fully known. None of these should ever be used without an extremely good reason. A study of the health effects of pepper spray (oleoresin capsicum or OC) was prepared by two physicians, C. Gregory Smith and Woodhall Stopford in 1999. They state that "there is no real scientific basis for the claim that OC sprays are relatively safe. In fact, several reports have associated serious adverse sequelae, including death, with legitimate use as well as misuse and abuse of these sprays,"[5] and they cite a 1993 warning by the U.S. Department of Labor's Occupational Safety and Health Administration that "OC spray posed significant health risks to exposed employees, that it could cause unpredictable, severe adverse health outcomes, and that it should not be intentionally sprayed on the skin, eyes, or mucous membranes of employees during training."[6]

To be effective, two other gases—chloroacetophenone (CN) and O-chlorobenzylidene malononitrile (CS)—are sprayed in the face and produce intense irritation of the eyes, mouth, nose, and sinuses. Patients with a history of glaucoma, eye disease, or past eye surgery; COPD, pulmonary disease, pulmonary infection, pulmonary surgery, or pulmonary trauma; myocardial infarction or angina pectoris; hypertension; diabetes; epilepsy; open skin wounds; and those who take cardiovascular medications or psychotropic medications are at elevated risk of serious harm from these toxic sprays.[7] These medical conditions are quite common—a fact that signals for great caution and restraint in the use of these chemicals. Both CS and CN are highly toxic. CS can cause severe damage to the lungs, heart, and liver.

OC or pepper spray is an irritant made from substances such as chili peppers. John Medici[8] provides a detailed description of the characteristics and toxic effects of various types of mace and oleoresins. Smith and Stopford say that serious adverse health effects, even death, have followed the use of OC sprays, pointing out that more than 70 deaths of people in custody involved the use of OC spray during arrest efforts, with positional asphyxia, drug intoxication, and other conditions causing or contributing to most of these deaths. They further note, "A review of reported injuries found that 61 of approximately 6,000 officers directly exposed to

OC spray during training experienced adverse effects . . . sufficiently severe to require medical attention."[9]

> It can never be ethical for health care professionals to approve the use of toxic sprays or to "medically clear" a prisoner (or a group of prisoners) to be sprayed.

Use of gas or mace in a punitive way—such as spraying prisoners in segregation if they attempt to talk with one another—is a serious misuse of this substance. Testimony of Craig Haney asserts that, in Florida's close management units,

[p]risoners report that these "gassings" occur with very little or no provocation and are not used to defuse otherwise difficult situations or potential conflicts. Instead they report that correctional officers use pepper spray as punishment—gassing prisoners for unpleasant but nonthreatening infractions, returning to gas them after a conflict has ended, and otherwise using this very painful and potentially physically damaging form of control to hurt and intimidate prisoners. Indeed, many prisoners reported that the gassings occur at night, when the prisoners are sleeping. They noted that they sleep with their clothes on to protect them from the gassings if they occur. . . . Several prisoners reported that prisoners were gassed for having declared psychiatric emergencies (presumably because correctional officers viewed the declarations as "manipulative").[10]

If true as reported, such usage would clearly exceed a legitimate or necessary penological purpose.

Whenever it is necessary to use toxic sprays, officers must decontaminate those sprayed as soon as possible, continuously monitor them for evidence of adverse effects, and seek medical attention immediately if serious symptoms develop. Decontamination involves a shower and change of clothing as soon as feasible. If the spraying occurred in an occupied cell, exposed surfaces will need to be washed because the toxic effects can linger.

In light of these facts, it can never be ethical for health care professionals to approve the use of toxic sprays or to medically clear a prisoner (or a group of prisoners) to be sprayed. Although they may reveal the fact that a particular inmate is especially vulnerable to these irritants, they should caution that other persons also may have similar conditions that may not have been identified.

Writing Tickets

Suppose an inmate, unobserved by correctional officers, makes obscene remarks to a nurse or touches her inappropriately, intentionally damages medical equipment, acts in a disorderly manner in the clinic, or expresses credible threats to injure someone. It would not be unethical for the health professional to report such behavior, even to the point of filing a formal complaint, knowing that this may lead to prosecution or punishment of the inmate. How does this square with *primum non nocere*—"Above all, do no harm"—the first rule of medical ethics. Reporting the incident under these circumstances cannot reasonably be perceived as an act of medical treatment. Medical professionals clearly are entitled to a safe working area. Were such behaviors to occur in a free world hospital or emergency room, the nurse would summon hospital security staff and possibly also the police. Staff would file formal charges. It is no different in a correctional institution. The doctor or nurse should immediately disengage from providing care to that patient until and unless the behavior is corrected and controlled. When such behavior is observed by an officer, it would be more appropriate for the officer to initiate the report rather than the nurse.

On the other hand, behavior that does not threaten safety or security such as swearing in the presence of staff ordinarily should not be written up by health care staff. Health professionals are not police and should not behave as such.[11] If a nurse is expected to write tickets, then she or he should object. It violates the intent of the nurse practice act and ethical standards. It also creates an inappropriate role conflict and undermines the trusting relationship between caregiver and patient. Clearly, there are exceptions. Profanity can be abusive and threatening and should not be tolerated. It is appropriate for health care staff to make it clear to inmates that profanity or unruly behavior is unacceptable in the clinic and that institutional policies will be enforced.

Some correctional administrators and their training divisions boldly proclaim that "Everyone who works here is 'security.' " Except in its loosest interpretation, such a statement is a misleading exaggeration. Although they must be alert and supportive of security concerns, nurses and doctors are not security staff. They do not have the training for security. Health care professionals have different duties and responsibilities.

Facility administrators want good nurses and doctors but will risk attracting and retaining only second-rate staff if they promote role confusion and create ethical dilemmas. Professionals willing to compromise their principles are not the type of staff you really want.

Use of Medication for Behavior Control

Certain medications are effective for altering mood or behavior. Some can render a person unconscious or so debilitated as to be unable to resist or be aggressive. It is unethical for these medications to be prescribed simply to control behavior. The use of such drugs always requires (1) informed consent (sometimes by a surrogate) and (2) a decision by a qualified provider that the patient has a diagnosed illness for which this is the appropriate treatment. Thus, a mentally ill patient whose aggressive behavior is a consequence of psychosis can be treated with a tranquilizer, but an assaultive, angry, or unruly inmate without a diagnosis of mental disorder should not be sedated in this way. This is the reason for the second principle of the codes of ethics of both the American Correctional Health Services Association (ACHSA) and the American College of Correctional Physicians (ACCP): "The correctional health professional shall . . . render medical treatment only when it is justified by an accepted medical diagnosis. Treatment and invasive procedures shall be rendered after informed consent."[12] Accordingly, every penal institution should have a policy that clearly prohibits the prescribing of medication except when appropriate for the treatment of illness.

In *Knecht v. Gillman* [488 F. 2d 1136 (1973)], a federal appellate court ruled on the question of mentally ill inmates being injected with apomorphine when they violated established behavior protocols. The medication caused vomiting and was explicitly administered as an aversive stimulus to achieve behavior control. The court declared this practice to be in violation of the Eighth Amendment.

A correctional official who pressures a physician to medicate a prisoner for behavior control is violating the essential principle of medical autonomy.

Shakedowns Performed by Health Professional Staff

Like writing tickets, witnessing the use of force, and granting medical clearance for punishment, equally distasteful and incongruous for the health professional is being assigned to perform shakedowns (intensive searches or frisks) of cells, persons, or property. The author does not believe this to be a widespread practice but is aware of a few locations where it occurs. Sound reasons for disallowing this practice include:

1. Its intent is not for the benefit and well-being of the patient.
2. It places the health professional in a role-conflict situation.
3. It creates an aura of ambiguity for patients. Is this a health professional whose job is to care for me or is his or her function to get me in trouble?
4. This behavior can constitute a violation of the ethical standards of the health professions and also (at least of the spirit) of the professional practice act.
5. Performing a shakedown is a security function, not a health care service.
6. The health professional has many more essential duties to perform and too little time in which to do them.
7. The health professional is not trained or experienced in how to conduct a thorough search or how to do so without risking injury.

Witnessing the Use of Force

Correctional authorities have sometimes requested health care professionals to stand by and observe instances when force is being used. This practice, which is now less frequent because of the widespread use of video cameras and surveillance, has been intended to lessen or prevent the excessive use of force and wanton brutality by having a humane and caring individual present. To the inmate, however, the health care professional may seem to be condoning and supporting the unwanted use of force and approving the violation of the inmate's liberty. Doctors, nurses, and psychologists must never let themselves be persuaded to participate in any manner in the use of force against inmates. Health professionals are really not qualified to monitor use of force for appropriateness and safety. Moreover, their presence has been known to "ratchet up" forcefulness as security staff see less need to exercise restraint, feeling that they can keep going until health staff intervene.[13]

American Public Health Association standards[14] explicitly prohibit health care staff from serving as witness to the use of force. So also do the codes of ethics of the ACHSA and the ACCP.

This practice should not be confused with the application of medically ordered physical restraint such as in the treatment of a severely disturbed psychotic or manic patient. Health care staff may participate in the application of restraints under these circumstances because their purpose is therapeutic and intended to protect the patient from harm.

Many jails and prisons have policies that require health care staff to check restraints that have been applied without any health care direction. The ACA explicitly prohibits the application of restraints as punishment.[15] The ACA code also requires the health authority to be notified to assess an inmate's medical and mental health condition whenever he or she is placed in a four- or five-point restraint. The health authority is to "advise whether, on the basis of serious danger to self or others, the inmate should be in a medical/mental health unit for emergency involuntary treatment with sedation and/or other medical management, as appropriate."[16] Further, in its Public Correctional Policy, the ACA requires policies that "prohibit the use of force as a retaliatory or disciplinary measure; establish strategies to reduce and prevent the need to use force; authorize force only when no reasonable alternative is possible; and advocate that force used be the minimum amount necessary . . ." Policies should also "provide ongoing specialized staff training designed to teach staff to anticipate, stabilize and diffuse situations that might give rise to conflict, confrontation and violence and that ensures staff's competency in the use of all methods and equipment in the use of force."[17]

For health care staff to check the health status of restrained prisoners is not objectionable. The purpose of this periodic monitoring is to ensure that the restraints do not constrict circulation or respiration and that the inmate's health is not threatened. The duty of health professionals is to their patients' clinical care, physical safety, and psychological wellness.

Participation in Executions

Participation in any aspect of capital punishment presents an essential and extreme ethical conflict for a physician or other health professional. In this activity, the skills and knowledge of the healer would be directed toward causing death.

The vast majority of physicians and other health professionals readily recognize this as an intrinsic conflict. The American Medical Association (AMA) strongly condemned physician participation in executions in its resolution of 1992,[18] and the American Public Health Association's standards (2nd edition) clearly state:

Medical and mental health personnel have a professional obligation to use their training and expertise to maintain the health and wellness of the patients. . . . Medical personnel must not participate in any aspect of the execution process. Medical and mental health personnel must not participate in the planning or carrying out of executions. They must not prepare medications to induce death or certify competence of the inmate for death.[19]

In its third edition of the Standards, the American Public Health Association concisely states: "Health care staff should not participate in any aspect of an execution."[20]

Numerous health care associations and medical practice boards have expressed opposition to any form of participation by clinical staff in capital punishment.[21] The American Nurses Association adopted a provision prohibiting participation by nurses and declared, "The American Nurses Association . . . is strongly opposed to nurse participation in capital punishment. Participation in executions, either directly or indirectly, is viewed as contrary to the fundamental goals and ethical traditions of the nursing profession."[22] In their codes of ethics, the ACCP and ACHSA state, "The correctional health professional shall not be involved in any aspect of execution of the death penalty."[23] The NCCHC explicitly states "The correctional health services staff do not participate in inmate executions" and makes clear that "[e]xecutions do not occur in the medical unit or area" and that "[h]ealth staff do not pronounce death."[24]

The World Medical Association's *Declaration of Tokyo* states:

It is the privilege of the physician to practice medicine in the service of humanity, to preserve and restore bodily and mental health without distinction as to persons, to comfort and to ease the suffering of his or her patients. The utmost respect for human life is to be maintained even under threat, and no use made of any medical knowledge contrary to the laws of humanity.[25]

Despite this strong consensus of opposition from professional, authoritative, and influential bodies, physician and writer Atul Gawande reported in 2006 that most of the states with the death penalty explicitly allowed physician participation in executions—and nearly half of them require it.[26]

Of 683 executions that took place in the United States from January 2001 to February 2014, 673 were accomplished by lethal injection. In 2016, the death penalty remained legal in 27 states, the U.S. government, and the U.S. military. Four states—Washington, Oregon, Colorado, and Pennsylvania—had governor-imposed moratoria even though the death penalty remains on the books. Nineteen states—Alaska, Connecticut, Hawaii, Iowa, Illinois, Maine, Maryland, Massachusetts, Michigan, Minnesota, Nebraska, New Jersey, New Mexico, New York, North Dakota, Rhode

Island, Vermont, Wisconsin, West Virginia—plus the District of Columbia and the Commonwealth of Puerto Rico are without the death penalty.

Some physicians have argued that it is an act of mercy for them to be present so as to ensure the comfort of the prisoner facing execution. However, in defense of the codes of ethics, the person being executed is not a physician's patient—indeed, usually the prisoner and his or her family are not even permitted to know the doctor's identity. The "medical assistance" that is rendered primarily serves the state's purposes, not those of the prisoner. Through this process, medicine is being made an instrument of punishment. Despite this, the American College of Physicians, Human Rights Watch, and other organizations have documented that a surprising number of physicians and other health practitioners have contravened these principles:

In the course of our research, we found that physicians are involved in all methods of executions, especially ones performed by lethal injection, in violation of professional ethical guidelines. Physicians continue to consult on lethal dosages, examine veins, start intravenous lines, witness executions, and pronounce death. The threat posed to the moral standing of physicians, and to the public trust that physicians hold, is great. It warrants immediate and decisive action to assure the public, and each patient, that physicians will not use their skills to cause immediate and irreparable harm. . . .

We also discovered that state law and regulation are in direct conflict with established ethical standards regarding physician participation in executions. The majority of death penalty states define a role for physicians in the execution process, from witnessing in an official capacity to monitoring vital signs and pronouncing death. Although many states declare execution methods are not medical acts, they seek to involve physicians to make the process more 'humane'; this is contradictory and a distortion of the physician's role in society.[27]

In January 2007, the North Carolina Board of Medicine ruled that any physician who assists in an execution will have sanctions applied to his or her license. State law, however, required a doctor's presence at the executions. Consequently, all executions in North Carolina were placed on hold. The legislature then attempted to enact a statute to declare that "the infliction of the punishment of death by administration of the required lethal substances under this Article shall not be construed to be the practice of medicine."[28] One North Carolina Supreme Court justice even suggested bringing in a doctor from out of state to resolve the conflict. In April 2009, the North Carolina Supreme Court ruled that the medical board cannot punish doctors who take part in executions. No executions have been carried out in North Carolina since 2006. However, in an effort to enable their resumption, the governor in August 2015 signed HB-744 into law, removing the requirement that a physician be present at executions and permitting state officials to hold in secrecy many elements of the lethal injection process, including the specific drugs to be used and the suppliers of those drugs. Physician assistants, nurse practitioners, registered nurses, emergency medical technicians (EMTs), and paramedics are now permitted by North Carolina law to be present at executions in lieu of a physician, but a licensed physician must pronounce death.[29]

The state of Florida similarly had to suspend executions because the AMA guidelines prohibit physicians from participating in the process. Hitherto, physicians had done so in secrecy, shrouded by a hood and goggles, until the state medical examiner's office released autopsy reports containing the names of these physicians. In an effort to shield health practitioners, Florida law states that "prescription, preparation, compounding, dispensing, and administration of a lethal injection does not constitute the practice of medicine, nursing, or pharmacy."[30]

Some proponents have argued that the act of pronouncing the prisoner dead does not violate any ethical code. Consider, though, what would be the situation if the physician were to find that the prisoner is not yet dead. What then is the physician's role? Is the doctor to initiate a heroic rescue attempt—or advise prison staff on how to complete the execution?

The medical practice boards and medical associations fundamentally echo the language of the Hippocratic oath taken by all physicians before commencing practice. It reads, in part, "I will prescribe regimen for the good of my patients according to my ability and my judgment and never do harm to anyone. To please no one will I prescribe a deadly drug, nor give advice which may cause his death."

The incongruously clinical appearance of the modern lethal injection chamber used in many jurisdictions—stretcher or gurney, intravenous apparatus, and medical monitoring equipment—belies the stark contradiction between the process of healing and the process of killing. The author recalls visiting one prison in a Midwestern state where, incredibly, the execution chamber itself was situated well inside the medical clinic of the facility, while the condemned man was at that moment being held in a room across the hall from the execution chamber, awaiting his death that same evening. Words cannot adequately express the utter contradiction represented by this practice. *Res ipsa loquitur* (The thing speaks for itself). Just as physicians and other health care staff must be healers, not killers or punishers, so also the clinic itself must be unambiguously a location where only healing activities take place.

Other methods of execution—death by firing squad, gas chamber, electrocution, and hanging—have all proved painful, cruel, and horrific experiences and have largely been rejected by American society in recent years. Lethal injection, although it appears painless and humane, can be anything but that when botched. A fundamental problem, however, is that it makes medicine the instrument of punishment.[31] An editorial on this subject appeared in the *New England Journal of Medicine*,[32] describing instances in which the physician acquiesced to play a limited role of just "being present" and of "pronouncing death," only to find that he would also be pressed into service to locate a suitable vein, insert a central line, or assist in other direct ways in the execution.

Employing any of the healing arts to inflict death on a condemned inmate is a direct contradiction of the proper code of conduct of health professionals. This applies to treatment to restore competence to undergo execution; advice on the amount of lethal force or material that will be required to inflict death to this person; positioning a target over the prisoner's heart; acquisition of, preparation, or supervision of preparation of the lethal injection or other means of execution; finding a suitable vein; inserting the needle; activating the injection mechanism; or advising when death has been accomplished and further lethal attempts are no longer necessary. As will be subsequently discussed, many hold that this applies also to the determination of competence to be executed.

In its compendium of ethical directives for physicians, the American Medical Association has included an explicit prohibition of any participation with capital punishment, and it defines an explicit set of actions that constitute participation. These include prescribing or administering agents or medications that are part of the execution procedure, monitoring vital signs, attending or observing an execution qua physician, and rendering technical advice regarding execution. Specifically with regard to lethal injection, the AMA prohibits physicians from engaging in any activity related to the process of execution by lethal injection such as selecting injection sites, starting intravenous lines, prescribing or preparing or supervising injection drugs or their dosages, inspecting or testing devices, and consulting with or supervising personnel.[33] The AMA makes clear that this prohibition is separate and apart from the individual practitioner's own sentiments and personal convictions regarding capital punishment.

On a related issue, the American Medical Association has also issued a statement regarding organ donation by condemned prisoners. This practice may be carried out only if the decision to donate the organ was made prior to the prisoner's conviction, and the organ may not be removed until after the prisoner is pronounced dead and the body has been moved from the place of execution. Finally, physicians may not provide any advice for modifying the process of execution so as to facilitate the organ donation.[34] In view of the obvious benefit to mankind that human organ donations represent, it is abundantly clear from the preceding that the AMA regards *any* involvement of physicians with the process of execution to be so horrific and untenable that it has intentionally set conditions that, for all practical purposes, render such a donation impossible.

People need to trust that their doctors, nurses, pharmacists, EMTs, phlebotomists, and other treatment and diagnostic professionals and technicians will have the patients' well-being as their first and highest care. Accordingly, it is fundamentally wrong for any health care practitioner—whether physician, midlevel practitioner, nurse, technician, phlebotomist, or medical assistant—to participate in any way in any action or event that has the purpose of inflicting death, whether by providing advice, technical information, supplies, materials, assistance, or personal involvement. Such participation promotes distrust of medical practice by the general public who have a right to believe and expect that all health care practitioners are guided by the principle of "Above all, do no harm." It is a betrayal of the essential trust that people place in nurses and doctors. Prison health care personnel should steadfastly refuse to participate in any way, even at the risk of losing their jobs. Medicine should not be made the instrument of punishment. As Gawande so tellingly concludes, "The hand of comfort that more gently places the IV, more carefully times the bolus of potassium, is also the hand of death. We cannot escape this truth. The ethics code seems about right."[35]

Employing any of the healing arts to inflict death on a condemned inmate is a direct contradiction of the proper code of conduct of health professionals.

In February 2006, a U.S. District Court in California issued an unprecedented ruling that ordered the state to have a physician, specifically an anesthesiologist, personally supervise an execution by lethal injection in California. The judge noted that evidence from execution logs showed that six of the previous eight prisoners executed in California had not stopped breathing before technicians gave the paralytic agent, raising a serious possibility that the prisoners experienced suffocation from the paralytic, a feeling much like being buried alive, and felt intense pain from the bolus of potassium. Such a death, in the opinion of the court, would be unacceptable under the Eighth Amendment's protection against cruel and unusual punishment. As Gawande related, the California Medical Association, the American Medical Association, and the American Society of Anesthesiologists strenuously opposed physician participation as a clear violation of medical ethics codes. The court subsequently added another requirement—that the anesthesiologist personally administer additional medication if the prisoner remained conscious or was in pain. This the assigned anesthesiologists would not accept; as a result, the execution of Michael Morales was postponed indefinitely because the federal court's order for supervision by licensed medical personnel could not be accomplished.[36]

The three-stage procedure that was commonly used for execution by lethal injection involves administering the anesthetic sodium thiopental in massive doses that are expected to arrest breathing and extinguish consciousness within one minute after administration. Then the paralytic agent pancuronium is given, followed by a fatal dose of potassium chloride.

The sole U.S. manufacturer of sodium thiopental ceased making the drug in 2011. When this supply was exhausted, European manufacturers refused to export more sodium thiopental to the United States for use in capital punishment; consequently, it was no longer available. Ohio then switched from sodium thiopental to pentobarbital in 2011 and then to an untested combination of midazolam and hydromorphone in 2014. (Pentobarbital is a drug commonly used to euthanize animals. In lower doses, it is used on humans as an emergency treatment for seizures or as a preanesthetic to cause sleep in preparation for surgery.) Since 2014, Ohio has postponed any further executions until the medication issue is resolved. Georgia switched from conventionally manufactured pentobarbital to a compounding pharmacy for pentobarbital. Texas also decided to use a compounding pharmacy for pentobarbital. Missouri went to a form of pentobarbital manufactured by a compounding pharmacy. Because compounding pharmacies are not subject to federal inspection, the quality of their products varies.

In July 2014, the Death Penalty Information Center reported that an execution in Arizona was botched, requiring nearly two hours before the man was finally pronounced dead. The state had used a combination of midazolam and hydromorphone (a narcotic). According to witnesses, he gasped more than 600 times during the course of the execution. The official report showed that he had been injected with 15 doses of the drugs. A reporter described him gulping like a fish on land and convulsing repeatedly. This same drug protocol had been used in Ohio's botched execution earlier that year. Witnesses to an October 2014 Florida execution using midazolam also reported that the death took longer than usual.[37]

It is true that the skills of physicians and other health professionals could likely avoid botched executions and render the process free of any physical pain. However, as Black and Sade[38] comment, although this argument may appear logical and compelling, it simply ignores the reality that the direct and unambiguous result of the lethal injection procedure is the death of a human being. Consequently, physicians may not ethically participate in or enable such proceedings, even when their intent in doing so is to prevent pain and provide comfort.

Position of the American Pharmaceutical Association

Curfman, Morrissey, and Drazen have concluded, "Physicians and other health care providers should not be involved in capital punishment, even in an advisory capacity. A profession dedicated to healing has no place in the process of execution."[39]

Virtually alone among medical professional societies, the American Pharmaceutical Association (APhA) has, until only recently, not prohibited its members from participating in executions and did not declare the provision of medications for lethal injection to be unethical. Yet, this profession is necessarily drawn into the inner orbit of executions that employ lethal injections of deadly combinations of drugs.

It is instructive to examine briefly the actual process of preparing and administering a lethal dose of pharmaceutical agents. Some states have recognized the inappropriateness of involving the medical profession in acts of execution and have thus created an exception so that prison administrators may order these drugs directly from the manufacturer without requiring a doctor's prescription, but this has not eliminated the need for the involvement of pharmacists.

In *Baze v. Rees* (2008), the petitioners' brief explains the effects of these chemicals:

It is undisputed that the administration of pancuronium bromide and potassium chloride, either separately or in combination, would result in a terrifying, excruciating death if injected into a conscious person. Consequently, inducing general anesthesia is "critical" . . . to ensuring humane execution. . . . If the intended dose of thiopental is not injected successfully, or does not bring about general anesthesia, the inmate will experience both the terror and agony of conscious suffocation and the excruciating pain caused by the potassium, but will appear peaceful and unconscious to observers.[40]

In fact, it is likely that the primary purpose of including the pancuronium bromide paralyzing agent in the three-drug cocktail is to prevent any manifestation of outward signs of pain or agony when the potassium is injected.

The petitioners' brief goes on to state that "[D]rug preparation involves getting medication from six separate kits of 0.5 gram of powder, each of which must be individually mixed with solution. . . . The combination of several thiopental kits and accompanying calculations are difficult tasks for those who do not prepare drugs in their day-to-day, and can lead to an insufficient dose."[41] The thiopental packaging specifies that "the only people who should mix or administer the sodium thiopental are those trained and experienced in the administration of intravenous anesthetics." The EMTs and phlebotomists responsible for mixing the thiopental in Kentucky had not been trained in this area. Moreover, under Kentucky law, EMTs are permitted to function only under the direct supervision of a doctor, and phlebotomists are not required to have a license. Even though phlebotomists may not require a license to practice, it is inconceivable that one could regard them as anything other than members of the healing profession. They are important members of the health care team and consequently have a duty to exercise care on behalf of their patient's best interests. As such, the ethical prohibition against participation in executions applies equally to them.

Despite all this, the U.S. Supreme Court, by a vote of seven to two, ultimately ruled in *Baze v. Rees* that the method of execution in Kentucky was constitutional.

The issue, then, is whether pharmacists may ethically provide the medications, mix them, administer them, or advise and instruct others on how to perform these functions in furtherance of an act of capital punishment. It is difficult to see how a pharmacist can comply with the APhA's ethical provisions that "a pharmacist respects the covenantal relationship between the patient and the pharmacist" or that "a pharmacist promotes the good of every patient in a caring, compassionate, and confidential manner,"[42] unless one construes the intent of these statements not to have included within its definition of "patient" the very person to whom the pharmaceutical substances are to be administered.

Certainly any of these actions (supplying, mixing, administering, advising, or instructing) can be viewed as intrinsic and indispensable to the execution function. Consequently, this use of the professional knowledge and skills of the pharmacist constitutes a significantly more direct and active role in causing the death of the condemned person than would the act of a physician who only observes the execution and pronounces that death has occurred.

The pharmacy profession's ethical standards include the promise "to help individuals achieve optimum benefit from their medications, to be committed to their welfare, and to maintain their trust."[43] Although pharmacists do correctly regard themselves as belonging to a healing profession, without a clear and explicit position on this subject from their professional associations, pharmacists were left to form their own conscience in each instance. They must determine whether such behavior is consistent with or in conflict with the essential character of their chosen profession and the duty they owe to the public, irrespective of their personal views about the death penalty.

This picture has recently changed. On February 11, 2015 a motion was introduced to the APhA's Board of Delegates to oppose pharmacist participation in executions, either directly or indirectly, on the basis that such activities are fundamentally contrary to the role of pharmacists as providers of health care.[44] A compromise was reached, and the language approved by the House of Delegates in March 2015 reads: "The APhA discourages pharmacist participation in executions on the basis that such activities are fundamentally contrary to the role of pharmacists as providers of health care."[45] The International Association of Compounding Pharmacists had adopted a similar resolution for its members a week earlier.[46]

The pharmaceutical manufacturer Pfizer[47] in May 2016 tightened its policies to prevent the use of any of its products for lethal injections. Earlier, in February 2015, Akorn Pharmaceuticals issued a statement that it will no longer sell the sedative midazolam to prisons in an effort to keep the drug from being used in lethal injections.[48]

The result of actions like these is that access to drugs for use in legal executions is becoming increasingly difficult, and this is having an effect in bringing the practice to an end.

Treatment to Render a Person Competent for Trial

May a physician ethically render treatment to a mentally ill patient for the purpose of restoring competence to stand trial? The issue revolves around whether medical ethics permit such treatment when it is known that the consequence may be conviction and punishment—possibly even the death penalty.

This question was answered from a legal perspective in *Sell v. United States* [539 U.S. 166 (2003)]. Here a basic assumption made by the Supreme Court was that Sell was not dangerous to himself or others; if he were, the *Washington v. Harper* ruling would have permitted an order for involuntary administration of medication.[49] The Court, however, declared that a pretrial detainee (one who is not imminently dangerous to self or others) may be forced to take antipsychotic medications in order to restore competence to stand trial—but only under the following stringent limits:

First, a court must find that *important* governmental interests are at stake. . . .

Second, the court must conclude that involuntary medication will *significantly further* those concomitant state interests. It must find that administration of the drugs is substantially likely to render the defendant competent to stand trial. At the same time, it must find that administration of the drugs is substantially unlikely to have side effects that will interfere significantly with the defendant's ability to assist counsel in conducting a trial defense, thereby rendering the trial unfair. . . .

Third, the court must conclude that involuntary medication is *necessary* to further those interests. The court must find that any alternative, less intrusive treatments are unlikely to achieve substantially the same results. . . .

Fourth, the court must conclude that administration of the drugs is *medically appropriate*, i.e., in the patient's best medical interest in light of his medical condition. The specific kinds of drugs at issue may matter here as elsewhere. Different kinds of antipsychotic drugs may produce different side effects and enjoy different levels of success.[50]

Dr. Douglas Mossman presents a strong ethical argument in defense of the administration of medication to restore competence to stand trial. He defines "medically appropriate" (the term used in *Sell*) as meaning that it is "in the patient's best medical interest in light of his medical condition." This interpretation, however, fails to take into account the full extent of the patient's best interest in view of the likely detrimental consequences once restored to competence. Instead, Mossman concludes that it is medically appropriate because competence-restoring treatment itself represents a potential benefit, even if the likely outcome of treatment is the defendant's conviction and punishment. Even using a utilitarian approach, an assessment of the best interest of the patient also must recognize the value to the patient of understanding his or her situation, cooperating in his or her defense, and seeing that justice is done. Following Kantian philosophy, Mossman reasons that:

"Because competence-restoring medical treatment makes prosecution allowable, it preserves the autonomy and humanity of accused criminals by letting them satisfy their obligations under the social contract," and, accordingly, "safe, effective, competence-restoring treatment is medically appropriate because it is the incompetent defendant's vehicle for exercising rationality and vindicating his autonomy."[51] Mossman goes on to say that if a psychiatrist refused to administer competence-restoring treatment, this would violate the defendant's personhood and fail to regard the patient as a responsible individual. Moreover, punishment "gives offenders the chance, at least, to identify their personal failings and accept responsibility for them." On the other hand, mere confinement of a psychotic individual without restoring competence deprives the patient of the chance to appreciate as well as experience the proper consequences of these actions.[52]

While this argument has some appeal, it appears to falter when confronted with the following reductio ad absurdum posed by Mossman himself. After pointing out that the ethical obligations of beneficence and nonmaleficence apply to all persons and not just to physicians, as for example, in the mandate "Thou shalt love thy neighbor as thyself," he concludes that punishment should pose a moral problem for everyone if all citizens are morally obliged to do only good and avoid harming others. "Thus the same arguments that would justify physician actions in competence restoration must all justify, *mutatis mutandem* [sic], the actions of jurors who convict, judges who sentence, jailers who effectuate sentences, and a society that, as a whole, collectively imposes suffering on its members through the actions of the criminal justice system."[53]

It is not suggested here that Dr. Mossman raised this point to contradict his main thesis. In fact, his obvious intent was to draw the exact opposite inference. In all fairness, therefore, interested readers are encouraged to read Mossman's lengthy and well-articulated treatise in order to remedy any inadvertent faulty interpretation or excessive summarization of his complex reasoning.

However, Mossman's argument as cited here accords insufficient weight to the fact that a physician's ethical responsibilities, although owed to the specific patient being treated, are also mandated by the importance of the trust that physicians must inspire in all potential patients—namely, the confidence that their physician will always and ever regard their well-being as the first and highest concern, and that the physician will never use the practice of medicine to cause them harm. In other words, society holds physicians to a higher ethical standard in their role as healing professionals, arguably placing the good of the patient above the important government trial-related interests.

Determination of Competence to Be Executed

The Supreme Court in *Ford v. Wainwright* held that execution of insane persons violates the Eighth Amendment's bar against cruel and unusual punishment: "The Eighth Amendment forbids the execution only of those who are unaware of the punishment they are about to suffer and why they are to suffer it."[54] This represents the standard of mental competence that is required before a person may legally be executed. The rationale for this conclusion, found in English common law, is that imposing the penalty of death on a prisoner who is insane and not aware of his impending execution and the reasons for it has questionable retributive and no deterrence value, and thus simply offends humanity. Hence arises the question: May a psychiatrist (or a psychologist) evaluate and render a determination concerning a person's competence to be executed?

Some psychiatrists such as Paul Appelbaum have argued that the forensic psychiatrist does not act qua physician and therefore is not bound by the traditional ethical principles of beneficence and nonmaleficence but is simply obligated to the ethical principle of truthfulness. "[T]he forensic psychiatrist in truth does not act as a physician. . . . If the essence of the physician's role is to promote healing and/or to relieve suffering, it is apparent that the forensic psychiatrist operates outside the scope of that role. . . ."[55] The argument is that a psychiatrist evaluating a defendant is not prohibited by medical ethics because that psychiatrist is not acting as a doctor. Consistent with this view, the American Academy of Psychiatry and the Law requires that "psychiatrists should indicate for whom they are conducting the examination and what they will do with the information obtained. At the beginning of a forensic evaluation, care should be taken to explicitly inform the evaluee that the psychiatrist is not the evaluee's 'doctor.' "[56]

But this position should be challenged because the forensic psychiatrist is nonetheless using the skills and knowledge of the medical profession to make the evaluation and is actually rendering a clinical judgment. She or he is thus acting like a physician. Moreover, this reasoning sets up a slippery slope that could permit physician participation in forceful interrogation, acts of torture, or any aspect of capital punishment on the grounds that the physician is not treating a patient and therefore is not "acting as a doctor."

"Under no circumstances should psychiatrists participate in legally authorized executions nor participate in assessments of competency to be executed."
—The World Psychiatric Association, in its *Declaration of Madrid* in 1996

D. A. Sargent has questioned the ethics of certifying competency for execution: "Psychiatrists should neither treat death row inmates to restore their competence nor diagnose their competence to be executed."[57]

Farber et al.[58] found that 41 percent of randomly selected practicing physicians indicated that they would perform at least one action disallowed by the American Medical Association, and 25 percent would perform five or more disallowed actions. Their perceived duty to society, approval of the death penalty, and approval of assisted suicide were highly correlated with their increased willingness to perform disallowed actions. The distressing conclusion was that so many physicians would be willing to be involved in carrying out executions despite the ethical prohibition of the medical society.

As suggested by this study, some might argue that, in the context of dual loyalty, physicians' duty to society outweighs their concerns over harming individual patients. But this approach, too, would open the door to medical personnel using their skills to assist in the interrogation of terrorist suspects or performing other roles in carrying out the judicial order of lethal injection. The American Medical Association holds that physicians may not conduct or directly participate in interrogation because doing so would undermine their role as healers and erode public trust in the medical profession.[59] This same logic would seem to argue convincingly against the ethics of assessing a condemned prisoner's mental competence to be executed.

The AMA, however, perhaps out of deference to the profession of forensic psychiatry, creates a subtle distinction and requires only that physicians should not *determine* "a prisoner's competence to be executed. A physician's medical opinion should be merely one aspect of the information taken into account by a legal decision maker such as a judge or hearing officer."[60] Moreover, among the actions that the same AMA code identifies as not constituting physician participation in an execution is "testifying as to medical diagnoses as they relate to the legal assessment of competence for execution."[61] Nonetheless, considered objectively, this action is clearly a necessary and enabling condition for the act of execution to proceed. It thus has the appearance of being and, in fact, *is* a proximate cause of death. The reasoning of the AMA—that it is the judge (not the psychiatrist) who determines competence and that this decision is based on the testimony of the psychiatrist along with other factors—is specious and does not alter this conclusion. If the combination of factors is not determinative without the psychiatrist's input, then the psychiatrist's input is clearly a necessary and enabling cause of death and therefore unethical. If, on the other hand, the psychiatrist's input were not necessary, then it should not be sought.

The NCCHC states that its "standards require that the determination of whether an inmate is 'competent for execution' should be made by an independent expert and not by any health care professional regularly in the employ of, or under contract to provide health care with, the correctional institution or system holding the inmate. This requirement does not diminish the responsibility of correctional health personnel to treat any mental illness of death row inmates."[62] Although the NCCHC explicitly prohibits the participation of correctional health care physicians, it understandably refrains from addressing the ethical obligation of physicians in general. In fact, it prefaces this statement with a note to the effect that the issue "continues to be fraught with difficulties stemming from unclear legal guidelines, lack of specific due process procedures, and issues of conflict of interest."[63]

As previously indicated, the American College of Correctional Physicians and the American Correctional Health Services Association expressly state that physicians shall not be involved in any aspect of execution of the death penalty. The United Nations General Assembly declares, "It is a contravention of medical ethics for health personnel, particularly physicians, to be involved in any professional relationship with prisoners or detainees the purpose of which is not solely to evaluate, protect or improve their physical and mental health." The U.N. General Assembly further states that "It is a contravention of medical ethics for health personnel, particularly physicians . . . to certify, or to participate in the certification of, the fitness of prisoners or detainees for any form of treatment or punishment that may adversely affect their physical or mental health. . . ."[64] In its *Declaration of Madrid* in 1996, the World Psychiatric Association held, "Under no circumstances should psychiatrists participate in legally authorized executions nor participate in assessments of competency to be executed."[65]

From the Canadian perspective, Dr. Frederic Grunberg calls it a vexing question for American psychiatry that the American Medical Association prohibits physician participation in the process of execution and yet exempts forensic psychiatrists from this principle on grounds that they are not governed by the same ethical code as treating psychiatrists. He says, "By implication, forensic psychiatrists are exempt from the obligation of beneficence and nonmaleficence. This is wrong. Even if one agrees that forensic psychiatrists need not always act in the best general interest of a patient, they must never jeopardize the health and life of the patient."[66] Grunberg then quotes Alfred Friedman and Abraham Halpern, two eminent American psychiatrists: "Many of us hold that clinical assessment of an inmate's competence to be executed is unethical because it gives the medical profession a decisive role with respect to the final legal obstacle to execution . . . [and that the very] proximity of this clinical role and the act of killing can and should be distinguished from other forensic activities."[67] This reasoning is persuasive.

Treatment to Render a Person Competent for Execution

May a psychiatrist treat a mentally ill patient who is facing execution when doing so would render the patient competent to be executed? In the light of all that has already been stated, this must be seen as an act that proximately enables the execution to go forward. As such, it is unquestionably contrary to ethical principles. The ethical psychiatrist in this case appropriately chooses to allow the patient to suffer from a treatable illness because rendering treatment would certainly lead to a greater harm—that is, the untimely death of the patient.

Treatment of medical conditions that would enable an execution to proceed is similarly prohibited. However, it is not difficult to imagine a situation in which the person facing imminent execution experiences acute appendicitis or a similar medical emergency where failure to treat will certainly entail extreme pain and suffering, extensive organ damage, and other adverse consequences, including death. But the act of treatment will inevitably be followed by capital punishment. This is by no means an easy decision, and many factors must be weighed—all of which, however, can be subsumed for the physician into a single question: what is in the best interest of the patient? If the decision to treat is made to relieve or prevent extreme pain and organ damage and this is judged to be in the best interest of the patient, then—even in view of the impending execution—it is ethical. To treat in order to enable the execution to take place would not be ethical. The treating physician has to balance the equation on the scale of what is best for the patient, above all other considerations.

Similarly, in the case of severe psychiatric illness in which pain and suffering is extreme and may include the potential for major self-injury, the psychiatrist might ethically determine that it is in the patient's best interest to treat the psychosis, even knowing that execution will follow. However, the psychiatrist would still be ethically prohibited from agreeing to state, having administered the treatment, that the patient is now fit for execution.

If the patient is capable of providing informed consent, the will of the patient must be taken into consideration.

Involvement with Acts of Torture

Little can be said to justify torture of human beings and even less can be said in support of physician participation in the process. This is a clear violation of our very humanity. Still, some people argue that torture is sometimes necessary to safeguard a nation from attack or acts of terrorism. Even under these circumstances, intentionally causing severe pain in another human being in order to extract information is diametrically opposed to the role of a healing professional and is therefore unethical.

History is replete with notable instances of ethically wrong physician involvement in prison settings. Among these, Nazi death camps represent perhaps the most well known. We are aware of more recent examples in various countries, such as in Central and South America, [68] where physicians, dentists, and psychologists participated in the torture of political prisoners or facilitated the psychiatric confinement of dissidents.[69]

Unfortunately, it is also true that some physicians in the United States have volunteered to assist in designing methods of capital punishment, to serve as witnesses to executions, to pronounce death, and, at times, to participate even more directly in causing a judicially ordered death. Moreover, disturbing allegations have arisen concerning the involvement of American physicians and psychologists in designing, monitoring, and enabling the torture—including waterboarding, stressful positions, and sleep deprivation—of alleged terrorists to elicit information during our recent history after the 9/11 attacks and the Iraq war. Regrettably, these allegations were revealed to be only too true.

In June 2016, the U.S. Central Intelligence Agency (CIA) released hundreds of declassified documents as required by law under the Freedom of Information Act. The documents showed that torture had been conducted by the CIA, principally to deter terrorist activities. Despite considerable redaction in the documents, there is clear and disturbing evidence of the significant role played by physicians and psychologists in the United States who enabled these unethical activities.[70] The following examples are just a few of the statements contained in these documents. Note the obvious role ambiguity and the almost contradictory positions being proclaimed:

The Medical Officer is expected to deliver the highest quality of care possible under the restrictive conditions usually encountered during rendition operations. The background and circumstances of the detainee do not override the obligation to maintain the highest professional and ethical standards and deliver appropriate care. Medical responsibilities include continued monitoring of the handling of the subject, and the medical officer has the authority to alter current handling if such handling may cause serious or permanent injury to the subject. . . .

A *cavity search with the intent of locating potential harmful devices must be performed during the acceptance medical evaluation.* . . . [italics in original]

At times it may be necessary to sedate a subject during the initial transfer or subsequent transport, to protect either the subject or the rendition security team. Sedatives are not to be used merely for the convenience of the security team. The decision to provide sedation is the responsibility of the Medical Officer. . . .

The Office of Medical Services is responsible for assessing and monitoring the health of all Agency detainees subject to "enhanced" interrogation techniques, and for determining that the authorized administration of these techniques would not be expected to cause serious or permanent harm. . . .

[T]echnique-specific advanced approval is required for all "enhanced" measures and is conditional on on-site medical and psychological personnel confirming from direct detainee examination that the enhanced technique(s) is not expected to produce "severe physical or mental pain or suffering."

"Psychological personnel" can be either a clinical psychologist or a psychiatrist. Unless the waterboard is being used, the medical officer can be a physician or a PA; use of the waterboard requires the presence of a physician.

Adequate medical care shall be provided to detainees, even those undergoing enhanced interrogation. . . . These medical interventions, however, should not undermine the anxiety and dislocation that the various interrogation techniques are designed to foster. . . .

Follow-up evaluations during this period may be performed in person, in the guise of a guard, or through remote video. All interventions, assessments and evaluations should be coordinated with the Chief of Site and interrogation team members to insure they are performed in such a way as to minimize undermining interrogation aims to obtain critical intelligence. . . . If during the initial phase of interrogation detainees are deprived of all measurements of time (e.g., through continuous light and variable schedules), a time-rigid administration of medication (or nutrition) should be avoided. . . .

The Office of Medical Services is responsible for assessing and monitoring the health of all Agency detainees subject to "enhanced" interrogation techniques, and for determining that the authorized administration of these techniques would not be expected to cause serious or permanent harm. . . . [71]

Even more troubling, amid these recent revelations, was that the set of guidelines issued by the Office of Medical Services outlined in detail methods to inflict pain, discomfort, anxiety, and disorientation on the detainees without causing serious physical injury or death. These guidelines describe the "correct technique" for effective application of each level of the enhanced interrogation methods. [72]

The AMA defines torture as "the deliberate, systematic, or wanton administration of cruel, inhumane, and degrading treatments or punishments during imprisonment or detainment." In its *Principles of Medical Ethics*, the association requires that physicians oppose and refuse to participate in torture for any reason. Moreover, they may not employ their services or their knowledge in any way to facilitate the practice of torture, nor may they even be present when torture is being used or threatened. [73] With respect to interrogation, AMA points out that the role of physician-interrogator undermines the physician's role as healer and erodes trust not only in the individual physician but also in the medical profession. Physicians are therefore prohibited from conducting or directly participating in an interrogation. Nor may they monitor an interrogation in order to intervene, if needed, because even this would constitute direct participation. [74] At the same time, the AMA did not intend to deprive torture victims of medical care and explicitly allows physicians to treat prisoners and detainees "if doing so is in their best interest" but cautions that this treatment may not consist of verifying that they are healthy enough for torture to be resumed. [75]

> A physician who perpetrates such crimes [acts of torture] is unfit to practice medicine.
>
> —World Medical Association

One can only react with shock and disbelief at this historical recital of horrors. Yet if we are to take effective measures to prevent ever again any recurrence of such events, we must pay close heed to what has gone before. Then we must reassess our own commitment to ethical principles.

In its *Declaration of Tokyo* in 1975, the World Medical Association specifically denounced the practice of torture and other forms of cruel, inhuman, or degrading procedures with prisoners:

1. The physician shall not countenance, condone or participate in the practice of torture or other forms of cruel, inhuman or degrading procedures. . . .

2. The physician shall not provide any premises, instruments, substances or knowledge to facilitate the practice of torture or other forms of cruel, inhuman or degrading treatment or to diminish the ability of the victim to resist such treatment. . . .

3. The physician shall not use nor allow to be used, as far as he or she can, medical knowledge or skills, or health information specific to individuals, to facilitate or otherwise aid any interrogation, legal or illegal, of those individuals.

4. The physician shall not be present during any procedure during which torture or any other forms of cruel, inhuman or degrading treatment is used or threatened.[76]

The World Medical Association reiterated its prohibition in 1997: "Physicians are bound by medical ethics to work for the good of their patients. Involvement by a physician in torture, war crimes, or crimes against humanity is contrary to medical ethics, human rights, and international law. A physician who perpetrates such crimes is unfit to practice medicine."[77]

Health professionals have an affirmative obligation to report abuses, acts of cruelty, or torture to the appropriate authorities—even if this reporting is perceived as being disloyal. There are sins of omission as well as sins of commission. One can do wrong by not doing right, if one has an affirmative duty to do the right thing. In other words, one can be complicit in wrongdoing, not only by acting, but by failing to act, and even by silence.

The NCCHC has consistently affirmed the components of a policy against torture and other cruel, inhuman, or degrading treatment of inmates. On October 14, 2007, the organization adopted a formal position statement on the "Correctional Health Care Professional's Response to Inmate Abuse." It reads, in part:

Correctional health care professionals should not condone or participate in cruel, inhumane, or degrading treatment of inmates. When such abusive treatment is either witnessed or suspected, they should identify and report such incidents to the appropriate authority.

Correctional health care professionals should refrain from participating, directly or indirectly, in efforts to certify inmates as medically or psychologically fit to be subjected to abusive treatment.

Correctional health care professionals should refrain from being present in the interrogation room, asking or suggesting questions, or advising authorities on the use of specific techniques of interrogation.

Correctional health care professionals should refrain from gathering health information for forensic purposes or sharing confidential health information or its interpretation to authorities for use in cruel, inhumane, or degrading treatment of inmates.

Correctional health care professionals should abstain from authorizing or approving any physical punishment of their patients, and should refrain from being used as an instrument of their employer to weaken the physical or mental resistance of inmates.

Correctional health care professionals should review their employer's policies and procedures, and work to ensure that they appropriately address how inmates are to be managed and what staff should do when abusive actions are suspected or witnessed.

Correctional administrators should ensure that policies and procedures address protections for employees who report the abusive actions of others.[78]

Health professionals have an affirmative obligation to report abuses, acts of cruelty, or torture to the appropriate authorities—even if this reporting is perceived as being disloyal. There are sins of omission as well as sins of commission. One can do wrong by not doing right if one has an affirmative duty to do the right thing. In other words, one can be complicit in wrongdoing, not only by acting, but by failing to act and even by silence.

Reporting Abuses by Staff

As stated previously, the vast majority of staff working in U.S. prisons, jails, and juvenile facilities adhere faithfully to the ethical tenets of their professions and do not participate in or condone abusive behavior toward inmates. Nevertheless, even though instances of abuse may be rare, we must know our ethical responsibility and take timely and appropriate action should such practices ever come to our attention.

Inmate abuse by staff can be difficult for supervisors to discover and prove. A "conspiracy of silence" often prevails, resulting in insufficient evidence to conclude an investigation in a satisfactory manner. An implied, although misdirected, the code of conduct deters employees from informing on their colleagues. In a correctional setting, this bond among peers can be extremely strong because these same coworkers must count on one another for protection in a disturbance or inmate-initiated attack.

Persuasive as these considerations may be, a higher ethical responsibility applies to situations in which the misconduct is abusive to prisoners. Any employee who is aware of such activity but fails to report its occurrence or to take appropriate action to prevent it from happening becomes a responsible party and shares in the blame for the injury or abuse inflicted.

Thus, a physician or nurse must report to the proper correctional authority any evidence that reasonably suggests that an inmate may have suffered a trauma or injury inflicted by an officer or when any abusive behavior is observed. Similarly, a worker on a mental health unit is obliged to report to proper authority any staff abuse of the rights of patients. The American Public Health Association states, "Health care staff are obliged to reveal medical evidence of staff brutality, including mental and physical abuse, to the appropriate authorities."[79] Furthermore, the NCCHC states, "Should correctional health staff witness or become aware of an inmate being subjected to harm in any of the forms described above [namely, mistreatment, abuse, torture, or sexual abuse], it is their duty to report this activity to the appropriate authorities to protect patients and other inmates."[80] When documenting injuries that could have been caused by violence or abuse, the documentation and reports should contain the inmate's account of how the injury occurred.

The health professional need not have conclusive evidence or certainty that the injury or trauma resulted from an act of abuse because it is not his or her role to render a judgment. The situation is analogous to a community physician reporting a suspicion of child abuse to protective services, even while conceding the reasonable possibility of a more benign explanation. Guidance on this matter is also supplied by the American Correctional Association's Code of Ethics: "Members shall report to appropriate authorities any corrupt or unethical behaviors in which there is sufficient evidence to justify review."[81] Examples of suspicious circumstances might be the prisoner who tells the doctor that his black eye was caused by bumping into a doorknob or who explains his bruises as caused by falling down the stairs.

Only in this way can abusive behavior patterns be stopped. Supervisors have an obligation to protect the informant from retaliatory action, and each facility should have a policy that ensures protection for employees who report the abusive actions of others. By the same token, false reporting or frivolous accusations should not be condoned. The responsibility to report abusive behavior of other employees should be taught in new employee school and regularly encouraged by supervisors. Every facility should make it clear that this is a zero-tolerance policy for abusive behavior.

Although reporting on colleagues may be difficult or repugnant for some—either out of a sense of loyalty to one's buddies or a fear of reprisal—this must be countered by a strong sense of duty and responsibility. Officers and health care staff are in positions of trust and have an obligation to protect their charges from harm, whether intentional or negligent. Therefore, true loyalty to all of their brethren and to their professional association requires taking this action.

Competing loyalties can create a conflict between health professionals' commitment to their patients' welfare and their institutional roles and responsibilities. It is not acceptable, however, for a health professional who observes abusive behavior toward a prisoner to remain silent. The basis of this obligation is the principle that medical professionals will "do no harm to the patient" (nonmaleficence), will remain autonomous from nonmedical authorities in making clinical judgments about their patients, and will honor their patient's trust. These are fundamental principles in the practice of medicine. This topic is also addressed in Chapter 9, "Corrections and Health Care Working Together," under "Speaking Out Loyally."

Because violence and assaultive behavior are harmful to health, their prevention clearly falls within the purview of correctional health care professionals who have an ethical duty to be supportive of the safe and secure management of prisons and jails.

A NOTE OF CAUTION—EROSION AND BURNOUT

Despite initial strong commitment to ethical principles, many health professionals begin to experience a blunting of these ideals after spending some time in corrections. The erosion is a gradual process and often appears proportional to the degree of direct contact with inmates. The erosion also will be greater the more the professional works in isolation from supportive peers.

Sometimes, the first signs are a growing tendency or willingness to deal punitively with patients such as putting "no shows" at the bottom of the list for rescheduled appointments, if at all, or identifying "malingerers" (those who report to sick call without legitimate medical problems) to correctional staff for punishment. Other signs may be the feeling that the inmates already are getting more than they are entitled to, given the nature of their crimes, or the belief or comment that "maybe going through withdrawal will teach him a lesson." Singling out perpetrators of socially disapproved behaviors as being less deserving of treatment reflects social prejudices rather than good logic.[82] Sometimes, too, correctional health care staff become callous and unresponsive to prisoners' complaints of chronic pain. Other evidence of the erosion may be reflected in the tone of voice adopted by nurses or doctors when addressing inmates. It is not customary in doctors' offices, outside of correctional institutions, for a nurse or receptionist to open the door to the waiting room and shout the patient's surname to summon him or her into the examination room. Insistence on habits of courtesy and respect, just as in community practice, serves as a reminder to staff and also will earn the reciprocal respect of inmates.

Dr. Robert Cohen, an experienced correctional physician, has observed this phenomenon and offers the following insight:

Prisons are places of violence, and they inure physicians and other health workers to the severe injuries caused by violence, sometimes involving them as participants. Prisoners are seen as less than persons, and their welfare becomes secondary to the welfare of the correctional institution.

There are many physicians whose daily practice contradicts this formulation. They deserve praise and tribute. Compassion is not easily taught but is effectively ground down by the daily experience of working in prison. Disrespect for prisoners is easily learned. The doctor/patient relationship is often fatally compromised by the transformation of the patient into a prisoner, with a consequent loss of sympathy and standing. It will not be possible to effectively apply the methods of quality assurance to correctional medicine unless health professionals working in prison identify the goal of quality solely as patient welfare. Health professionals must identify with the welfare of their patients, not with the needs of the prison.[83]

Contact with fellow health professionals, regular attendance at professional conferences, and periodic discussion of ethical considerations among health care staff are therefore to be encouraged. Coworkers also can be a strong source of support and encouragement in maintaining and sharpening the awareness of medicine's lofty principles.

As detailed in Chapter 7, "A Patient or a Prisoner?," terminology is important. If correctional health professionals persist in calling their patients *inmates, prisoners,* or *offenders,* they will soon conceptualize them as such and begin to treat them differently. How contrary to their training and professional preparation, when they were taught how to care for *patients!* Although this distinction in terminology may appear to be trivial, it is a combination of many small things that makes us what we are and influences what we do. And for those who work in the correctional environment with its strong focus on punishment and restriction of freedom, one can too easily learn to disrespect one's own patients. There are sound ethical and practical reasons to insist that health care professionals refer to their patients (clients) as such. This applies to references made in speech, in written reports, and in medical records.

What we have been exploring in this section—namely, the gradual erosion of professional ethical values among correctional health care staff—cannot be properly understood without also recognizing the broader phenomenon of employee burnout, which is so common among healing professionals in general and among correctional custody staff and law enforcement personnel. It should thus not be regarded solely or even primarily as a consequence of disparity between the medical world and the world of corrections, although these factors certainly come into play and cannot be overlooked.

By the same token, the solution or treatment must address more than bolstering one's moral compass and needs to look also to balancing one's lifestyle, dealing appropriately with stress, securing adequate rest and relaxation, and, in some instances, availing oneself of counseling or psychotherapy. Interested readers are encouraged to explore recent research and writings that discuss burnout among health professionals and correctional staff.

Burnout syndrome is a special type of job stress and consists in a state of mental, emotional, or physical exhaustion that may be combined with doubts about one's own competence and even the value of the work being performed. People in such situations can become cynical and overly critical and behave irritably and impatiently with coworkers and patients (or clients). Sometimes this is partly the result of poor job fit, but many other factors can be involved.

"It [burnout] can destroy some of the most highly motivated, selfless people in the helping professions," according to a literature review on the subject of burnout.[84] Common symptoms, according to García-Arroya and Domínguez-López, include "detachment from work, depersonalization, insensitivity to the people being helped, lack of empathy, etc."[85]

Lorry Schoenly summarizes the situation for nurses, and the picture she describes can be applied with few alterations to physicians, psychologists, dentists, and other health care staff in corrections. "Moral distress in nursing is described as a psychological imbalance or disequilibrium that occurs when nurses find themselves in situations where they feel unable to do the right thing. This conflict can cause physical, emotional, and spiritual suffering. The residual build up of continuing moral distress can lead to burnout and burden."

Schoenly continues:

Correctional nurses have unique situations that lead to moral distress. Examples include conflict with custody over inmate access to care, a higher volume of healthcare needs than resources available to meet them, and continuing need for guarded evaluation of potential manipulative patient behaviors. Other potential sources of moral distress include nurse-physician conflict, disrespectful interactions, workplace violence, and clinical ethical dilemmas.[86]

According to Bonnie Sultan, a social worker and criminologist, "Correctional environments take their toll on all who pass through the gates," referring explicitly to the staff who work there and not just to the inmates who are required to live there.

There is something superhuman in law enforcement and first response work. When the urge to run away is overtaken by the urge to run towards, these people become something more than even they once thought they could be. With this ability comes great responsibilities and stresses. We ask a lot of our law enforcement officers. We ask for superhero strength and superhuman heart. The balance is a difficult one. It causes much strife in personal and professional lives. How does one take off the cape and, once again, become human?[87]

For correctional health providers, burnout can be occasioned or potentiated by overwork, staffing or resource shortages, obvious inmate patient need, and limited coping resources. In some cases, it can be linked to compassion fatigue.

Compassion fatigue is a form of secondary traumatic stress that "refers to the emotional distress and PTSD-like symptoms that result when professional helpers hear about the firsthand traumatic experiences of persons whom they are helping. . . . [It] mimics the symptoms of PTSD, but to a lesser extent and without meeting all criteria for the disorder."[88]

A well-researched paper by Spinaris, Denhof, and Morton develops the definition of "correctional fatigue" as a further specification of compassion fatigue, "to better capture the nature and impact of traumatic exposure on correctional professionals (whether indirect or direct) and its interactions with organizational and operational stressors." The authors state that correctional fatigue is "fueled by repeated exposure to traumatic and other high-stress events, potentially manifesting in a negatively altered outlook on self and others, functional impairments, and, in more severe cases, in the development of psychiatric disorders." They term it "an unavoidable occupational hazard. No one who works in corrections is completely immune to it." They also point out how the organizational culture of correctional agencies can be affected over time by the attitudes and behaviors characteristic of trauma-affected correctional staff, including cynicism, pessimism, disrespectful behaviors, a negative mood, emotional callousness, indifference, mistrust, a susceptibility to conspiracy theories, disproportionate or extreme vigilance, hostility, and aggression. "The 'normalized' behaviors can drastically affect staff wellness and functioning, and counter what new employees are taught at the training academy."[89]

Correctional health professionals should take great comfort and encouragement in the realization that their efforts to serve the incarcerated are worthwhile and noble, representing the highest and best ideals of their chosen profession. Difficult though it may seem at times, they can take satisfaction in the knowledge that they have contributed to humanizing and elevating the lives of persons who are otherwise consigned to a life of humiliation, deprivation, confinement, and often despair. Moreover, in the day-to-day interactions with their correctional counterparts, many health professionals demonstrate an understanding of the stresses and situations with which the officers are coping each day, offering support and help through word and example.

CONCLUSION

Finally, a word to those well qualified and highly ethical health care professionals who begin a career in the world of corrections but quickly become disillusioned and frustrated at the gap between what they see and what they know should be. They fear that they may compromise their own ethical principles if they remain. They feel the pressures of role conflict. They dislike the conditions of confinement in which they find their patients. They feel their evaluations and patient interviews are being rushed. They want to see their patients more frequently, but their caseloads are too great. They are not allowed to make the changes they feel important. They are faulted by supervisors for being too caring. They feel powerless to influence the tone and direction of the correctional system in which they work. Ultimately, they ponder the question, "Should I quit my job?"

To people like these, this author has said, "Don't give up. If good and caring health professionals leave, who will be left? It will be only those who do not care as much as you do. While correctional health care in many places is less than ideal, imagine that it could get much worse. The only hope of improving conditions and eventually making the authorities aware of needed changes is to get enough good people working in the field. By staying there, at least you have a chance to make things better—to provide relief where you can, and to serve as a patient advocate."

These ideas and admonitions are eloquently expressed by correctional psychologist Joel A. Dvoskin:

Some ethicists argue that participating in unacceptable systems is wrong. They argue that the participation of credentialed professionals legitimizes and thus perpetuates these systems. They admonish such professionals to simply walk away. . . . And these arguments seem reasonable. But when I meet the people who have stayed, I do not find them less ethical or less moral for it. . . . To maintain one's standards of decency and professionalism in the face of an apparently uncaring political system takes courage and tenacity and goodness of heart. . . . Watch what happens when a psychologist quits in moral indignation. See if the place closes down. It won't, and no matter how good the quitter feels about having quit, if he or she were any good, it is the clients who have been hurt, not the system. . . . Your jail or prison or hospital or free clinic is a little better each day because you are there. You leave each of your clients a little better than you find them, and occasionally foster hope in people for whom hope is but a distant memory.[90]

Should you find that you are required to compromise your principles and to act in an unethical manner, then it may be time to leave. Do not just walk out, however. In a polite and respectful manner, let the person in charge know how you feel and why you are obliged to leave, so as not to violate the principles of your profession. Or respectfully but firmly refuse to comply when directed to administer a sedative for behavior control, reveal confidential information, witness the use of force, or perform duties that fall outside the scope of your license. If you take this route, seek support and assistance from your professional association. You may be inviting dismissal, but at least you can appeal that action up to the highest levels and perhaps your point of view will prevail.

Chapter 3

Other Challenging Topics in Ethics

ETHICAL REASONING

This chapter continues the presentation of ethical issues in correctional health care by discussing several largely unrelated topics that can pose special and challenging ethical conflicts for correctional health professionals. These are:

- biomedical research and experimentation involving prisoners as human subjects,
- housing mentally ill prisoners in conditions of extreme isolation and segregation,
- chemical castration as an alternative to prison, and
- a compelling ethical challenge to initiate preventive measures.

Other topics could logically be included here because of their signal importance, complexity, or controversial nature, including issues of physician participation in executions, the use of torture, and the use of mace, but these are addressed in other chapters.

The ethical reasoning surrounding these topics can involve complex and difficult issues, so there are controversial aspects to each. Strong feelings may exist on both sides. As the standards of human decency continue to evolve, these issues should be carefully reexamined. This chapter discusses a few such concerns and proposes pathways toward their resolution. Ethicists, practitioner associations, criminal justice experts, and relevant others are encouraged to explore these ethical challenges with candor and honesty so as to reach, if possible, a new consensus or at least a reasonable degree of clarification.

Opponents to biomedical research on prisoners argue for a ban on all experimental studies involving prisoners as human subjects. Their reasons are persuasive and cogent in view of a horrendous history of abuse. Others argue, however, that humanity, including incarcerated persons, could benefit by well-designed research involving prisoners. Can reasonable safeguards be devised to facilitate such beneficial research in a completely humane and ethical manner?

Housing prisoners for prolonged periods under conditions of extreme segregation and isolation has been championed or defended by numerous correctional experts, as evidenced by the construction of supermaximum (or supermax) facilities and security housing units (SHUs) across the country. The declared need for these high-security settings is to prevent violent attacks on staff and other inmates while safely confining these dangerous prisoners away from the public—a concern highlighted by the reality of gangs and terrorist organizations. On the other hand, it is well known that prolonged isolation tends to induce and exacerbate mental illness. Can the legitimate interests of the criminal justice system be accommodated while safeguarding inmates from serious and unconstitutional risks to their health? Can the needs of corrections be satisfied without housing mentally ill prisoners in these settings?

Depo-Provera or similar medications to bring about chemical castration is a treatment sometimes ordered by trial courts for sex offenders as an alternative to incarceration. The American Medical Association (AMA) has made strong statements about unethical aspects of physician participation in this practice, while at the same time creating finely nuanced distinctions to overcome objections to the element of coercion. Autonomy is highly regarded as a basic human right by all medical professionals. Is the consent of a person voluntary when he is under judicial order to submit to chemical castration or other treatment in lieu of prison time? Does cooperation in this treatment square with the ethical obligation of health professionals to treat involuntarily only in cases where an incompetent person is at imminent risk of causing serious harm to self or others and there is no less intrusive alternative available? Does it avoid the ethical fault of maleficence?

The final topic to be discussed in this chapter does not present an ethical concern to correctional health professionals precisely in terms of performing their daily routines, but it does encourage them to become eloquent advocates for change in view of their heightened awareness of a tragic reality.

As will be stressed in the following discussions concerning these topic areas, our application of ethical principles should be consistent and clear, and we should take care to identify and question any fuzzy reasoning or self-serving faux defenses by interested groups.

BIOMEDICAL RESEARCH AND EXPERIMENTATION

Working in the Context of a Blemished History

Not far back in U.S. history, numerous shameful and unethical experiments were conducted on unknowing prisoners to test treatments for malaria, learn more about the effects of radiation, advance the science of dermatology, explore the effects of deprivation of ascorbic acid, and pursue other types of medical and biological research. In many cases, the prisoners were intentionally misinformed about the

nature and risks of the experiments, were offered inappropriate or excessive inducements to participate, were not properly treated or compensated for injuries sustained,
and were not provided reasonable pain relief. At Holmesburg Prison in Philadelphia, for instance, subjects were able to earn up to $1,500 a month, roughly 40 times
as much as inmate workers were being paid there.[1]

> It is simply unethical for doctors, when acting qua doctors and using the knowledge
> and skills of their profession, to harm or injure others intentionally.

The following are just a few instances of biomedical research on prisoners that
took place in the United States, roughly during the third quarter of the 20th
century:

- *Malaria*—In 1973, the author toured the basement of the infirmary at the Illinois State
  Penitentiary at Joliet-Stateville and was shown numerous screened cages containing
  malaria-infected mosquitoes. These were being used to infect prisoner volunteers who
  then became subjects for testing of various treatments to prevent or cure malaria. The
  prison medical director explained that this research had begun in 1944 during World War
  II and proved helpful to the U.S. military when conducting operations in malaria-infested
  regions of the world.[2]
- *Radiation*—At state penitentiaries in Oregon and Washington between 1961 and 1973,
  inmates' testicles were biopsied and heavily x-rayed by Doctors Carl G. Heller and C.
  Alvin Paulsen to determine the impact of repeated doses of radiation on the male reproduc-
  tive system.[3]
  - In another example, blood samples were taken from 10 Utah State Prison inmates in
    1961 and 1962, mixed with radioactive chemicals, and then injected back into their
    bodies.[4]
- *Dermatology*—Between 1951 and 1974, inmates at Holmesburg Prison were exposed to
  toxic chemicals such as dioxin, hallucinogens, radioactive drugs, and skin-blistering
  agents by dermatologist Dr. Albert M. Kligman and others. Dioxin was the main poison-
  ous ingredient in Agent Orange, a powerful defoliant used in the Vietnam War.[5] Studies
  funded by Dow Chemical Company in the 1960s and performed by Kligman on prisoners at Holmesburg Prison sought to determine the threshold of toxic effects in humans
  from dioxins and resulted in cancers in some of the human subjects.
  - Although nearly 300 inmates sued the University of Pennsylvania, Dr. Kligman, Dow
    Chemical, and Johnson & Johnson in 2000, the suit was dismissed because the statute
    of limitations had expired.[6]
- *Ascorbic Acid*—The paper by Dr. Robert E. Hodges et al. reports on their research to
  define the metabolism of vitamin C (ascorbic acid) in the face of severe dietary deficiency.
  Five prisoners at the Iowa State Penitentiary were placed in a cold-climate room for four
  hours a day and were fed a liquid formula free of ascorbic acid through a stomach tube.
  After about three months, the prisoners developed severe scurvy, resulting in extremely
  painful bone and tissue loss and irreversible damage.[7]

• *Other Experiments*—Among other experiments, some of the most well known were those conducted by Dr. Leo Stanley, chief surgeon at the San Quentin Penitentiary in California from 1913 to 1951. Stanley performed experiments on hundreds of prisoners—many of them testicular transplants from other men or from animals.[8]

To be fair, not all of these physicians were depraved and evil people who took pleasure from the torture, maiming, and suffering of other human beings. Some, at least, performed a balancing calculus and concluded that the "greater good" they might achieve for all humankind outweighed the harm done to a few individuals. Furthermore, a good many of these physicians did not hold themselves out as caregivers of the prisoners, thus possibly avoiding a direct role conflict. Yet there remains a tragic and troubling ethical dissonance because none of these behaviors can be squared with the essential caring function of the healing profession. It is simply unethical for doctors, when acting qua doctor and using the knowledge and skills of their profession, to harm or injure others intentionally.

As these unfortunate examples demonstrate, potential conflicts of interest can arise when a physician becomes involved as an agent of the state in the correctional setting. In such circumstances, the penological interest standard and the medical interest standard often collide. A psychiatrist who refuses the order of a warden to subdue an unruly prisoner with medication, or who refuses to share with the warden the confidences of a patient, will likely not retain his or her job. How does the doctor act who knows financial loss may follow adherence to ethical principles? Is that decision influenced at all by the fact that the injured party is "only a prisoner" and not a patient in the free world?[9]

First Steps toward Regulation of Biomedical Research in U.S. Prisons

In 1994, President William Clinton commissioned the Advisory Committee on Human Radiation Experiments (ACHRE) to investigate and report on the use of human beings as subjects of federally funded research using ionizing radiation. The extensive report documents the history of such experiments from the 1940s to the 1970s and provides a detailed and candid acknowledgement of these events and what led to them. This welcome transparency lifted the veil of stealth and secrecy that had shrouded these experiments and affords us a better understanding of what happened so we can take responsible steps to ensure such mistakes do not recur. In reviewing the history of this research, the ACHRE says that some:

. . . doctors viewed prisoners as ideal subjects. They were healthy, adult males who were not going anywhere soon. In 1963 few if any researchers had moral qualms about using them as subjects, although there seems to have been a consensus in the research community on the rules that should govern such experimentation. By 1973, however, some ethicists, researchers, and others, such as the investigative journalist Jessica Mitford, pointed out that incarcerated people were not well placed to make voluntary decisions. In 1976, the National Commission for the Protection of Human Subjects of Biomedical and Behavioral Research recommended the banning of almost all research on prisoners. Prison experimentation effectively came to an end in this country a few years after the commission offered its recommendations.[10]

These past errors and abuses should not have happened, and strenuous safeguards must be implemented to ensure they never happen again. Blind trust in the benevolence and ethics of medical professionals, government agents, and the academic world is clearly not sufficient, especially given the sad lesson of history and the lucrative incentives available from pharmaceutical and other corporate interests as well as from government. Several different approaches have been taken with respect to biomedical research on prisoner subjects. Despite their complexity, the history of our nation's response to these abuses merits discussion here.

The National Commission for Protection of Human Subjects of Biomedical and Behavioral Research was formed in 1974 and published its *Belmont Report* in April 1979, spelling out the basic ethical principles that should underlie the conduct of biomedical and behavioral research involving human subjects. The *Belmont Report* formulated the following thoughtful principles for the use of any human subjects in the conduct of biomedical research:

- *Respect for the Person*: "[I]ndividuals should be treated as autonomous agents" and "persons with diminished autonomy are entitled to protection." (This is a recognition that, "under prison conditions, [persons] may be subtly coerced or unduly influenced to engage in research activities for which they would not otherwise volunteer.")
- *Beneficence*: Researchers are obliged to "(1) do no harm and (2) maximize possible benefits and minimize possible harms" to the research subject. It is essential "to decide when it is justifiable to seek certain benefits despite the risks involved, and when the benefits should be foregone because of the risks."
- *Justice*: "An injustice occurs when some benefit to which a person is entitled is denied without good reason or when some burden is imposed unduly." The research provider must be nonexploitative, and the costs and benefits should be administered fairly and equally to potential research participants. In publicly funded research, "justice demands both that these not provide advantages only to those who can afford them and that such research should not unduly involve persons from groups unlikely to be among the beneficiaries of subsequent applications of the research."[11]

In providing this moral framework for decision makers, the *Belmont Report* does not specify how these three principles should be weighted or prioritized, leaving this determination to the Institutional Review Board (IRB) in each case.

An earlier report of the same commission dealt explicitly with prisoners. Its results were published by the U.S. Department of Health, Education, and Welfare (DHEW) in 1976 and recommended against the use of prisoners in research on human subjects except under the strictest of conditions. These conditions include:

[A]dequate living conditions, separation of research participation from any appearance of parole consideration, effective grievance procedures and public scrutiny at the prison where research will be conducted or from which prospective subjects will be taken; importance of the research; compelling reasons to involve prisoners; and fairness of such involvement. Compliance with these requirements must be certified by the highest responsible federal official, assisted by a national ethical review body."[12]

The National Commission for the Protection of Human Subjects expressed two chief ethical concerns in its 1976 *Report and Recommendations*:

(1) whether prisoners bear a fair share of the burdens and receive a fair share of the benefits of research; and (2) whether prisoners are, in the words of the Nuremberg Code, "so situated as to be able to exercise free power of choice"—that is, whether prisoners can give truly voluntary consent to participate in research. . . . These two dilemmas relate to two basic ethical principles: the principle of *justice*, which requires that persons and groups be treated fairly, and the principle of *respect for persons*, which requires that the autonomy of persons be promoted and protected.[13]

The Nuremberg Code of 1947 cited by the commission was developed for use in the postwar military tribunals following World War II to establish a standard against which the conduct of Nazi officials, including physicians and scientists, could be measured. Its message remains vitally relevant today and is included here.

The Nuremberg Code

1. The voluntary consent of the human subject is absolutely essential. This means that the person involved should have legal capacity to give consent; should be so situated as to be able to exercise the power of choice, without the intervention of any element of force, fraud, deceit, duress, over-reaching, or other ulterior form of constraint or coercion; and should have sufficient knowledge and comprehension of the elements of the subject matter involved, as to enable him to make an understanding and enlightened decision. This latter element requires that, before the acceptance of an affirmative decision by the experimental subject, there should be made known to him the nature, duration, and purpose of the experiment; the method and means by which it is to be conducted; all inconveniences and hazards reasonably to be expected; and the effects upon his health or person, which may possibly come from his participation in the experiment. . . .

2. The experiment should be such as to yield fruitful results for the good of society, unprocurable by other methods or means of study, and not random and unnecessary in nature.

3. The experiment should be so designed and based on the results of animal experimentation and a knowledge of the natural history of the disease or other problem under study, that the anticipated results will justify the performance of the experiment.

4. The experiment should be so conducted as to avoid all unnecessary physical and mental suffering and injury.

5. No experiment should be conducted, where there is an a priori reason to believe that death or disabling injury will occur; except, perhaps, in those experiments where the experimental physicians also serve as subjects.

6. The degree of risk to be taken should never exceed that determined by the humanitarian importance of the problem to be solved by the experiment.

7. Proper preparations should be made and adequate facilities provided to protect the experimental subject against even remote possibilities of injury, disability, or death.

8. The experiment should be conducted only by scientifically qualified persons. The highest degree of skill and care should be required through all stages of the experiment of those who conduct or engage in the experiment.

9. During the course of the experiment, the human subject should be at liberty to bring the experiment to an end, if he has reached the physical or mental state, where continuation of the experiment seemed to him to be impossible.

10. During the course of the experiment, the scientist in charge must be prepared to terminate the experiment at any stage, if he has probable cause to believe . . . that a continuation of the experiment is likely to result in injury, disability, or death to the experimental subject.[14]

Even though many prisoners interviewed by the National Commission for the Protection of Human Subjects reported that they had willingly—even eagerly— volunteered to be research subjects and had not been coerced, the commission in 1976 expressed its concerns that this may yet not constitute true informed consent:

When persons seem regularly to engage in activities which, were they stronger or in better circumstances, they would avoid, [the ethical principle of] respect dictates that they be protected against those forces that appear to compel their choices. . . . [Further,] the conditions of social and economic deprivation in which they live compromise their freedom. The Commission believes, therefore, that the appropriate expression of respect consists in protection from exploitation.[15]

In November 1978, the Department of Health and Human Services (DHHS) approved strict regulations limiting prisoner experimentation to four narrow categories of nonintrusive, low-risk, and individually beneficial research but failed to call a complete halt to the use of prisoners in nontherapeutic experimentation.[16] These important categories of restrictions are summarized in the *IRB Guidebook* as follows.

Only certain kinds of research conducted or supported by DHHS may involve prisoners as subjects: (1) studies (involving no more than minimal risk or inconvenience) of the possible causes, effects, and processes of incarceration and criminal behavior; (2) studies (involving no more than minimal risk or inconvenience) of prisons as institutional structures or of prisoners as incarcerated persons; (3) research on particular conditions [for example, vaccine trials and other research on social and psychological problems such as alcoholism, drug addiction, and sexual assaults] affecting prisoners as a class (providing the Secretary, HHS, has consulted with appropriate experts and published [his or her] intent to support such research in the *Federal Register*); and (4) research involving a therapy likely to benefit the prisoner subject (and if the therapeutic research also involves nontherapeutic research with a control group, the Secretary, HHS, must also consult with appropriate experts and publish [his or her] intent to support the research in the *Federal Register*).[17]

Last updated in 1993, portions of these regulations are now obsolete. The four permitted categories of research, however, have been adopted verbatim and without change in the Human Research Protection Program's "Standard Operating Procedure/Policy Approval & Implementation."[18]

During the Carter administration (1977–1981), DHEW Secretary Joseph Califano was charged with enacting and implementing new regulations and even considered a prison accreditation scheme to ensure the possibility of voluntary consent. Much of this complex history is summarized in the ACHRE report. Following the settlement of a lawsuit[19] brought by inmates at the State Prison of Southern Michigan in Jackson, Michigan in 1980 (*Henry Fante v. Department of Health and Human Services*), federal regulations concerning research on prisoners were based on Office of Human Research Protections law rather than on U.S. Food and Drug Administration (FDA) law and therefore apply only to federally funded, conducted, or supported research.[20]

"When persons seem regularly to engage in activities which, were they stronger or in better circumstances, they would avoid, [the ethical principle of] respect dictates that they be protected against those forces that appear to compel their choices. . . . [Further,] the conditions of social and economic deprivation in which they live compromise their freedom."
—National Commission for the Protection of Human Subjects

Nevertheless, by the 1980s drug companies had discovered that students, poor people, and third world populations were viable alternative groups from which to draw participants for nontherapeutic experiments if the cash rewards were sufficient. Considerations of expediency, rather than of ethics or law, largely led drug companies to abandon virtually all nontherapeutic biomedical prisoner research.[21] In addition to using students and poor people, pharmaceutical companies also transferred much of their biomedical research effort to developing countries that lack regulatory protections.

As reported by President Clinton's Advisory Committee on Human Radiation Experiments in 1995:

Joseph Califano . . . spent nearly a year formulating his response regarding the use of prisoners in medical research. Califano explored the possibility of an accreditation scheme as suggested by the [National Commission for the Protection of Human Subjects of Biomedical and Behavioral Research]. However, in a letter to the commission, Califano reported that the American Correctional Association [ACA], "the one currently qualified [prison] accrediting organization," had no interest in "accrediting correctional institutions as performance sites for medical research." "On the contrary," Califano went on to explain, the ACA had recently decided it "would not fully accredit any institution which permitted research on prisoners." After his interchange with the ACA, Califano ultimately decided to issue regulations that, for almost all intents and purposes, brought an end to federally funded nontherapeutic medical research in American prisons.[22]

Secretary Califano then directed the FDA to issue similar rules governing the use of prisoners in research. These were published in the spring of 1980. However, before they were scheduled to take effect,

a group of prisoners at the State Prison of Southern Michigan filed suit against the federal government. These inmates claimed that the impending FDA regulations threatened to violate their "right" to choose participation in medical research. The case was settled out of court when FDA attorneys decided to reclassify the agency's prison drug-testing regulations as "indefinitely" stayed. The FDA's regulations still exist in this bureaucratic limbo.[23]

Note that subpart A (the portion of 45 CFR §46 known as the "Common Rule" because it is more widely applicable than subpart C, which applies to prisoners) includes language granting exemptions from full IRB committee review for categories thought to present little or no risk to subjects. These exemptions, however, are not available to research involving prisoners as human subjects. Examples of these exemptions are research in educational settings involving normal educational practices such as instructional effectiveness and research involving the collection of existing pathological specimens where an investigator removes all identifying information from the specimens so that subjects cannot be identified. Even research of this type involving prisoners is subject to full review by the IRB when conducted by studies funded or sponsored by the DHHS.

Much of subpart C follows the recommendations made by the National Commission for the Protection of Human Subjects of Biomedical and Behavioral Research in its 1976 report entitled *Research Involving Prisoners*.

As indicated, the protective language of 45 CFR §46 subpart C applies to research involving prisoner subjects only when that research is "conducted or supported by DHHS." This has resulted in a situation lamented by Lawrence O. Gostin, chair of the prestigious Institute of Medicine (IOM) Committee for Research Involving Prisoners:

The most glaring problem is that the federal rules cover only a small fraction of the research being undertaken in prisons. . . . There appears to be no morally defensible reason for excluding a large number of prisoners from human subject protection, as is currently the case.[24]

The *IRB Guidebook* issued by the Office of Human Research Protections offers this advice:

Prisoners should neither bear an unfair share of the burden of participating in research, nor should they be excluded from its benefits, to the extent that voluntary participation is possible. . . . To the extent that prisoner-subjects are found able to voluntarily consent to participation, and to the extent allowable under applicable regulations, prisoners should be allowed the opportunity to participate in potentially beneficial research.[25]

The ACA standards explicitly prohibit "the use of offenders for medical, pharmaceutical, or cosmetic experiments."[26] The accompanying commentary explains that "experimental programs include aversive conditioning, psychosurgery, and the application of cosmetic substances being tested prior to sale to the general public." The standard itself goes on to allow "offender participation in clinical trials that are approved by an institutional review board based on [his or her] need for a specific medical intervention," and it adds that institutions electing to perform research must be in compliance with all state and federal guidelines. Moreover, the ACA public correctional policy prohibits "the use of offenders as experimental subjects in medical, psychological, pharmacological and cosmetic research except when warranted and prescribed for the diagnosis or treatment of an individual's specific condition in accordance with current standards of health care."[27]

The standards of the National Commission on Correctional Health Care (NCCHC) do not prohibit research but affirmatively require that "biomedical, behavioral, or other research using inmates as subjects is consistent with established ethical, medical, legal, and regulatory standards for human research."[28] Although not explicit in the language of this standard, it seems appropriate to apply the guidelines of 45 CFR §46 to any research conducted on prisoners and not solely to research sponsored or funded by DHHS.

The compliance indicators of NCCHC (2014) Standard P-I-06 require a written policy and defined procedures that specify the process for obtaining approval to conduct research and the steps to be taken to preserve the subject's rights. The discussion on this standard states that it intends to support legitimate research initiatives and that:

[the] Code of Federal Regulations (45 CFR §46, revised) has established provisions that protect inmates involved in research activities. These regulations allow, under proper conditions and with appropriate external reviews and approvals, for the participation of inmates in studies of the possible causes, effects, and processes of incarceration; studies on conditions particularly affecting inmates as a group; and research on practices, both innovative and established, that are intended and reasonably likely to improve the health and well-being of the subject.[29]

Another relevant pronouncement is the World Medical Association's *Declaration of Helsinki*, whose language includes the following:

5. Medical progress is based on research that ultimately must include studies involving human subjects. . . .

7. Medical research is subject to ethical standards that promote and ensure respect for all human subjects and protect their health and rights.

8. While the primary purpose of medical research is to generate new knowledge, this goal can never take precedence over the rights and interests of individual research subjects.

9. It is the duty of physicians who are involved in medical research to protect the life, health, dignity, integrity, right to self-determination, privacy, and confidentiality of personal information of research subjects. . . .

15. Appropriate compensation and treatment for subjects who are harmed as a result of participating in research must be ensured.

16. In medical practice and in medical research, most interventions involve risks and burdens. Medical research involving human subjects may only be conducted if the importance of the objective outweighs the risks and burdens to the research subjects.

17. All medical research involving human subjects must be preceded by careful assessment of predictable risks and burdens to the individuals and groups involved in the research in comparison with foreseeable benefits to them and to other individuals or groups affected by the condition under investigation. Measures to minimise the risks must be implemented. The risks must be continuously monitored, assessed and documented by the researcher.

18. Physicians may not be involved in a research study involving human subjects unless they are confident that the risks have been adequately assessed and can be satisfactorily managed. When the risks are found to outweigh the potential benefits or when there is conclusive proof of definitive outcomes, physicians must assess whether to continue, modify or immediately stop the study.

19. Some groups and individuals are particularly vulnerable and may have an increased likelihood of being wronged or of incurring additional harm. All vulnerable groups and individuals should receive specifically considered protection.

20. Medical research with a vulnerable group is only justified if the research is responsive to the health needs or priorities of this group and the research cannot be carried out in a non-vulnerable group. In addition, this group should stand to benefit from the knowledge, practices or interventions that result from the research. . . .

26. In medical research involving human subjects capable of giving informed consent, each potential subject must be adequately informed of the aims, methods, sources of funding, any possible conflicts of interest, institutional affiliations of the researcher, the anticipated benefits and potential risks of the study and the discomfort it may entail, post-study provisions and any other relevant aspects of the study. The potential subject must be informed of the right to refuse to participate in the study or to withdraw consent to participate at any time without reprisal. . . .

35. Every research study involving human subjects must be registered in a publicly accessible database before recruitment of the first subject.[30]

In 1982 the World Health Organization and the Council of International Organization of Medical Societies promulgated the *International Ethical Guidelines for Biomedical Research Involving Human Subjects*. Its statements include the following:

Guideline 9—When there is ethical and scientific justification to conduct research with individuals incapable of giving informed consent [". . . because, as in the case of prisoners, their autonomy is limited, or because they have limited cognitive capacity"—from the commentary to Guideline 9], the risk from research interventions that do not hold out the prospect of direct benefit for the individual subject should be no more likely and not greater than the risk attached to routine medical or psychological examination of such persons. Slight or minor increases above such risk may be permitted when there is an overriding scientific or medical rationale for such increases and when an ethical review committee has approved them.

Guideline 19—Investigators should ensure that research subjects who suffer injury as a result of their participation are entitled to free medical treatment for such injury and to such financial or other assistance as would compensate them equitably for any resultant impairment, disability or handicap. In the case of death as a result of their participation, their dependents are entitled to compensation.

Subjects must not be asked to waive the right to compensation.[31]

The International Covenant on Civil and Political Rights, adopted by the United Nations in 1966, states in Article 7: "No one shall be subjected to torture or to cruel, inhuman or degrading treatment or punishment. In particular, no one shall be subjected without his free consent to medical or scientific experimentation."[32]

Institute of Medicine Recommendations and Some Critical Responses

At the behest of the Office of Human Research Protections (OHRP) of the U.S. Department of Health and Human Services, the IOM issued a 2006 report outlining an updated ethical framework for conducting research in jails and prisons, including expanded oversight of prison experimentation. Its recommendations are summarized as follows:

The Committee boldly recommends five paradigmatic changes in the system of ethical protections for research involving prisoners. First, expand the definition of the term *prisoner* to include a much larger population of persons whose liberty is restricted by virtue of sentence, probation, parole, or community placement. Second, ensure universal, consistent standards of protection so that safeguards based on sound ethical values apply to prisoner research irrespective of the source of funding. Third, shift from a category-based to a risk–benefit approach to defining ethically acceptable research so that prisoners are never exposed to research risks unless there is a distinctly favorable benefit-to-risk ratio. Fourth, update the ethical framework established by the National Commission to include collaborative responsibility— the concept that research should be conducted in meaningful collaboration with the key stakeholders—notably prisoners and prison staff. Finally, enhance systematic oversight of research involving prisoners so that human subject protections are more rigorous and more reliable than those that exist under the existing institutional review board (IRB) mechanism.[33]

Comments are in order with reference to these five IOM recommendations. Because these have not been codified into regulations, the definition of *prisoner* as used in the first IOM recommendation has not been expanded. For example, "The OHRP does not interpret 45 CFR §46.303(c) to include subjects living in the community and receiving court mandated drug treatment."[34] IOM wants to expand the reach of the regulations to the fuller population of persons whose liberty is restricted by the criminal justice system. Note that 45 CFR §46.303(c) states "*Prisoner* means any individual involuntarily confined or detained in a penal institution." This definition is unchanged in the February 25, 2016, "Standard Operating

Procedure/Policy Approval and Implementation" issued by DHHS's Office of Human Subjects Research Protections.

In its second recommendation, the Institute of Medicine called for a national registry to serve as a central database so as to enable better monitoring of the benefits and burdens of research among prisoners, echoing the *Declaration of Helsinki.*

The third recommendation of IOM would require, as does the *Declaration of Helsinki*, that ethically permissible research offer potential benefits to prisoners that outweigh the risks. Thus, cosmetic product testing that offers no potential benefits to the human research subjects would be precluded, and studies offering considerable benefit with low risk would be allowed. Biomedical research in correctional settings would thus be severely limited. Phase I (safety) and phase 2 (effectiveness) studies would be disallowed, but phase 3 (after effectiveness is shown) studies would be permitted as long as the ratio of prisoner to nonprisoner subjects does not exceed 50 percent (to ensure a fair distribution of research burdens). The only benefits considered are those accruing to the subjects themselves. This emphasis on a risk–benefit approach echoes the *Declaration of Helsinki*.[35]

By requiring active collaboration of relevant stakeholders (prisoners, correctional officers, medical staff, and administrators) in the design, planning, and implementation of the research, the IOM intends in its fourth recommendation to facilitate openness and transparency of the research environment and the creation of ethical conditions that favor respect and disfavor exploitation.

High-risk research and highly restrictive correctional settings require stronger design and monitoring safeguards, according to IOM's fifth recommendation. Approval of research by the IRB is a necessary step, but throughout the course of the study, close ongoing monitoring, preferably by a prison research subject advocate, would be needed to ensure that approved procedures are being followed and that adverse events or problems are being promptly detected. To ensure that protections apply to all research involving prisoners, the enhanced OHRP model would have to be replicated for all agencies and for privately funded research.[36]

None of these recommendations have yet been codified into U.S. law or regulation. Some commentators, including Osagie K. Obasogie,[37] feel that the IOM position is unwise and ill conceived. According to Obasogie, these recommendations unduly relax the ethical considerations restricting research on prisoners, which were based primarily on justice (fair share of burdens and benefits) and respect for persons (principle of autonomy). He criticizes IOM for arguing that modern ethical principles have evolved over the past three decades and for substituting a more subjective standard of risk–benefit analysis.

A critical review by Keramet Reiter generally concurs with the IOM recommendations, although she sharply disagrees with their central recommendation concerning risk–benefit analysis.

Implementing a risk–benefit analysis standard of review requires two preconditions. First, minimum human rights standards must exist in U.S. prisons and be incorporated into standards of review. Otherwise, a risk–benefit approach cannot feasibly and accurately determine the risks or the benefits of any individual prisoner's participation in medical experimentation. Second, any risk–benefit analysis must focus solely on the risks and benefits to the individual prisoner participant, and not on any potential benefit to general scientific knowledge or society-at-large. Until these two conditions are met, regulatory agencies should seek to curtail severely, rather than to expand, human subjects research on prisoners.[38]

In addition, Reiter holds that replacing categorical limitations with risk–benefit analyses is premature: "First, further research is needed to determine the prevalence and scope of prisoner subjects experimentation. . . . Second, further research is needed to explore the relationship between current U.S. prison conditions and prisoners' abilities to provide informed consent, participate in experimentation, and challenge inhumane practices."

Prisoners probably face exceeding difficulties in mounting effective challenges to inhumane research practices because the degree of control exercised in prisons can be so extreme and pervasive and because of the nearly insurmountable obstacles posed by the Prisoner Litigation Reform Act of 1996 (PLRA) when prisoners seek judicial relief or review. The severe burdens imposed on prisoners by the PLRA are described in detail in Chapter 4, "Legal Issues in Correctional Health Care," under "Prison Litigation Reform Act of 1996." In view of the history of ethically reprehensible biomedical experiments conducted in U.S. prisons, Reiter concludes:

Sanctioned by universities and federal agencies alike, these nontherapeutic biomedical experiments took place across the United States until the late 1970s. These experiments do not represent isolated instances of human subjects experimentation gone wrong but rather widespread abusive practices with abusive results in the years leading up to the 1976 DHEW Report. Indeed, the DHEW Report Commission found . . . that many government agencies were involved in a wide variety of biomedical experiments in prisons in the 1970s.[39]

As indicated, the Institute of Medicine's 2006 report called for significant changes in the procedures and protections governing medical experiments on prisoners, including streamlining and expanding oversight of prisoner experimentation. To avoid a return to the horrific abuses that were so prevalent before 1980, it is critically important, especially in any form of biomedical research involving prisoners, to ensure knowledgeable and informed consent, absence of any element of coercion or excessive inducements or exploitation, and close watchful monitoring by an IRB that is duly constituted and includes prisoner advocates. "Prisoners still need to be protected from the risk of coercion, undue inducement, and exploitation."[40] The IOM study recommended that biomedical research on prisoners be "severely limited" and only involve phase 3 studies and that the ratio of prisoner to nonprisoner subjects not exceed 50 percent.

IOM's recommendations for establishing a mandatory national database of all research involving prisoners, broadening the applicability of the safeguards to all such research regardless of funding source, defining "prisoner" to mean "all persons whose liberty has been restricted by decisions of the criminal justice system,"[41] and placing a new emphasis on collaborative responsibility are all commendable and should be implemented.

The regulations and declarations of virtually all these organizations emphasize the ethical obligation deriving from the principle of *justice* so that the risks and burdens of research are allocated equitably with its expected benefits. They also require protecting the health, well-being, autonomy, and other human rights of prisoners in the context of research.

Encouraging Appropriate Research

Lawrence O. Gostin, chair of the IOM study, said that although we must heed history's warning about prisoner exploitation in research, prisoners might benefit by a modern approach to research with proper safeguards, and he suggests the importance of achieving a better understanding of the kinds of issues that prisoners face, including mental illness, substance abuse, and transition back to their communities.[42]

As a consequence of the legitimate concerns over egregious excesses perpetrated in the past, many formidable barriers that served to discourage systematic research among correctional populations now exist, including federal guidelines for protecting the incarcerated, requirements for institutional review board approvals, and the many logistical and procedural burdens and inconveniences faced by the correctional agency. At the same time, however, there is an increasing recognition that many critical questions related to inmate populations remain largely unstudied and unanswered. Dr. Newton Kendig[43] cited a few examples, including the fact that certain diseases that disproportionately affect incarcerated populations—including hepatitis C and the devastating oral health consequences of methamphetamine abuse—are not captured by large-scale epidemiologic studies such as the National Health and Nutritional Examination Survey. These populations are largely unstudied in community-based clinical trials, so are we optimally treating ethnic minorities with chronic infectious diseases related to injection drug use? Could we improve ambulatory care in the United States by critically evaluating different models of health care delivery in the highly structured environment of corrections? Other topics for needed research[44] include the effectiveness of harm-reduction strategies in the context of preventing the transmission of blood-borne pathogens, outcomes and effectiveness of patient health education in prisons and jails, how correctional health programs can be more relevant to culture and gender, validation of mental health screening and diagnostic tools used with prisoners, and defining and assessing functional behavior in correctional settings.

Even research on topics such as these, which can be reasonably expected to significantly benefit prisoners, should conform to the requirements and protections embodied in the *Belmont* and Institute of Medicine reports so as to ensure that the process is always ethical, fair, and nonabusive. The wording and intent of the ACA standard,[45] properly understood, do not seem to categorically prohibit this kind of research. An important definitional nuance should be recognized here. The range of experimental programs that ACA is explicitly and appropriately prohibiting— those involving aversive conditioning, psychosurgery, or the application of cosmetic substances—does not embrace what Kendig and others are suggesting. However, the wording of the ACA standard may nevertheless discourage correctional administrators from seriously entertaining any proposal that is called "research" on grounds that it might interfere with accreditation. This would be unfortunate because prisoners, their families, and the free community might all potentially benefit from well-designed research investigations that involve partnership with academic institutions and incorporate appropriate ethical safeguards in the quest for answers to important questions that directly or disproportionally affect criminal justice populations.

Nevertheless, in this highly complex area, ACA auditors or NCCHC surveyors could not be expected—within the limited time available during an accreditation visit—to even begin to assess the evidence for compliance with this standard and the regulations. However, this matter could be assessed in other ways during an accreditation so that it would not deter legitimate and beneficial research. For example, a detailed preaudit questionnaire could be completed in advance by the correctional facility, portions of which might require input from the IRB and from the responsible physician, to vouch for having satisfied all of the legal and ethical requirements. The visiting team could then randomly select a few persons from a roster of current research participants for a brief personal interview. Alternatively, for audits of facilities engaging in prisoner research, the NCCHC or ACA could include a person with relevant qualifications on the visiting committee. This situation, in the foreseeable future, will not likely apply to more than a small number of correctional facilities nationwide.

How Do We Bring It All Together?

This author believes with Reiter[46] and others that the Belmont requirements remain essentially sound and applicable and that IOM recommendations one, two, four, and five should be adopted and enacted into law or regulation. These would (1) expand the definition of *prisoner* to include probationers and parolees in the context of research subjects; (2) ensure consistent ethical protection regardless of funding source or sponsorship and also establish a public database to track all research involving prisoners; (3) [see below]; (4) incorporate *collaborative responsibility* into the ethical principle of justice so that relevant stakeholders participate actively in the design, planning, and implementation of the research in order to open the research environment and create ethical conditions favorable to respect and unfavorable to exploitation; and (5) enhance systematic oversight of research so that protections are more rigorous and relevant than those that exist under the current IRB mechanism.

The third IOM recommendation, however—calling for a shift from a category-based to a risk–benefit approach to research review—raises important concerns. Given the tragic history of abusive research on prisoner subjects in this country, it seems advisable to retain for the present the four previously cited categories[47] of permissible research on prisoners that are established in subpart C of 45 CFR §46 and not allow them to be substituted or bypassed by the risk–benefit analysis.

In itself, the idea of a risk–benefit analysis is not objectionable and is explicit or implicit in other formulations of ethical principles for human subject research. This point is made, for example, in the *Declaration of Helsinki*: "17. All medical research involving human subjects must be preceded by careful assessment of predictable risks and burdens to the individuals and groups involved in the research in comparison with foreseeable benefits to them and to other individuals or groups affected by the condition under investigation."[48]

> The benefits must outweigh the risks for the human research subjects and the subpopulation they represent. However, for prisoners, because of their impaired liberty and disadvantaged status and the history of past abuses, suitable categorical protections appear to be needed at this time since these are less subjective than a balancing of risks and benefits.

In other words, the benefits must outweigh the risks for the human research subjects and the subpopulation they represent. However, for prisoners, because of their impaired liberty, disadvantaged status, and history of past abuses, suitable categorical protections appear to be needed at this time because these are less subjective than a balancing of risks and benefits.

The rationale advanced by the Institute of Medicine Report is that abandonment of the categorical approach is necessary to enable research that is beneficial and desirable to prisoners. However, the current regulations already appear to permit legitimate and useful types of research, including experimental treatments designed to benefit their individual health and well-being as is done with similarly afflicted persons in the free world. The regulations likewise impose no impediment to prisoner participation in nonintrusive behavioral research involving only voluntary confidential interviews. Virtually all of the studies suggested by Kendig,[49] Paar et al.,[50] Appelbaum,[51] and Hale et al.[52] would probably allow the use of prisoner subjects following the categorical restrictions, rules, and protections required by 45 CFR §46, and therefore should be encouraged. The risk versus benefit criterion proposed by IOM is relevant and should always be applied by the IRB as a necessary, although not sufficient, condition for approving the study.

We should recognize some important efforts being made by university-based research programs to investigate topics relevant to correctional populations. Some of this work is being done under the auspices of the University of Massachusetts Medical School's Health and Criminal Justice Program, the University of Texas-Medical Branch, and the University of Miami. Such projects, in the author's view, whether or not receiving DHHS funding, should follow the 45 CFR §46 revised provisions of the Code of Federal Regulations and satisfy the IRB requirements.

HOUSING THE MENTALLY ILL IN ISOLATION OR SUPERMAX SETTINGS

Some mentally ill patients can cope well on an outpatient basis in the general population of a prison or jail as long as they receive any needed psychotherapy, counseling, and periodic follow-up for their medications. Many, however, require considerably more than this as described in Chapter 6, "Conceptualizing Mental Illness as a Chronic Condition," under "Jail and Prison Environments Are Countertherapeutic." They can readily decompensate in the outpatient setting of a correctional facility but may find an intermediate level of care helpful to mitigate the adverse impact of the correctional environment.

Most correctional systems have far too few intermediate mental health beds available to house the large number of persons who need them. Because the mentally ill present significant management problems for correctional officers and administrators, it is not surprising that they are commonly found in segregation units, security housing units (SHUs), and maximum security (or supermax) facilities where they encounter even greater stress. Their behavior is often unpredictable and nonconforming; their attitudes can be argumentative and confrontational, and they tend to be loud and sometimes violent. They get into fights or fail to follow orders. They receive disciplinary reports and are sent to segregation. Their stay in segregated housing can become prolonged when one sanction is repeatedly added to another.

Correctional staff regard these persons as extremely dangerous and place them in handcuffs and leg irons whenever the cell door must be opened or they need to be transported for any reason. This perception of danger is not misplaced or erroneous, but it is akin to the phenomenon of a pressure cooker that will discharge an explosive burst of steam if opened while under pressure. These people have been caged for long periods without social contact; with no frame of reference other than the four walls of their cell; often without books, magazines, radio or TV, or other distractions; and without orientation to time or place or events. Prolonged exposure to these conditions is disorienting, exacerbates whatever mental illness already exists, leads to despair and suicidal behavior, and presents the potential for violent behavioral outbursts when they are unrestrained. Some mentally ill prisoners voluntarily remain in their cells rather than participate in dayroom or outdoor activities, perhaps because they do not want to be taunted or pestered by other inmates. This, too, can have deleterious consequences because it is not healthy to remain closeted in a cell for extended periods without exercise, fresh air, sunshine, or social contact.

When this occurs, therapeutic intervention may be helpful, but it would be more effective to transfer such patients to an intermediate environment where they will feel safer and can be encouraged to participate regularly in guided therapeutic activities.

Keeping with the metaphor of the pressure cooker, it would be unwise to insist that the lid must be kept tightly on the pot to prevent the dangerous steam from venting. In fact, covering the pot is what brings the internal pressure to a dangerous level. It is instructive to recall that in 1793, Philippe Pinel, a French psychiatrist, was the first to insist on removing the chains that bound the arms and legs of "lunatics" to the wall. Though he had been warned that these people had to be chained because they were dangerous and assaultive, he argued that the cause of their violent behavior was their continuous confinement with chains. History has proved Pinel to be correct, but perhaps this important lesson again needs to be learned.[53]

As Dr. Jeffrey L. Metzner explains, "Clinicians generally agree that placement of inmates with serious mental illnesses in settings with extreme isolation is contraindicated because many of these inmates' psychiatric conditions will clinically deteriorate or not improve. In other words, many inmates with serious mental illnesses are harmed when placed in such settings."[54] The American Psychiatric Association has made a similar declaration: "Prolonged segregation of adult inmates with serious mental illness, with rare exceptions, should be avoided due to the potential for harm to such inmates. If an inmate with serious mental illness is placed in segregation, out-of-cell structured therapeutic activities (i.e., mental health or psychiatric treatment) in appropriate programming space and adequate unstructured out-of-cell time should be permitted."[55]

Disruption of the circadian rhythm—the built-in 24-hour body clock whose timing is normally adjusted by the natural onset of day and night—can be disorienting for prisoners whose housing affords little or no access to natural lighting (or when the bright fluorescent lighting in their cell is never turned off). This disorientation can be a common feature of conditions such as depression, posttraumatic stress disorder, anxiety, and obsessive–compulsive disorder. Prolonged deprivation of sunshine is also well known to bring about a condition called *seasonal affective disorder* (SAD), which is often termed "winter depression" or "winter blues."

Although other factors may play a role, the overall quality and effectiveness of the mental health program in a prison system will tend to be inversely proportional to the percentage of its mentally ill prisoners housed in segregation. The better the mental health program, the less need to place these inmates in segregation. An effective mental health policy begins with prevention strategies that are targeted toward eliminating unnecessary sources of stress and aggravation.

In testimony before the Commission on Safety and Abuse in America's Prisons, Fred Cohen spoke of the prevailing types of isolation in many penal settings:

Isolation is not a fixed, invariable condition of penal confinement. It is variable in its extremes of deprivation and at its most extreme should be banned and in its less onerous forms sharply limited, very closely regulated, and closely monitored. . . . Isolation or solitary confinement, then, conveys a set of circumstances beyond life in a single, quiet cell and includes all manner of deprivation of life's most basic components. . . . The greater the deprivation, then, the more suspect the practice and the greater the obligation on proponents to produce evidence of benefits outweighing liabilities.[56]

Dr. Kenneth L. Appelbaum, acknowledging the importance of the American Psychiatric Association's declaration and similar recommendations made by psychiatrists and others, makes an eloquent appeal for a broader prohibition of the use of extended segregation or isolation for anyone, even those not known to be mentally ill. Appelbaum points out how much of the rest of the world has pulled back from placing persons into extreme isolation, while the U.S. mostly had not. He also states that "[m]any, if not most, inmates housed in segregation units . . . are not even assaultive," citing considerable evidence to support this assertion.[57]

A nation-wide survey of corrections department policies on segregation, conducted by the Liman Public Interest Program at the Yale Law School in 2013, states:

Reading the many policies makes plain the degree of discretion accorded to correctional officials. At the formal policy level, most permit placement in segregation based on a wide range of rationales. The elasticity suggests that administrative segregation may be used for goals other than incapacitation. In exchanges about our inquiry into administrative segregation, several commentators referred to the potential for its overuse based on what is colloquially known as being "mad" at a prisoner, as contrasted with being "scared" of that individual.[58]

The tragedy of housing the mentally ill in segregation units is not only the intense human suffering that this environment causes. It also includes the associated depression and self-harmful activity, the monumental impediments to access to timely and appropriate health care, the difficulty of attempting any meaningful monitoring of symptoms, the utter lack of control over one's own life situation, and the resulting long-term physical and mental deterioration. A mental health professional or nurse faces a formidable challenge when attempting to pass medications, conduct a sick call visit, perform an evaluation, or conduct therapy through a closed door and inch-thick Plexiglas window. Sometimes health professionals even try to perform these tasks in a crouched or kneeling position and talking through the waist-high food slot in a steel door. Officers are loath to bring the patients out to another room to meet health professionals because this practice is time consuming and not without risk. The ethical challenges to delivering health care under such circumstances are many.

"Clinicians generally agree that placement of inmates with serious mental illnesses in settings with extreme isolation is contraindicated because many of these inmates' psychiatric conditions will clinically deteriorate or not improve. In other words, many inmates with serious mental illnesses are harmed when placed in such settings."
Jeffrey L. Metzner, MD

On occasion, the author has observed mental health professionals attempting to provide care to prisoners who were individually confined in small iron cages or were shackled to a pole during one-on-one or group therapy sessions. Treatment staff explained that they felt this arrangement, although unsatisfactory, was a decided improvement over cell-side interactions in segregation, and they expressed the belief that their custody officials would strongly resist any further normalization of the treatment setting for this type of patient. Granted that these strategies had been creatively adopted in a desperate and well-intentioned effort to enable treatment without being exposed to harmful behavior, their use is so patently inhumane and degrading that it could only be justified as a temporary measure, such as during transition from maximum confinement to a less restricted treatment setting.

It is ethically imperative that those who hold responsible positions at prisons where these practices exist do not simply accept the situation as inevitable. The fact that it has been this way for years does not mean that it must remain so. Correctional and health officials need to confer and discuss how to improve the conditions of segregation and, especially, how to avoid its use for housing the mentally ill. The American Correctional Association stipulates in its public correctional policy that "[c]omprehensive correctional mental health services shall include . . . continued access to mental health services while housed in disciplinary or administrative segregation."[59] This principle is not often fulfilled because access is usually intermittent and subject to highly unsatisfactory conditions.

According to correctional psychologist Dean Aufderheide, approximately one-third of mentally ill inmates are found in segregation. Whether these are "seriously" mentally ill depends on whether the definition being used is based on diagnosis, symptom severity, functional impairment, or some combination. Aufderheide prefers the functional definition, saying: "In my clinical opinion, if a mental illness impairs adaptive functioning to the extent that it requires ongoing mental health treatment, it is serious!"[60] For those in segregation, a post-placement screening evaluation by a mental health professional should be conducted within one week, and weekly rounds thereafter by mental health staff are essential. Furthermore, a behavioral risk assessment should be conducted "periodically and especially after a critical incident such as a use of force, threats to the safety of others or institutional security, etc."

A Vicious Cycle

Once a seriously mentally ill patient is placed in conditions of extreme segregation, it is extremely difficult for that patient to get out. The placement occurs because of unruly behavior, which may be due to the illness itself. Then the severe sensory and social deprivation and lack of treatment exacerbate the patient's symptoms, causing extreme pain and suffering and resulting in uncontrolled outbursts that are answered with new disciplinary infractions—further extending the time in segregation.

Psychologist Craig Haney reports the assertion of a segregated mentally ill prisoner in Florida: "Once you get back here, you get madder and madder. So you get DRs [disciplinary reports] and unsatisfactories, and that means you can't get out." He described another patient who had begged repeatedly for psychiatric help and finally went to the extreme measure of setting himself on fire to get that help. The outcome was that he was written up for arson, put in a strip cell for 21 days, and given no psychiatric assistance.[61]

Psychologist Keith Curry explains in detail why this form of discipline is so ineffective with the mentally ill:

Whether or not this system effectively serves as a deterrent to the typical administrative segregation inmate, its deterrence value for seriously mentally ill inmates is dubious. Inmates suffering from schizophrenia, schizoaffective disorder, bipolar disorder, psychotic depression, and severe forms of personality disorders have, as a part of their illness, poor impulse control, delusional thinking, volatile emotions, distorted perceptions of their environments, as well as gross social skills deficits. They typically suffer serious disabilities in terms of planning for future events and learning from experience. Once segregated, they may lose the ability to track the passage of time. Disoriented and confused psychotic inmates often misinterpret the muffled voices of staff and other inmates in ways that confirm their fantasies and fears, or they may suffer outright hallucinations. Those suffering from paranoia typically misconstrue the motives of others in ways that prevent them from acting in their own best interest. Once cut off from external reality cues due to social and sensory deprivation, psychotic inmates may become autistic and lose the ability to differentiate events occurring inside versus outside of themselves.[62]

Although many of these symptoms could be ameliorated through aggressive mental health treatment, mental health services in these settings are so extremely limited and unsatisfactory that inmates who most need such services are least able to get them. As Curry points out, these are the "bottom dwellers," and many remain hopelessly stuck in segregation for the duration of their sentences.

Despite the widely held view of mental health professionals that prolonged exposure to segregation and isolation can have deleterious effects on prisoners' mental health, a somewhat different finding was suggested by a recent study[63] funded by the National Institute of Corrections. Focusing on a sample of 247 persons in the Colorado prison system over a period of one year, a group of persons housed in administrative segregation were compared with persons in the general prison population and residents of a psychiatric care prison. The subjects, who were not randomly assigned to the study groups, were given standardized tests at three-month intervals to measure states such as anxiety, depression, and psychosis. These test results were supplemented by psychological functioning observations from clinical staff and ratings of behavior from correctional staff. The results showed that the mental health of 20 percent of persons in administrative segregation improved,[64] that of 7 percent deteriorated, and no significant change was detected for the remainder. This study, however, did not include persons with serious mental illness and was limited to adult males who were literate and could self-administer the psychological test instruments. Moreover, the conditions of isolation were, relatively speaking, benign, with 80 square feet of floor space in each cell, five hours of out-of-cell recreation each week, three 15-minute showers each week, a visit from a mental health professional each month, scheduled mental health appointments in the visiting room (rather than cell-side), the opportunity to select books and magazines from the library cart each week, and a 20-minute phone call and one noncontact visit each month. These and other concerns about the validity of this study's findings were pointed out by Philip Bulman,[65] a writer for the National Institute of Justice, which funded the study. Clearly, these conditions do not constitute the extremes of isolation as practiced in supermax and some other settings. The researchers themselves emphasize that the findings should not be generalized to systems that are more restrictive and have fewer treatment and programming resources, nor should they be generalized to periods of isolation lasting longer than one year or to patients who are seriously mentally ill.

Just as there is a proper procedure for safely removing a pressure cooker's lid, there needs also to be a carefully thought-out method for transitioning mentally ill persons believed to be dangerous out of long-term segregation and extreme isolation into a less restrictive setting. Expert advice from experienced mental health professionals is imperative. Strategies might include one or more intermediate step-down living arrangements, additional staff (therapeutic and custody) so as to permit gradual relaxation of restrictions, appropriate rules for daily operation of the unit, concomitant introduction of a variety of active and passive therapeutic activities, and supervised introduction to structured social interaction with peers.

Not every patient will progress at the same pace, and individualized treatment planning and a team approach are essential. The environment should be nonthreatening and as pleasant as possible. Appropriate color, décor, furnishings, and peaceful background music could promote relaxation and confidence and reduce anxiety, paranoia, and fear. Because the intense condition was built up and maintained over a long period, the passage out may be lengthy. Treatment efforts will be more effective when a therapeutic environment is maintained.

Given that a high percentage of these inmates have been victims of closed head injuries and physical and sexual abuse, many have low intellectual functioning. Cognitive limitations affect the ability to function normally, and individual and group cognitive behavioral treatment interventions may prove beneficial.

Extreme Segregation, Isolation, and Supermax Settings

Conditions of extreme isolation are not new as this excerpt from the proclamation of Daniel Rose,[66] a physician and the first warden of the Maine State Prison, noted at its opening in 1824:

Prisons should be so constructed that even their aspect might be terrific and appear like what in fact they should be, dark and comfortless abodes of guilt and wretchedness. No more of degree of punishment . . . is in its nature so well adapted to purposes of preventing crime or reforming a criminal as close confinement in a solitary cell, in which, cut off from all hope of relief, the convict shall be furnished a hammock on which he may sleep, a block of wood on which he may sit, and with such coarse and wholesome food as may best be suited to a person in a situation designed for grief and penitence, and shall be favored with so much light from the firmament as may enable him to read the New Testament which will be given him as his sole companion and guide to a better life.[67]

Since the late 1980s, the United States has trended toward constructing supermax facilities. The use of the redundant superlative was intended to show that increasing security levels significantly beyond what was already regarded as maximum security was indeed possible.

"Many of the inmates who end up confined in the most severe conditions of confinement are precisely the group least capable of tolerating such conditions."

Stuart Grassian, MD

During this prison building boom, 41 of the 50 United States, as well as the federal government, built at least one supermax institution. Arizona was the first in 1986.[68] These prisons are essentially escape proof, and inmates' movement is severely restricted and controlled. Each inmate is housed alone and remains in the cell at least 23 hours a day. The hour out of the cell can be used to exercise alone in a long and narrow fenced pen, to shower, and perhaps to make a telephone call. All meals are eaten alone in the cell. Visual barriers prevent inmates from observing what is happening in adjacent building interiors, let alone in the world outside. Lighting is controlled by officers, and they tend to be on most or all of the time. Boredom is enforced, without companionship, and typically without reading material, television, or other distractions. Visits are rare and of the noncontact variety. Steel and concrete block construction magnifies sounds so that sleep can be extremely difficult. Typically, the cell doors have a small Plexiglas window that can be fully shuttered by the officer. Waist-high food slots allow for the passage of serving trays, papers, and medicines and for affixing or removing handcuffs. An ankle slot permits the attaching or removing of leg irons when the inmate exits or enters the cell. Some supermax facilities incorporate a tiered behavior modification program whereby sustained compliant behavior can earn restoration of some privileges and removal of certain restrictions.

Many segregation units in state prisons resemble or are modeled after supermax facilities. Their stated purpose is to house the "worst of the worst," the "incorrigible," those believed to be the most dangerous of the inmate population. The length of stay varies but tends to be long. Almost no opportunity exists for interpersonal contact or conversation, either among prisoners or between staff and prisoner. This creates a great deal of sensory deprivation and social isolation. Communication by medical or mental health personnel with persons confined in these circumstances is limited and difficult.

A court's (*Jones 'El v. Berge*) graphic description of the conditions prevailing at a supermax prison is revealing:

Inmates on Level One at the State of Wisconsin's Supermax Correctional Institution in Boscobel, Wisconsin spend all but four hours a week confined to a cell. The "boxcar" style door on the cell is solid except for a shutter and a trap door that opens into the dead space of a vestibule through which a guard may transfer items to the inmate without interacting with him. The cells are illuminated 24 hours a day. Inmates receive no outdoor exercise. Their personal possessions are severely restricted: one religious text, one box of legal materials, and 25 personal letters. They are permitted no clocks, radios, watches, cassette players, or televisions. The temperature fluctuates wildly, reaching extremely high and low temperatures depending on the season. A video camera rather than a human eye monitors the inmate's movements. Visits other than with lawyers are conducted through video screens.[69]

Mental health experts who have studied these facilities report that extended confinement under such conditions can destabilize even healthy inmates, but they most often cause mentally ill and vulnerable individuals to decompensate and manifest severe psychotic symptoms. Dr. Stuart Grassian, a forensic psychiatrist at Harvard, testified as follows:

It has in fact long been known that severe restriction of environmental and social stimulation has a profoundly deleterious effect on mental functioning. . . . The prison setting is a particularly toxic environment, and there is a particular problem associated with it. Many of the inmates who end up confined in the most severe conditions of confinement are precisely the group least capable of tolerating such conditions. These often include individuals with long histories, beginning in childhood, of emotional lability, hyperactivity, impulsivity, or other indications of subtle central nervous system dysfunction. As a result of this dysfunction, such individuals are almost pathologically stimulation-seeking, and pathologically incapable of tolerating stimulus deprivation. When placed in stringent conditions of confinement, they become agitated and paranoid, their emotional state and behavior deteriorates, and finally they "max out"—many become floridly psychotic, or so agitated that they engage in awful, grotesque behaviors: they cover themselves and their cells with feces, they mutilate themselves, they try to kill themselves. . . . Unfortunately, the prison system has traditionally had little capacity to understand or cope with this problem. Instead, once such an individual gets into this downward spiral of disturbed behavior and punishment, he cannot get out. He just stays there, being punished more and more for his behavior, and he mentally rots.[70]

Dr. Grassian further described the severe psychiatric harm that can be caused by solitary confinement:

This harm includes a specific syndrome which has been reported by many clinicians in a variety of settings, all of which have in common features of inadequate, noxious and/or restricted environmental and social stimulation. In more severe cases, this syndrome is associated with agitation, self-destructive behavior, and overt psychotic disorganization. In addition, solitary confinement often results in severe exacerbation of a previously existing mental condition, or in the appearance of a mental illness where none had been observed before. Even among inmates who do not develop overt psychiatric illness as a result of confinement in solitary, such confinement almost inevitably imposes significant psychological pain during the period of isolated confinement and often significantly impairs the inmate's capacity to adapt successfully to the broader prison environment. . . .

The restriction of environmental stimulation and social isolation associated with confinement in solitary are strikingly toxic to mental functioning, producing a stuporous condition associated with perceptual and cognitive impairment and affective disturbances. In more severe cases, inmates so confined have developed florid delirium—a confusional psychosis with intense agitation, fearfulness, and disorganization. But even those inmates who are more psychologically resilient inevitably suffer severe psychological pain as a result of such confinement, especially when the confinement is prolonged, and especially when the individual experiences this confinement as being the product of an arbitrary exercise of power and intimidation. Moreover, the harm caused by such confinement may result in prolonged or permanent psychiatric disability, including impairments which may seriously reduce the inmate's capacity to reintegrate into the broader community upon release from prison.[71]

Thomas Conklin, psychiatrist and medical director at the Hampden County Jail in Massachusetts, wrote the following after evaluating mental health care in a Texas supermax facility: "All suicide gestures by inmates [were] seen as manipulating the correctional system with the conscious intent of secondary gain. In not one case was the inmate's behavior seen as reflecting mental pathology that could be treated."[72]

A U.S. Department of Justice evaluation of the goals, impacts, and costs of supermax prisons was conducted by the Urban Institute in 2006 and described numerous shortcomings and concerns. It did not find such prisons to be an effective management tool, stating that their effectiveness "remains unknown and questionable" and noting that some reported unintended effects "such as increased mental illness, raise substantial concerns."[73]

Conditions of confinement in supermax facilities have been repeatedly brought to the attention of the courts—particularly in terms of their harmful effects on mentally ill prisoners. For example, an extensive discourse on the special psychiatric and psychological problems that arise in the course of isolated confinement in supermaximum security prisons can be found in the amicus curiae brief filed in support of the respondent in *Reginald A. Wilkinson v. Charles E. Austin*, which was written by several well-respected psychiatrists and psychologists who are thoroughly familiar with the conditions of extreme isolation and supermax confinement.

Their compelling report to the court stated, in part:

. . . [S]upermax confinement imposes a significant "hardship" in the form of grave psychiatric and psychological risks to prisoners. No study of the effects of solitary or supermax-like confinement that lasted longer than 60 days failed to find evidence of negative psychological effects. Moreover, research raises significant doubts about the ability of supermax prisons to achieve their goal of reducing violence in prison systems. . . . [p. 4]

Methods of psychological torture include stimulus deprivation, of which solitary confinement is an example, as well as so-called "constraint" techniques in which "[v]ictims are submitted to a detailed set of regulations and rules, resulting in close supervision where everything (including completely insignificant details) is controlled."[74] When used in this way as a method of torture, solitary confinement has been recognized as contributing to cognitive impairment, including the inability to think coherently and logically, as well as producing anxiety, anger and depression in its victims. . . . [p. 13]

All other things being equal, the more prolonged and complete the isolation, the greater the risk of harm. . . . [p. 14]

In more systematic research involving hundreds of in-depth interviews with isolated prisoners, psychologist Hans Toch concluded that "isolation panic" was a serious problem among prisoners in solitary confinement. Symptoms reported included rage, panic, loss of control and breakdowns, psychological regression, a build-up of physiological and psychic tension that led to incidents of self-mutilation.[75] Toch noted that this kind of confinement marked an important dichotomy for prisoners: the "distinction between imprisonment, which is tolerable, and isolation, which is not."[76] [p. 17]

Craig Haney's study of a random sample of prisoners housed in a "state-of-the-art" supermax prison in California had these findings: This study found extraordinarily high rates of symptoms of psychological trauma. More than four out of five of those evaluated suffered from feelings of anxiety and nervousness, headaches, troubled sleep, and lethargy or chronic tiredness, and over half complained of nightmares, heart palpitations, and fear of impending nervous breakdowns. Equally high numbers reported specific psychopathological effects of social isolation—obsessive ruminations, confused thought processes, an oversensitivity to stimuli, irrational anger, and social withdrawal. Well over half reported violent fantasies, emotional flatness, mood swings, chronic depression, and feelings of overall deterioration, while nearly half suffered from hallucinations and perceptual distortions, and a quarter experienced suicidal ideation.[77] [pp. 21–22]

The report concludes, "Severe conditions of isolated confinement such as those found in supermax prisons inflict psychological pain and distress and, if prolonged, create a serious risk of harm for prisoners" (p. 30). Nevertheless, the courts have tended to avoid any finding that the concept and practice of a supermax facility is itself unconstitutional. Still, issues of cruel and unusual punishment have been raised, and some have resulted in prohibiting the housing of mentally ill patients in supermax facilities.

In 1994, a federal district court lawsuit against California's Pelican Bay isolation unit ruled that the mentally ill should not be made to endure supermax conditions. The court found that for certain categories of mentally ill prisoners, confinement in SHUs, which are typically segregated units characterized by extremes of isolation, was unconstitutional. "[F]or these inmates, placing them in the SHU is the mental equivalent of putting an asthmatic in a place with little air to breathe" [*Madrid v. Gomez*, 889 F. Supp. 1146, N.D. Cal. (1995) at 1265].

In Wisconsin in 2002, an out-of-court settlement in a federal court case [*Jones 'El et al. v. Berge et al.*, 164 F. Supp. 2d 1096, 1098, W.D. Wis. (2001)] resulted in an agreement that mentally ill prisoners and juveniles will no longer be imprisoned at the supermax facility—the Boscobel prison. This facility was subsequently down-graded in 2007 from supermax to maximum security. The state of Michigan in 2004 downgraded its only supermax facility to a level-five maximum security prison. The federal penitentiary at Marion, Illinois, was downgraded from a supermax to medium security in 2006 when the new federal ADX Supermax facility opened in Florence, Colorado.

In assessing solitary confinement and a severely restrictive behavioral manage-ment plan for a mentally ill inmate, the Montana Supreme Court said in 2003 that this is an "affront to the inviolable right of human dignity and . . . constitutes cruel and unusual punishment. . . ." [*Walker v. Montana,* 68 P. 3d 872 and 885, Mont. (2003)].

Ohio now has a policy that mentally ill prisoners will not be placed in its super-max facility. In 2005, a unanimous Supreme Court affirmed that prisoners do have a protected liberty interest under the Fourteenth Amendment to due process before being placed in a supermax setting. Because supermax isolation imposes such "atypi-cal and significant hardship," it is different enough that prisoners may not be denied a due-process hearing before being imprisoned in such a facility.[78]

No one who is psychologically vulnerable or has serious mental illness should be housed in punitive or administrative isolation. According to David Fathi, "every federal court order to consider the question has held that *supermax* confinement of the seriously mentally ill is unconstitutional" (*Wilkinson v. Austin*).[79]

Many, if not most, of the mentally ill persons now housed in extreme isolation units could be safely and more humanely housed in therapeutic settings where a combination of behavioral and medication approaches is used. A token economy that provides rewards and incentives for acceptable behavior, along with cognitive behavioral skills training and, as appropriate, use of psychotropic medication, can be helpful. These patients benefit from structured therapeutic activities and inter-action with care staff and fellow patients.[80]

By definition, one who requires acute inpatient or intermediate level treatment needs more than outpatient care. The only mental health service available in seg-regation, however, is outpatient care, and this is often extremely limited in fre-quency, individuality, intensity, and duration. As described by Keith Curry,

Outpatient care provided within administrative segregation units is inadequate in its own right, but would not even under the best of circumstances be sufficient to meet the needs of inmates requiring sub-acute care. The deficiency is not in the quality but in the type of treat-ment provided. Outpatient care is appropriate for relatively healthy inmates having difficulty adjusting to prison life or chronically ill inmates who have become essentially asymptom-atic. . . . As a result, inmates in this group of sub-acutely mentally ill inmates are harmed by their long-term assignment to a housing status where the appropriate level of care necessary to treat their serious illness does not exist.[81]

The Society of Correctional Physicians, now the American College of Correc-tional Physicians, proclaims "that prolonged segregation of inmates with serious mental illness, with rare exceptions, violates basic tenets of mental health treatment." Further, the group recommends "that correctional systems provide mental health input into the disciplinary process in order to appropriately shunt some of these inmates into active mental health housing and programming rather than disciplinary segregation when the mental condition is a mitigating factor in the commission of the infraction."[82]

The evidence of severe harm inflicted by extreme isolation, particularly to the mentally ill, is abundant and compelling. Given the availability of better ways to handle mentally ill prisoners safely and humanely, there is no longer any reasonable excuse for failing to implement whatever measures are necessary to correct this problem. Close collaboration of mental health professionals and correctional officials will be required. For those unsure how to proceed, expert consultation and technical assistance can be readily obtained.

CHEMICAL CASTRATION BY COURT ORDER

Is It Legal?

In the criminal trials of chronic sex offenders, pedophiles, and serial rapists, some courts have ordered chemical castration by use of the drug Depo-Provera (an injectable contraceptive) or other antiandrogen hormone medications. This alternative has been offered to convicted persons in lieu of some or all of the prison time levied. Although this book will not directly address the constitutionality of this type of punishment, let it be said that castration, whether chemical or surgical, is indeed a form of maiming. The Eighth Amendment prohibits "cruel and unusual punishment." Other forms of maiming practiced in some nations—such as the loss of an eye for causing the loss of another person's eye and cutting off a hand for crimes of theft—would not pass the test of constitutionality in this country. As a society, we do not condone physical beatings and whipping or use of the rack or thumb screws, burning, public dissection, or other horrendous means of punishment. We also note that the federal maiming statute (18 U.S. Code §114)[83] makes it a crime for someone who "with intent to torture, maim, or disfigure, cuts, bites, or slits the nose, ear, or lip, or cuts off or disables a limb or any member of another person."

John Stinneford argues convincingly that chemical castration fails to meet the two basic requirements that a punishment must meet to be constitutional: "First, it must not be designed to control or negate the interior capacities of the defendant considered most integral to human dignity, such as reason and free will. Second, it must not impose conditions that treat the offender's suffering as either a matter of indifference, or something to be enjoyed."[84]

Thus far, however, even capital punishment has not been declared "cruel and unusual" in the United States, though it is more severe and final than castration, flogging, or cutting off of limbs. Therefore, for purposes of this discussion, we will not challenge the legality of a court order for chemical castration as a punishment for crimes of sexual violence.

Nevertheless, we should examine the process. The state legislature enacts enabling legislation, although specific provisions of state laws differ. Typically, a court orders the punishment, leaving it to the convicted to accept it or refuse, with the consequence of refusal being lengthy incarceration. What has happened? Did the judge (or perhaps the legislature) practice medicine by prescribing the drug? Did the judge assess the convicted person's health status and evaluate the risk of unintended adverse side effects that might ensue from the use of this medication? Clearly, the judge is not a medical practitioner and is not licensed to diagnose, prescribe, or treat.

Consequently, even though involvement of a physician or other medical professional is not usually required by statute, once the sentence has been issued by the court, there would be a logical need for a practicing physician to examine the patient, assess his health status, determine which drug would be appropriate to achieve the desired effect, evaluate the risk of adverse side effects, prescribe the medication, and conduct appropriate follow-up. Should there be a high risk of serious adverse side effects, then the doctor might prescribe an alternative drug if available or would advise the court of this finding. Monitoring might involve taking periodic blood levels to ascertain that the proper dosage is being ingested, and other tests would be performed to detect any adverse effects. It is immediately obvious that the performance of any or all of these functions by a physician would constitute the practice of medicine as an agent of the state in order to incapacitate or inflict harm on the patient, not for the benefit of the patient. The physician would thereby become an intrinsic and essential part of the process of carrying out the sentence of maiming. Although a physician might argue that the convicted person is not his or her patient, this would contradict both the reality and appearance of what is occurring. Why is this different than if a surgeon, using sterile and efficient techniques, were to carry out a court's order to cut off the hands of a convicted thief?

Regrettably, our nation's history attests to the practice of involuntary surgical castration and sterilization of mentally defective men and women, especially in the late 1800s and early 1900s, carried out in state-operated mental hospitals. In fact, this procedure was found constitutional by the U.S. Supreme Court in *Buck v. Bell* 274 U.S. 200 (1927) when Justice Oliver Wendell Holmes justified the eight-to-one decision thus: "It is better for all the world, if instead of waiting to execute degenerate offspring for crime, or to let them starve for their imbecility, society can prevent those who are manifestly unfit from continuing their kind. The principle that sustains compulsory vaccination is broad enough to cover cutting the Fallopian tubes. Three generations of imbeciles are enough."[85]

Such a practice would surely be rejected today as inhumane, and it would be deemed unethical for any physician to participate. Does the fact of a court order alter the situation? Recall that an action can sometimes be legal even though unethical and immoral.

In 1984, a Michigan circuit court sentenced an heir of the Upjohn Pharmaceutical Company who had been convicted of the serial rape of his stepdaughter to one to five years in prison plus a requirement to take Depo-Provera to quell his sex drive. Despite a public outcry that this sentence was too lenient, the Michigan

Supreme Court ruled that the chemical castration portion of the sentence was illegal. Chemical castration with Depo-Provera had been first introduced by psychiatrist Dr. Fred S. Berlin at Johns Hopkins Hospital where he treated many sex offenders with this drug. The first chemical castration law was enacted in California in 1996. Chemical castration involves injecting massive doses of a synthetic female hormone that mimics the effects of surgical castration by eliminating almost all testosterone from the offender's system. It alters the brain and body function by reducing the brain's exposure to testosterone, thus depriving offenders of the capacity to experience sexual desire and engage in sexual activity. Severe side effects include irreversible loss of bone mass (leading to osteoporosis), diabetes mellitus, pulmonary embolism, depression, excessive weight gain, nightmares, headaches, and muscular cramps.[86] It is also believed to be carcinogenic.

This law has not been struck down as cruel and unusual. However, because most criminal cases are resolved by plea bargains, relatively few persons sentenced to chemical castration have a right to appeal. Stinneford points out that the Supreme Court has not declared a noncapital sentence to be inherently cruel since *Trop v. Dulles* in 1958, when the Court held that the "dignity of man" is the essential foundation of the Eighth Amendment and that the Eighth Amendment should be interpreted in accordance with "evolving standards of decency."

Is Physician Participation Ethical?

Although chemical castration is clearly a form of punishment that affronts the basic human dignity of sex offenders, whether this punishment violates contemporary standards of decency is less clear given the great public hatred of sex offenders—a fact that would probably not change significantly even if the side effects of this treatment were widely known and understood. However, in terms of physician participation in this process, the ethical principles of beneficence, nonmaleficence, autonomy, and respect for persons are clear and should ensure that the skills and art of medical practitioners do not assist in inflicting harm on patients. These same principles should prevent healing practitioners from being suborned by the state to carry out an agenda of social control in conflict with the goals of the medical profession.

Not a single state statute requires that the offender suffer from a sexual disorder before imposing this punishment. California, moreover, has no statutory requirement that a doctor determine the treatment to be medically appropriate or even medically safe. There is no informed consent requirement. A patient does not have the right to refuse chemical castration. Accordingly, it would appear that neither legislatures nor courts have regarded this procedure as a medical treatment.

Dosages of the drug given to men are eight to 43 times greater than doses given to women for contraception. Yet pharmaceutical manufacturer Pfizer has warned women not to use it for more than two years because it deprives the body of bone mineral density, which could result in crippling osteoporosis or bone fracture.[87] The court-imposed treatment is potentially for a lifetime.

In its Code of Medical Ethics, the American Medical Association sets forth the fundamental principle that physicians are bound to providing competent medical care with respect for human dignity; it admonishes physicians to respect the law while maintaining a responsibility to seek changes in laws that "are contrary to the best interests of the patient," and it declares the physician's responsibility to the patient to be paramount.[88]

These important principles must guide our response to the issue of physician participation in court-mandated medical treatment.

The AMA asks whether linking medical treatment to a criminal sentence might confuse treatment with punishment, and it questions whether physicians can ethically cooperate in administering or overseeing such treatments.[89]

The AMA's position can be summarized as follows: physicians can ethically participate in court-initiated medical treatments only if the procedure being mandated is based on a sound medical diagnosis and is therapeutically efficacious and consistent with scientific evidence and nationally accepted clinical practice guidelines. It must offer a direct medical benefit for the health condition from which the patient suffers. Thus it would be unethical for physicians to follow through with a court-initiated medical procedure unless such a benefit exists because otherwise the procedure without proven therapeutic benefits appears to be mandated as a form of punishment and not treatment. Furthermore, the patient must render informed consent despite an inevitable element of coercion.[90]

Although it could appear that the AMA has opened a small window for accepting this practice as ethical, in fact it exacts an especially tight set of difficult-to-achieve criteria. Chemical castration is only questionably efficacious and can be construed as both a form of punishment and a mechanism of social control. If the court is unable to diagnose or treat, then the practice can only be ethical if the physician finds this treatment to be appropriate based on a sound medical diagnosis. This author is not aware of any national medical society that has yet approved preestablished scientifically valid treatments involving chemical castration for medically determined diagnoses. If any were to do so, however, the third criterion of AMA would be satisfied only if the finding were able to withstand critical peer review and indeed was consistent with nationally accepted practice guidelines.

An argument can be made that the physician is not participating as an agent of the court in carrying out the ordered punishment but is serving as the physician voluntarily chosen by the patient to assist him in exercising his free choice to accept the chemical castration in lieu of extended incarceration, which he sees as a less desirable consequence. On this premise, the convicted person is asking the doctor to examine him, prescribe the drug, monitor its effectiveness, help alleviate any adverse side effects, and assist him in every way to remain in good standing with the court so he can continue to enjoy freedom from prison. Would the physician in this scenario be harming the patient or, on the contrary, be doing good to the patient by serving his well-being and his informed choice? The author here asserts his own view to attempt an answer to this question, namely, that the act itself constitutes a maiming, an injury to the body and to the person, and is therefore a harm, even though it may indeed be a harm freely chosen by the patient and one decreed by law. A physician is not justified in excising a healthy limb or organ, even if requested to do so by a competent patient or by a judge. This is decidedly different from excising a gangrenous limb or a cancerous organ because the removal of infected or diseased tissue results in a net benefit to the body and to the person, who is now able to survive, while the harm that is avoided—death—would have been the natural alternative to the treatment, not one arbitrarily imposed by the court.

May a physician ethically condone or cooperate in involuntary treatment of a competent patient? If we were to concede that the coercion is a legitimate act of the judiciary and antecedent to the free choice made by the convicted person who prefers the maiming to prolonged incarceration, then we might conclude that the physician is "treating" with informed patient consent. In other words, it is the court who coerces the treatment, not the physician, and given the options decreed by the court, the patient freely expresses his informed choice among available alternatives, leaving the physician free to treat. The AMA appears to support this logic in asserting that the physician must determine the voluntariness of the informed choice (between castration and incarceration) that is being made, recognizing the element of coercion that is inevitably present. Because people will weigh risks and benefits differently, some may prefer a court-mandated medical procedure to incarceration. The AMA thus concedes the possibility of voluntary consent under coercive circumstances.[91] Nevertheless, as we have already seen, it would be a form of treatment that is more accurately depicted as harm. It indirectly benefits the patient with respect to the goal of avoiding prison but does so by directly inflicting physical and mental harm to the patient. Accordingly, any participation by physicians or other health professionals in court-ordered chemical castration would appear to contravert the principles of medical ethics.

Fundamental differences can be seen between court-ordered chemical castration and court-ordered substance abuse treatment. In the former case, the "treatment" ordered by the court constitutes a physical and mental maiming, causes harm to the recipient, and is intended as punishment as well as a deterrent. In the second case, the "treatment" ordered by the court is beneficial to the patient and is intended primarily as a rehabilitation. In both cases, an additional intent of the court is protection of the public. Thus, it is easier to accept the ethical decision of a health professional to treat the addicted person because this does not violate the requirement to "do no harm," as it does in the instance of castration.

It is the judge, not the therapist, who coerces treatment. But in this scenario, who is the person who diagnosed the medical condition requiring treatment, and who is the person who has prescribed the appropriate medical treatment indicated for this diagnosis? Clearly, as the AMA indicates, it cannot be the judge because a court is qualified neither to make a medical diagnosis nor prescribe medical treatment. And the patient does not even have a medical diagnosis but rather a judicially determined condition. How then can it be appropriate and ethical for a physician to prescribe the chemical or surgical castration or a therapist to administer rehabilitative treatment as a cure for a judicially imposed sentence?

The American Medical Association sounded a caution when it concluded that physicians who cannot secure adherence to these criteria may be liable for medical malpractice or charges of battery, but warns that such a practice could do great harm to the ethical position and the integrity of the medical profession. Physicians must cling to their role as providers of treatment and never allow themselves to become agents of social control.[92]

Finally, even if studies should demonstrate chemical castration to be effective in preventing recidivism, would that serve to justify the practice? A coerced appendectomy or hemodialysis also works. Yet for both ethical and legal reasons, we do not enforce such treatment on a competent but unwilling patient. Only treatment for which there is sound evidence of efficacy may be ethically rendered, but the reverse is not true. To argue logically that coerced treatment is ethical because it is found to be effective would also assert that the end can justify the means.

RETROSPECTIVE CLUES FOR A CURRENT ETHICAL IMPERATIVE

We are indebted to Carl C. Bell,[93] a highly respected correctional psychiatrist, for his brief but thought-provoking and stimulating editorial in 2012 that identified for us a significant ethical challenge facing correctional health professionals. After recounting the high prevalence of intellectual deficit and mental disorder among inmates of adult and juvenile correctional facilities, citing in particular the frequent occurrence of mild mental retardation among low-income African Americans, and describing similar problems among the First Nations population of Canada, Bell concludes that this phenomenon is largely due to fetal alcohol exposure with its two subcategories of fetal alcohol syndrome and fetal alcohol spectrum disorder (FASD). Among these intellectual challenges are attention deficit hyperactivity disorder, specific learning disorders, and various speech and language disorders.

The telling inference drawn by Bell is that correctional health professionals not only have an ethical responsibility and professional duty to care for the health and well-being of their current slate of incarcerated patients but also are duty bound to advocate proactively for the prevention of this eminently preventable disorder in the future. From a public health perspective, the implications are obvious and compelling. Prevention is so much less costly than the cure—not only in terms of dollars but also especially in terms of human life and societal well-being.

We live in a culture that inexcusably but ostentatiously promotes and extols the pleasure and benefits of alcoholic drink. When a pregnant woman consumes alcohol, there is a known and well-documented risk to the mental and physical health of her unborn child. Clarke and Gibbard[94] indicate that FASDs are the most common form of developmental disability and birth defects in the Western world. Alcohol is a known teratogen that can disrupt fetal brain development in all three trimesters—in other words, at any point in gestation—even before the mother becomes aware that she is pregnant.

According to the National Institute on Alcohol Abuse and Alcoholism,[95] persons with FASD can have trouble with learning and remembering, understanding and following direction, controlling emotions, communicating and socializing, and performing daily life skills. In support of Bell's conclusion, these specific indicators suggest a pattern that is so typical among persons involved in the criminal justice system. It may also be that prenatal alcohol exposure predisposes unborn infants to a lifelong susceptibility to addiction, facilitating their devastating abuse of heroin, methamphetamines, and other drugs. In addition to the physiological reality of alcohol's effect on fetal brain development, environmental and familial factors concerning behavior and nutrition can also be relevant. Children who grow up watching their father and mother drinking alcohol and smoking tobacco tend to learn addictive behaviors.

These disorders from fetal alcohol exposure last a lifetime. There is no cure, although medication and behavior therapy can alleviate some symptoms. No amount of alcohol is safe for pregnant women to drink. Heavy drinking puts the fetus at greatest risk for severe problems.

In view of all this, who can speak out more convincingly on this subject than the nurses and doctors, psychiatrists and mental health professionals, and substance abuse therapists who work in correctional health settings? They know perhaps better than others from day-to-day experience the ravages that fetal alcohol exposure has wrought on the lives and destinies of so many of their patients. These are stories that need to be told to our high school and college students. In addition, health professionals working in women's correctional facilities have a unique opportunity to impress this important lesson on their patients.

Our society has glamorized the consumption of alcohol, drugs, and tobacco. Reversing this trend requires that we do something. None of us can alter what has already occurred, but everlasting shame be upon us if we do not learn from the past and do what we can to prevent such mistakes in the future. If fetal alcohol syndrome and addiction are major root causes of our unconscionable and bloated prison population, then we who are "in the know" can claim no excuse for remaining silent about this eminently preventable problem.

CONCLUSION

We have completed the trilogy of chapters explicitly devoted to a presentation of the foundational notion of ethics and an exploration of some common or significant ethical issues. Chapter 1 dealt with topics such as informed consent, a caring approach, DNA testing, body cavity searches, evaluation of competence, patient assessment through a closed door, harm-reduction strategies, food loaf, and hunger strikes. In Chapter 2 we discussed several significant areas of ethical role conflict for correctional health professionals, including medical clearance for punishment, use of medicine for behavior control, and participation in capital punishment or acts of torture, and we touched on the need to report abuse of prisoners by staff. In Chapter 3 we reviewed the tragic history and the subsequent regulation of biomedical research involving prisoners as human subjects, the all-too-common practice of housing mentally ill and other prisoners in conditions of severe and extended isolation, and physician participation in court-ordered medical procedures such as chemical castration. We also examined the ethical duty of correctional health care professionals to recognize and share their insights to help prevent future fetal alcohol exposure that, for so many prisoners, was a factor leading to their subsequent involvement in the criminal justice system.

As to this latter point, it would be interesting to speculate on whether other insights gained through the practice of our profession in the correctional context could, if shared appropriately, likewise bring benefit to society. In a sense, the prison is like a laboratory magnifying the effect of certain stimuli or phenomena because of the density of concentration, the atmosphere of control, and the unique ability to observe. One such example is mentioned in Chapter 6, "Conceptualizing Mental Illness as a Chronic Condition," under "Conclusion: An Ethical Impera-tive." There it is suggested that correctional mental health professionals, based on their profound understanding of the countertherapeutic impact that prison and jail settings have on seriously mentally ill persons, should advocate in the community for effective strategies to minimize the number of mentally ill persons being arrested and brought into the criminal justice system in the first place.

Future chapters will raise some other particular obligations of correctional health care professionals—also within an ethical framework. These things should be done (or avoided) precisely because they are the right (or wrong) thing to do. Sometimes the law, by legislation or court ruling, tells us what to do, and this area will be explored especially in Chapter 4. However, in general our behavior must reflect the thoughtful and mature conviction of our personal and professional codes of con-duct. We will look at the factors to consider (or not consider) in deciding whether to treat (Chapter 5), the value of recognizing the chronic nature of mental illness (Chapter 6), the subtle influence of words and language on our attitude and behav-ior (Chapter 7), and the importance of medical autonomy and the public health role of corrections (Chapter 8). The ninth and final chapter will emphasize the need for mutual respect, dialogue, and cooperation between correctional staff and health care professionals to ensure the ethical delivery of humane health care for all prisoners.

Our review of ethical challenges reveals that subtle but consistent pressures to engage in unethical behavior can stem from the divergent objectives and methods of corrections and medicine. They can also be occasioned by fiscal scarcity, the profit motive, societal vindictiveness, or a dual loyalty to the ethical standards of our profession on the one hand and a competing sense of obligation to our employer, colleagues, country, or the good of society. We continue to examine how these con-flicting pressures can sometimes be reconciled by thoughtful and candid dialogue and sometimes by a careful and honest balancing of benefits and risks, always with due reflection and regard for the basic tenets of our ethical standards.

Not everyone will immediately agree with each of the conclusions that were drawn. Some people never will. If, however, these matters were uncomplicated and the answers were obvious, perhaps all would be of the same mind and this book would not need to have been written.

At the risk of oversimplification, the message of this book may be summarized as generally requiring correctional health care professionals to conceptualize and treat their patients in exactly the same way that they would if they were not pris-oners at all.

Chapter 4

Legal Issues in Correctional Health Care[*]

WHAT THE COURTS HAVE DONE

We do not need to look back far in history to discover almost unbelievably inadequate and shameful health care services in correctional facilities throughout the United States. As recently as the late 1970s, most health care services delivered to U.S. prisoners were provided by fellow inmates. Only a handful of civilian health care professionals worked in prisons and jails, and not all of these were fully reputable, competent, or licensed. Female employees were not allowed to work inside the secure perimeter, thereby excluding the majority of qualified health professionals, particularly nurses. Some of the inmate "nurses" developed fairly good skills and worked with dedication and care. But serious abuses abounded. There were no formal policies or procedures or protocols for health care. When they even existed, medical records were woefully inadequate. Some indication of "the way it used to be" in correctional health care may be found in Chapter 1, "Ethics in the Context of Correctional Health," under "A Brief Historical Perspective."

The momentous and revolutionary changes in correctional health care during the 1970s and 1980s did not begin in a vacuum. To understand how these changes came about, we must begin our review a bit earlier to look at important events and precedents. Prisoners would not have been accorded a constitutional right to health

[*] The author is immensely grateful for the helpful advice and insights provided by William J. Rold, JD, CCHP-A, who graciously consented to provide a general review of an earlier draft of this chapter and of excerpts from several other chapters that touch on legal matters. Bill is an experienced civil rights attorney and has practiced and taught in the field of correctional health care litigation for many years.

(Note: The author reminds the reader that no book can capture the entire evolution and progression of particular cases, whether they are historical or continue to unfold, and cautions the reader to seek specific legal advice when presented with a particular factual problem.)

care if prisoners were still held to be "slaves of the state," if the courts had maintained their "hands-off" posture, or if what transpired behind prison walls continued to escape public attention. It is therefore appropriate to touch briefly on a series of enabling events that opened the way for the groundbreaking court decisions of the 1970s that brought prison health care out of its callously inhumane and primitive status to one that today begins to approach the community standard of care.

HANDS-OFF POLICY

Contrary to popular belief, the Thirteenth Amendment to the U.S. Constitution did not abolish all slavery in the United States when it was ratified in 1865. The amendment reads as follows: "Neither slavery nor involuntary servitude, except as punishment for crimes whereof the party shall have been duly convicted, shall exist within the United States, or any place subject to their jurisdiction." Thus, the effect of this amendment was not to abolish slavery in its entirety but to limit it to persons convicted of crimes.

In an 1871 case (*Ruffin v. Commonwealth*), the Supreme Court of Virginia declared that prisoners were "slaves of the state":

The bill of rights is a declaration of general principles to govern a society of freemen, and not of convicted felons and men civilly dead. Such men have some rights it is true, such as the law in its benignity accords to them, but not the rights of freemen. They are the slaves of the State undergoing punishment for heinous crimes committed against the laws of the land. While in this state of penal servitude, they must be subject to the regulations of the institutions of which they are inmates, and the laws of the State to whom their service is due in expiation of their crimes.[1]

In many other states at that time, prisoners were officially deemed "civilly dead slaves of the state." Persons sentenced to prison typically lost all legal identity. Even when their liberty was restored after release from prison, convicted felons at that time had no right to vote, hold office, make contracts, own property, or compose a will because those rights remained forfeited to the state. This was an era when the Constitution stopped at the jailhouse wall.

In recent years, courts tend to follow the important proposition enunciated in *Coffin v. Reichard* [143 F. 2d 443, 6th Cir. (1944)] that incarceration deprives a prisoner "only of such liberties as the law has ordained he shall suffer for his transgressions." Thus, the government has a duty to protect prisoners from harm. *Coffin* is the first instance in which a federal appellate court declared that a person does not lose all civil rights on becoming a prisoner.

The Eighth Amendment to the U.S. Constitution, containing its prohibition of "cruel and unusual punishment," was ratified in 1791. Surprising though it may seem, however, the courts took no interest in the plight of prisoners. (There were exceptions. In a 1926 opinion, one judge explained the public's responsibility to provide medical care for prisoners: "It is but just that the public be required to care for the prisoner, who cannot by reason of the deprivation of his liberty, care for himself"—*Spicer v. Williamson*).[2]

Even though the Civil Rights Act under which so many prisoner lawsuits have been filed in recent years was enacted in 1871, the courts for another century consistently declared that conditions inside correctional institutions were outside their scope of interest and were best left in the capable hands of prison administrators. Part of the reason for this noninterventionist policy was the matter of separation of powers. Federal and state legislatures had delegated the responsibility for managing prisoners to the executive branch. Because the Constitution was silent on the issue, courts were reluctant to intervene. Another reason federal courts were reluctant to interfere in the cases of state prisoners was concern for states' rights. There is now broad agreement that involvement of the federal courts is not barred where alleged deprivations are of constitutional dimension.

When prisoners would on occasion attempt to file lawsuits, these might be intercepted by prison officials and discarded by wardens before they ever could reach a court or attorney.[3] Occasionally, a prisoner's pleadings would reach the attention of a judge, but the typical response was that the court does not interfere in the internal affairs of prisons or that the court defers to prison officials as the correctional experts in these matters. This approach came to be known as the "hands-off" doctrine and prevailed in this country until the 1970s. Moreover, if prisoners had no rights, it was easy for the courts to avoid the burden of overseeing correctional agencies.[4]

A BREAK IN THE HANDS-OFF ERA

As part of a growing trend toward increased protection of individual rights in the United States, the 1940s witnessed judicial decisions that augured an opening of the doors to prisoner litigation. In 1941, the U.S. Supreme Court (*Ex parte Hull*) held that inmates had a right to unrestricted access to federal courts and that "the state and its officers may not abridge or impair petitioner's right to apply to a federal court for a writ of habeas corpus. Whether a petition for writ of habeas corpus addressed to a federal court is properly drawn and what allegations it must contain are questions for that court alone to determine."[5]

State officials cannot enact regulations that "abridge" or "impair" an inmate's right of access to the courts. They cannot, for example, interfere with the right of inmates to file petitions in court. In 1944, a federal district court (*Coffin v. Reichard*) expanded the scope of habeas corpus to include lawsuits filed by inmates that challenged the conditions of their confinement but not the confinement itself. The same court held that "[t]he Government has the absolute right to hold prisoners for offenses against it, but it also has the correlative duty to protect them against assault or injury from any quarter while so held."

Although these decisions paved the way, change began in earnest in the early 1960s in the context of widespread social unrest that played a direct role in ending this hands-off policy. The courts began to chip away at the jailhouse wall, granting an expanding list of important constitutional protections to prisoners. Several events, in particular, deserve mention.

First, in 1961, the Supreme Court (*Monroe v. Pape*)[6] ruled that citizens could bring Title 42 U.S.C. §1983 suits against state officials without first exhausting all state judicial remedies. Although this court ruling strictly addressed only the rights of free citizens, other cases subsequently reasoned that it applied equally to prisoners. Thus, Section 1983 became a vehicle that prisoners could use to challenge the constitutionality of prison conditions. It will be discussed further in this chapter under "*Estelle v. Gamble.*"

Second, in 1962 in *Robinson v. California* [370 U.S. 660 (1962)] the Supreme Court extended the Eighth Amendment prohibition against cruel and unusual punishment to the states by reason of the due process clause of the Fourteenth Amendment.

Third, black Muslim prisoners who were experiencing blatant religious discrimination were successful in persuading the courts that their constitutional right to religious freedom was being violated. For example, *Fulwood v. Clemmer* [295 F. 2d 171 (1961)] in 1967 established that the Muslim faith must be recognized as a religion and that prison officials may not restrict members from holding services.

Fourth, during the civil rights movement of the 1960s, many white, middle-class citizens came into conflict with the law for the first time, largely through deliberate acts of civil disobedience. Liberal groups and foundations sponsored legal aid societies staffed with competent attorneys to defend persons arrested in connection with civil rights demonstrations. Heretofore, prisons and jails had been filled chiefly with society's outcasts and rejects—mostly black people and other minorities and poor people with little education or influence. Prisons were located far from population centers; the inmates were locked up and quite forgotten. At this juncture, however, the composition of the inmate population was changing. Many of these new prisoners were affluent and had influential connections on the outside, so a stream of effective, articulate, and credible reports disclosed the intolerable, shocking, and inhumane conditions of incarceration. The news media began to report the plight of inmates, and courts were no longer able to reject the allegations of inmates out of hand. Referring to this period, Margaret Wishart and Nancy Dubler wrote, "[F]or the first time since the American Revolution, political activism brought large numbers of well-connected, middle-class people to jail. This atypical prison population contributed to a growing awareness of prison conditions, legislative committee reports, and exposés in the national media."[7]

Fifth, the 1960s and early 1970s were times of widespread civil unrest and protest against the war in Vietnam. Having achieved major gains in the mid-1960s, civil rights activists began to turn their attention to the struggle for peace. Dr. Martin Luther King Jr. and the Southern Christian Leadership Conference, for example, used the effective tactics of civil disobedience and nonviolence. Influential and well-educated professionals and religious leaders championed the cause of draft resisters, organized boycotts of the draft, invaded federal draft centers and destroyed files, publicly burned draft cards, and conducted protests at munitions factories. Again, correctional facilities encountered educated, articulate, influential, credible, and compassionate inmates such as Angela Davis, Huey Newton, and the Catholic priests Daniel and Philip Berrigan who eloquently recited their tales of injustice and inhumane conditions to the courts and the press.

Sixth, the conscience of the nation was awakened in 1972 by a deadly riot at a state maximum security prison in Attica, New York. Millions of Americans watched their television sets each evening as network media vividly portrayed the atrocities and violence of the Attica uprising and the equally violent retaking of control by the authorities. The McKay Commission was established to review the events and noted that "medical care was one of the primary inmates' grievances."[8] The plight of inmates, so long successfully hidden, had come suddenly and dramatically to public view and attention.

Seventh, a phenomenon of the 1960s and early 1970s that facilitated an active role for the courts in prison reform arose from the so-called War on Poverty. This federally funded program of the Office of Economic Opportunity in the administration of President Lyndon Johnson directed attention to weak, defenseless, and powerless groups in the country and promoted an awareness of their rights and entitlements.

In 1968, California amended its penal code to grant prisoners certain rights, including the right to inherit real estate and personal property; to correspond confidentially with attorneys, holders of public office, and the media; to receive most books and printed material available to the public; and to own written material that they produced while imprisoned. As a result, both the press and public officials began to hear of inhumane conditions and physical abuse inside the state's prisons. What followed were decades of investigation, scandal, and court oversight of California prison practices.

Holt v. Sarver

This period also saw a change in membership of the U.S. Supreme Court. Under Chief Justice Earl Warren (1953–1969), the Court extended many protections to criminal defendants, including the exclusionary rule, *Miranda* warnings, and the right to counsel at any "critical stage" in a defendant's prosecution. This led to the focus on protection of the individual rights of persons convicted of crimes. The Warren Court's liberal rulings generally remained in effect throughout the tenure of Chief Justice Warren E. Burger (1969–1980). The much more conservative court of Chief Justice William Rehnquist (1986–2005), however, granted correctional officials considerable discretion to decide what restrictions should be placed on inmates, consistent with Rehnquist's belief that the Fourteenth Amendment had been misapplied with regard to prisoners' rights.

One important decision was *Holt v. Sarver* [442 F. 2d 304 (1971)]. A federal district court in Arkansas determined that inmates could challenge as unconstitutional not merely individual practices but also the totality of a prison's conditions.

This form of suit became known as the "conditions of confinement" lawsuit. The judge enjoined the prison system from inflicting cruel and unusual punishment as prohibited by the Eighth and Fourteenth Amendments and from interfering with access to court. This set the stage for other successful challenges of the cumulative effect of confinement conditions by prisoners in several Southern states, especially Alabama and Texas.

Newman v. Alabama

An early case involving the medical care of prisoners attracted national attention in 1974. In *Newman v. Alabama*,[9] which was tried in the Alabama federal court of Judge Frank M. Johnson, plaintiffs alleged the existence of inhumane conditions and deprivation of health care throughout the Alabama state correctional system. The court found inter alia that "unsupervised prisoners without formal training regularly pull teeth, screen sick-call patients, dispense as well as administer medication, including dangerous drugs, give injections, take x-rays, suture, and perform minor surgery." Among examples of abuse cited were the case of a quadriplegic whose bedsores had become infested with maggots because his bandage had not been changed in the four weeks before his death and the case of a patient whose prescribed intravenous feeding had not been administered during the three days prior to his death.

In 1974, Judge Frank Johnson declared that the overall health care delivery system in Alabama prisons was constitutionally impermissible. The court also held that "disorganized lines of therapeutic responsibility" contributed to an Eighth Amendment violation. The court ruled:

[F]ailure of board of corrections to provide sufficient medical facilities and staff to afford inmates basic elements of adequate medical care constituted willful and intentional violation of rights of prisoners guaranteed under Eighth and Fourteenth Amendments and intentional refusal by correctional officers to allow inmates access to medical personnel and to provide prescribed medicines and other treatment was cruel and unusual punishment in violation of the Constitution.

"Excessive bail shall not be required, nor excessive fines imposed, nor cruel and unusual punishments inflicted."

—Eighth Amendment to U. S. Constitution

Estelle v. Gamble

Not long after the *Newman* decision, the now famous *Estelle v. Gamble* [429 U.S. 97 (1976)] case was decided in the U.S. Supreme Court in 1976. Gamble, a state prisoner in Texas, was assigned the job of unloading bales of cotton from boxcars.

He injured his back and received treatment from prison medical staff. He later filed suit in federal court, alleging inadequate medical care and treatment and complaining that he had been punished for his inability to work. The case eventually went to the Supreme Court. Indeed, Gamble had been seen 17 times by prison health care staff and had been treated for his injury. Therefore, the court declared that no constitutional right had been violated, but it acknowledged that Gamble might have a valid claim of tort liability (medical malpractice) in a state court. The criterion proclaimed by the Supreme Court in *Estelle v. Gamble* to determine whether a case involved a constitutional issue was whether "there was deliberate indifference to the serious medical needs of inmates." It went on to say that the Constitution is violated if care is intentionally denied, if access to care is prevented, or if physicians' orders and prescriptions for care are not followed. The celebrated passage, written by Justice Thurgood Marshall, reads as follows:

We therefore conclude that deliberate indifference to serious medical needs of prisoners constitutes the "unnecessary and wanton infliction of pain," proscribed by the Eighth Amendment. This is true whether the indifference is manifested by prison doctors in their response to the prisoner's needs or by prison guards in intentionally denying or delaying access to medical care or intentionally interfering with the treatment once prescribed. Regardless of how evidenced, deliberate indifference to a prisoner's serious illness or injury states a cause of action under §1983.

The floodgates were now open. Prisoner-initiated lawsuits were filed in great numbers. Many lawyers and legal aid societies were eager and willing to bring these pleadings to court. The times had radically changed during the decade from the late 1960s to the late 1970s. Before then, the walls of correctional institutions were as effective in keeping the public from seeing what occurred behind the gates as they were in preventing prisoners from escaping. But 10 years later, much of the secrecy was gone. The courts emphatically and with determination had stepped in and made a difference.

Change never comes easily, and there was stubborn and prolonged resistance. States' rights issues were raised. For a time, most state and local jurisdictions stonewalled the courts, tried all manner of delaying tactics, and steadfastly refused to acknowledge or fix the problems. Little by little, however, the courts gained ground. In some cases, wide-ranging consent decrees were wrested from the correctional systems in which compromise agreements were reached, often promising to improve conditions beyond what the Constitution itself guaranteed.

Today, most correctional jurisdictions have been sued successfully by one or more inmates who alleged improper care or conditions of confinement. The majority of suits continue to be brought in federal court, although some are filed in state courts. Many are class action suits, often filed under the Civil Rights Act, Title 42 U.S.C. Section 1983, alleging violation of civil rights.

Section 1983 reads in part, "Every person who, under color of any statute, ordinance, regulation, custom, or usage, of any State or Territory, subjects, or causes to be subjected, any citizen of the United States or other person within the jurisdiction thereof to the deprivation of any rights, privileges, or immunities, secured by the Constitution and laws, shall be liable to the party injured in an action at law, suit in equity, or other proper proceeding for redress."

The Civil Rights Act was intended to give federal protection against the ineffectiveness or unwillingness of states in protecting newly enfranchised blacks from the Ku Klux Klan. It gives the right to sue persons acting "under color of state law" for deprivation of "rights, privileges or immunities secured by the Constitution."

As Ian Forsythe explains: "In *Monroe*, the Supreme Court held that a police officer was acting "under color of state law" even though his actions *violated* state law. This was the first case in which the Supreme Court allowed liability to attach where a government official acted outside the scope of the authority granted to him by state law. In the years since *Monroe v. Pape* was decided, an extensive body of law has developed to govern Section 1983 claims."[10]

As remedies, the act allows money damages, equitable relief (injunctions), or other proper proceedings for redress. In 1961, the U.S. Supreme Court held that Section 1983 creates a remedy that is "supplementary" to state remedies, and therefore the existence of alternate state remedies does not require dismissal of the federal complaints. Thus, a litigant may choose whether to resort to a state court or a federal court for such relief.

Most prisoner plaintiffs expect to have a more receptive audience in lifetime-appointed federal judges who are further removed from local pressures than are elected state judges.

"If a State elects to impose imprisonment as a punishment for crime, I believe it has an obligation to provide the persons in its custody with a health care system which meets minimal standards of adequacy. As a part of that basic obligation, the State and its agents have an affirmative duty to provide reasonable access to medical care, to provide competent, diligent medical personnel, and to ensure that prescribed care is in fact delivered. For denial of medical care is surely not part of the punishment which civilized nations may impose for crime."

—Justice John Stevens (who cast the sole dissenting vote in *Estelle v. Gamble*)

Tort Liability

Lawsuits come in many varieties. Perhaps the most common is a suit for negligence or malpractice. This is under the concept of tort liability, the word *tort* meaning a civil wrong as opposed to a criminal wrong. Although this approach is not frequently used in the area of correctional health care, it can occur, so the concept should be understood.

There are some variations across different states with regard to what can affect the success or outcome of a malpractice lawsuit, but some general requirements must be met to bring a suit based on negligence.

1. There must be a *duty* owed to the person who claims to have been harmed, and this duty must be evident from the relationship between the parties.
2. There must be *negligence*—that is, the failure to exercise *due* care, defined as the care that a reasonably prudent and careful person would use under similar circumstances.
3. There must be *harm* done to someone as a result of *failure* to use *due* care. In other words, a person must have suffered some damages that a court could then remedy by an award of money if the negligence is proved.

By definition, negligence is not the same as deliberate or intentional harm done to someone. Some legal defenses, such as the contributory negligence of the person making the claim, specify that if the person who is harmed has some fault in the harm, then the claim may be prohibited or reduced by the extent of that person's participation in causing the harm.

In the medical context, doctors owe a duty of care to their patients. As long as the doctor exercises due care in making a diagnosis or giving a treatment, there would be no negligence even if harm occurs because of the doctor's actions. But a doctor who fails to exercise due care would be negligent and liable if the negligence causes damage. This is a civil wrong, or tort.

Malpractice suits are usually directed at a single act or omission and are governed by the laws of individual states. They are also rare occurrences in correctional litigation. In contrast, federal civil rights suits often attack the totality of medical care and conditions. These are the ones that have forced prison and jail administrators to begin revamping their health care systems.

Deliberate Indifference

The Supreme Court has noted that "(n)o static 'test' can exist by which courts determine whether conditions of confinement are cruel and unusual" [*Rhodes v. Chapman*, 452 U.S. 337 (1981) at 146]. Further, "[t]he basic concept underlying the Eighth Amendment is nothing less than the dignity of man. While the State has the authority to punish, the Amendment stands to assure that this power be exercised within the limits of civilized standards. . . . The Amendment must draw its meaning from the evolving standards of decency that mark the progress of a maturing society" [*Trop v. Dulles*, 356 U.S. 86 (1958)].

Deliberate indifference involves a reckless disregard of a known risk. It differs from intentional denial. In *Estelle v. Gamble* [429 U.S. at 104, 105 (1976)], the Supreme Court ruled that the proper standard to be applied in considering prisoners' medical cases was whether the action or nonaction of prison officials showed "deliberate indifference to serious medical needs of prisoners." This was defined as the "wanton infliction of unnecessary pain" that can be "manifested by prison doctors in their response to the prisoner's needs or by prison guards in intentionally denying or delaying access to medical care or intentionally interfering with the treatment once prescribed."

The Court noted that Gamble's treatment might constitute medical malpractice under state law but ruled that mere malpractice did not amount to deliberate indifference and a violation of the Constitution. Disagreement with prison officials about what constitutes appropriate medical care does not state a cognizable claim under the Eighth Amendment.

In *Todaro v. Ward* [565 F. 2d 48 (1977)], the Court stated:

While a single instance of medical care denied or delayed, viewed in isolation, may appear to be the product of mere negligence, repeated examples of such treatment bespeak a deliberate indifference by prison authorities to the agony engendered by haphazard and ill-conceived procedures. . . . When systematic deficiencies in staffing, facilities or procedures make unnecessary suffering inevitable, a court will not hesitate to use its injunctive powers.

As Ellen J. Winner explains, "By permitting or engaging in a *pattern* of delay, neglect, or refusal to provide medical care, those in a position of responsibility may be found to be deliberately indifferent to the needs of a class of prisoners as a whole, even without a specific motive against any particular prisoner."[11] A subjective test is required for deliberate indifference. The plaintiff must prove that defendant was aware of the serious need and ignored it. Missing a medication occasionally is not deliberate indifference, but a pattern of missing medications for a number of inmates might be enough evidence to rise to a claim of deliberate indifference. As an example, Winner cites the situation in *Todaro v. Ward* in which the court found that the screening system for women prisoners' medical complaints, conducted by nurses from behind a barred door, in a residence building lobby, without privacy, adequate record keeping, or medical equipment inevitably caused delay and denial of needed medical care and unnecessary suffering.

"The basic concept underlying the Eighth Amendment is nothing less than the dignity of man. While the State has the authority to punish, the Amendment stands to assure that this power be exercised within the limits of civilized standards. . . . The Amendment must draw its meaning from the evolving standards of decency that mark the progress of a maturing society."

—*Trop v. Dulles*

The sole dissenting vote in *Estelle v. Gamble* came from Justice John Stevens. Time has shown that his criticism of the majority was quite appropriate: "I believe the Court improperly attaches significance to the subjective motivation of the defendant as a criterion for determining whether cruel and unusual punishment has been inflicted. Subjective motivation may well determine what, if any, remedy is appropriate against a particular defendant. However, whether the constitutional standard has been violated should turn on the character of the punishment, rather than the motivation of the individual who inflicted it."[12] The reasoning of Justice Stevens, as expressed in his dissent, is instructive:

If a State elects to impose imprisonment as a punishment for crime, I believe it has an obligation to provide the persons in its custody with a health care system which meets minimal standards of adequacy. As a part of that basic obligation, the State and its agents have an affirmative duty to provide reasonable access to medical care, to provide competent, diligent medical personnel, and to ensure that prescribed care is in fact delivered. For denial of medical care is surely not part of the punishment which civilized nations may impose for crime. Of course, not every instance of improper health care violates the Eighth Amendment. Like the rest of us, prisoners must take the risk that a competent, diligent physician will make an error. Such an error may give rise to a tort claim but not necessarily to a constitutional claim. But when the State adds to this risk, as by providing a physician who does not meet minimum standards of competence or diligence or who cannot give adequate care because of an excessive caseload or inadequate facilities, then the prisoner may suffer from a breach of the State's constitutional duty.

Qualified Immunity

Qualified immunity is "a legal concept applied in civil rights cases, which says that when a government official, exercising a discretionary power, violates the federally protected rights of someone, such as an inmate, the official is not liable for damages if the official's actions do not violate clearly established statutory or constitutional rights of which a reasonable person would have known" [*Babcock v. White*, 102 F. 3d 267, 7th Cir. (1996)]. Note that qualified immunity only protects against damage claims. Injunctive relief is not foreclosed.

Ian Forsythe points out that a government official is entitled to qualified immunity unless his "act is so obviously wrong, in the light of preexisting law, that only a plainly incompetent officer or one who was knowingly violating the law would have done such a thing."[13] Although the qualified immunity defense has some similarity to the "good faith" defense, the official's subjective good faith is virtually irrelevant in deciding whether the official is protected by qualified immunity. Saying "I was simply following policy" will not normally suffice if the policy is inconsistent with the law.

Only "persons" under federal statute are subject to liability. A state is not a person subject to suit under §1983. Municipalities and local governments are "persons" subject to suit for damages as well as prospective relief, but the United States government and individual states are not. Employees of federal, state, and local government may be sued in their individual capacities for damages, declaratory, or injunctive relief.

"Both state and federal courts have jurisdiction over §1983 suits," ruled the U.S. Supreme Court in *Haywood v. Drown* [556 U.S., 129 S. Ct. 2108 (2009)] in 2009. The court struck down a New York statute that barred all damages lawsuits brought under Section 1983 against prison officers. "Whatever its merits, New York's policy of shielding corrections officers from liability when sued for damages arising out of conduct performed in the scope of their employment is contrary to Congress' judgment that *all* persons who violate federal rights while acting under color of state law shall be held liable for damages."

A prisoner was handcuffed to a metal hitching post and left shirtless, virtually without water, and without bathroom breaks in the Alabama sun for seven hours. The Supreme Court [*Hope v. Pelzer,* 536 U.S. 730 (2002)] ruled in 2002 that officers should have known that their actions were unlawful, and therefore the defense of qualified immunity did not apply. Their actions were such an obvious violation of the plaintiff's Eighth Amendment rights that the Court's prior cases put the correctional officials on notice that using the hitching post would violate the Eighth Amendment. The Supreme Court found that "respondents knowingly subjected [plaintiff] to a substantial risk of physical harm, unnecessary pain [caused by the handcuffs and the restricted position of confinement for a seven-hour period], unnecessary exposure to the sun, prolonged thirst and taunting, and a deprivation of bathroom breaks that created a risk of particular discomfort and humiliation."

Independent-contractor physicians probably do not have "qualified immunity," but state officials do. The Supreme Court in *West v. Atkins* [487 U.S. 42 (1988)] ruled that a contractor paid by the state to provide medical services is a state actor and that the contractor also becomes liable for constitutional violations, commenting: "It is the physician's function within the state system, not the precise terms of his employment, that is determinative."

Farmer v. Brennan

The concept of awareness was further clarified in the unanimously decided case of *Farmer v. Brennan* [511 U.S. 825, 837 (1994)]. There must be *subjective* awareness. It is not enough that the prison official *ought to have known* about the excessive risk to a prisoner, but the official must *be subjectively aware* of the risk. "Prison officials may not be held liable if they prove that they were unaware of even an obvious risk or that they responded reasonably to a known risk, even if the harm ultimately was not averted." The prison official must *know of and disregard* an excessive risk to inmate health or safety. "The official must both be aware of facts from which the inference could be drawn that a substantial risk of serious harm exists, and he must also draw the inference." A deliberate indifference finding requires that the responsible person acted in reckless disregard of a risk of which he or she was aware, as would generally be required for a criminal charge of recklessness.

Farmer points out that "use of the subjective test does not foreclose prospective injunctive relief, or require a prisoner to suffer physical injury before obtaining prospective relief. The subjective test adopted today is consistent with the principle that '[o]ne does not have to await the consummation of a threatened injury to obtain preventive relief.'"

Dee Farmer, a transgender inmate of a federal prison, was housed with male prisoners and within two weeks was beaten and raped by her cell mate. The Court ruled that prison officials showed deliberate indifference to a substantial risk of serious harm, as long as they were subjectively aware of the risk and disregarded it. The *Farmer* decision was approved unanimously by the Court. Although Justices Harry A. Blackmun and John Paul Stevens concurred, they also expressed the opinion that inhumane conditions violated the Eighth Amendment regardless of the state of mind of prison officials.

For state officials to be found liable in their personal capacity under Section 1983, it must be shown that there was some personal involvement in the alleged violation. In civil rights suits, the issue is *personal* liability. The doctrine of *respondeat superior* or vicarious liability is not applicable [*Hays v. Jefferson County, Ky.*, 668 F. 2d 869, 874, 6th Cir. (1982)]. The appellant must show that the official participated directly, failed to remedy the wrong after being informed of the violation through a report or appeal, created a policy or custom under which unconstitutional practices occurred or allowed the continuance of such a policy or custom, or was grossly negligent in supervising subordinates who committed the wrongful acts. Supervisors become involved only for their failure to supervise, failure to train, or failure to budget or staff. In tort liability, however, the principle of *respondeat superior* applies.

Civil Rights of Institutionalized Persons Act

In 1980, Congress passed the Civil Rights of Institutionalized Persons Act (CRIPA),[14] which enables the U.S. attorney general to investigate and intervene to remedy a "pattern and practice" of unlawful conditions in public institutions.

The Civil Rights Act of 1871 and more notably its Section 1983 substantially altered the relationship between the federal government and states. States had long been considered sovereign, independent, and ultimately in charge of protecting the rights of all their citizens. This statute, however, altered states' power by empowering the federal government and the federal courts with the authority necessary to prevent and remedy violations of federal rights.[15]

With passage of CRIPA, a new mechanism became available for redressing wrongs in penal institutions. The attorney general of the United States was empowered to initiate suit in federal court, acting on behalf of institutionalized persons who are presumed—because of mental illness, mental retardation, prisoner status, youth, or orphan status—to not have the capability (or are impaired in their ability to) file a suit on their own behalf. The office of the attorney general must make a determination, so as to have standing to file suit under CRIPA, that under color of state law, the jurisdiction is depriving institutionalized persons of their civil rights guaranteed under the Constitution or laws of the United States.

Cases were filed by the attorney general's office and pursued vigorously for several years by competent plaintiff attorneys employed by the federal government.

The enthusiasm and aggressive prosecution of these cases, so evident during the Carter administration, waned under subsequent administrations but did not completely vanish.

Bivens v. Six Unknown Agents of the Federal Bureau of Narcotics

No federal statute, including the Civil Rights Act of 1871, authorizes the courts to hear suits or grant relief against federal officers who violate the U.S. Constitution. Section 1983 applies to states and local officers but not to the federal government or federal officials. However, in 1971, the Supreme Court ruled in *Bivens*[16] that a plaintiff could seek monetary damages from individual federal officers for their alleged violation of the plaintiff's Fourth Amendment right to be free from unjust search and seizure. The Court thus found that a federal law cause of action could be inferred directly from the Fourth Amendment.[17] Although the Court placed limitations on the application of *Bivens*, the case can serve as a parallel to Section 1983 suits when federal officials are involved.

See, however, the issue of private prisons housing federal inmates that was raised in *Minneci v. Pollard*; this is discussed later in this chapter under "Some Important Legal Cases."

PULLING IN THE REINS

A 1995 National Institute of Justice report[18] gave voice to the concern that although the courts established a floor under health care for prisoners, they have failed to define an appropriate ceiling. The courts have ordered the provision of many services, but they have not placed or defined limits on what must be provided. As a result, an inexorable and unrestrained pressure to raise costs and escalate the quality of health care services for prisoners was alleged.

On the other hand, intervention by the courts has been and remains necessary to ensure that inmates are guaranteed care that is not "cruel and unusual punishment" and is consistent with the contemporary standards of professional practice in the community. Little political advantage accrues to elected officials who increase expenditures for prisoners, but the desire to avoid lawsuits can provide a necessary measure of motivation. In addition, the view that the very large costs incurred by prison systems in accomplishing the improvements ordered by the courts were indeed excessive must be tempered by two important facts:

1. The vast majority of these improvements were basic, fundamental, and long overdue given the centuries' old neglect.
2. The cost of these improvements was substantially escalated by long protracted and drawn-out litigation and by sluggish implementation of court orders because jurisdictions typically planted their feet in a stubborn adversarial stance and actively resisted every step of the way. This increased both legal and monitoring costs far beyond what could have been the case if medical experts from both sides had been permitted to meet

and hammer out what community standards require of an adequate health care system—that is, what was necessary and appropriate—and then move ahead. This has happened in state after state.

Correctional health care administrators can and should develop a reasonable and fair strategy, consistent with community standards and practice, to ration or limit access to unnecessary health care services. The difficult and somewhat daunting task of defining appropriate and necessary health care is both timely and legitimate. Courts have not implied any prohibition of such efforts. See Chapter 5, "How Much Care Is Appropriate and Necessary?," for an extensive discussion about how a correctional system can determine what health care procedures are necessary.

The last word has not been heard on this subject. Recent decisions have signaled a much more conservative interpretation than what the Supreme Court pronounced in *Estelle v. Gamble*. In *Wilson v. Seiter* [501 U.S. 294 (1991)], the Court made it more difficult to hold correctional institutions and their officials liable for bad confinement conditions because the plaintiff must now show a culpable state of mind on the part of prison officials.[19] Justice Clarence Thomas even challenged the "deliberate indifference" standard of *Estelle v. Gamble* in 1993, although none of the other justices shared his views.[20] In *Helling v. McKinney* [509 U.S. 25 (1993)], Justice Thomas argued that there are "substantial doubts" whether prison conditions are within the scope of the cruel and unusual punishments clause at all, and stated that he "might vote to overrule *Estelle*" if the issue were squarely presented. He reached this conclusion based on his reasoning that the Eighth Amendment referred to *punishment* as the penalty ordered by a judicial tribunal, not the prison conditions and deprivations. Given these developments, what the court will do in the third and fourth decades of the 21st century is open to speculation.

Prison Litigation Reform Act of 1996[21]

On April 26, 1996, the Prison Litigation Reform Act (PLRA)[22] was signed into law, radically affecting both individual and class action suits brought by or on behalf of prisoners. It provided new procedural requirements and restrictions on bringing actions and limited the ability of courts to order relief. This law extends only to prison, jail, and juvenile facility cases. Lawsuits brought by inmates of mental institutions, for example, are not affected. It also applies only to the federal courts and not to an action in a state court unless it is a civil rights case brought under Title 42 U.S.C. Section 1983.

Administrative remedies now must be exhausted in any federal action involving prison conditions, including civil rights actions under Section 1983. The law also amends Section 7 of the Civil Rights of Institutionalized Persons Act to provide that "[n]o action shall be brought with respect to prison conditions under Section 1983 of this title or any other Federal law, by a prisoner confined in any jail, prison, or other correctional facility until such administrative remedies as are available are exhausted."

Josh Kurtzman offers some helpful advice to plaintiffs on how to overcome the exhaustion requirement of the PLRA, namely, challenging whether administrative remedies were truly available. He suggests that valid reasons for questioning availability include lack of remedies, improper guidance from prison staff, and intimidation and fear of reprisal by prison staff.[23]

The same act provides that defendants need not reply, unless so ordered by the court, to any action by a prisoner under Section 1983 or any other federal law and that failure to reply will not constitute an admission of the allegation of the complaint. Further, the court can grant no relief to the plaintiff until the defendant responds. A judge can order the defendant to reply only if the court finds that the plaintiff has a reasonable opportunity to prevail on the merits.

The PLRA also provides that inmate plaintiffs may not recover damages for mental or emotional injury sustained while in custody without a prior showing of physical injury [42 U.S.C. § 1997e(e) (2007)]. Many courts have held that this provision applies even to all personal injuries—including proven violations of prisoners' religious rights, free speech rights, and due process rights—so that none of these are compensable because their violation is not accompanied by physical injury. Some courts have even ruled that sexual assault, including forcible rape and sodomy, do not constitute "physical injury" within the meaning and intent of the PLRA.

For example, in *Hancock v. Payne* [2006 WL 21751 at *3, S.D. Miss. (2006)], the U.S. magistrate judge in the Southern District of Mississippi dismissed a lawsuit that had been filed by several male inmates who alleged they had been sodomized. The judge wrote: "The plaintiffs do not make any claim of physical injury beyond the bare allegation of sexual assault."

This provision of the PLRA would make even severe psychological trauma exempt from judicial scrutiny. As noted in Chapter 3 under "Housing Mentally Ill in Isolation or Supermax Settings," long-term confinement in segregation as in the isolated conditions of a supermax facility can result in real and serious injuries. In an interview with Human Rights Watch in 2008, Dr. Terry Kupers stated: "What we know is that long-term isolated confinement causes difficulty thinking, cognitive impairment, and difficulty with memory. A very frequent, almost universal symptom is that they've stopped reading, because it's useless to read—they can't remember what they read three pages ago. . . . I've never met anybody who hasn't been damaged by long-term confinement in segregation."[24]

These provisions of the law have placed most violations of prisoner rights outside the reach of the courts—a major step back toward the hands-off era from which we had so recently emerged.

In addition, the PLRA terminated then existing settlements and consent decrees in cases that were final and required all actions to be dismissed where there had been no finding by the court that the relief "extends no further than necessary to correct the violation of the Federal Right, and is the least restrictive means necessary to correct the violation of the Federal Right" (PLRA § 802, amending 18 U.S.C. § 3626). If prospective relief was ordered by a court with respect to prison conditions, such relief automatically was to be terminable on the motion of any party or intervener two years after it was granted or one year after the court entered an order denying termination. Previously, many prisoner suits were settled between the parties without any finding or admission of liability. Such settlements, according to the PLRA, also are subject to dismissal.

Another serious problem with the PLRA is the inclusion of juvenile institutions within its scope. Because of their immaturity and limited education, persons confined in juvenile institutions are even less able to comprehend and navigate the cumbersome and often vague administrative labyrinth of the grievance and administrative redress system. And the courts, under PLRA, have refused to allow their parents or guardians to plead on their behalf on grounds that the child had failed to exhaust the administrative remedies available. In one such case (*Minix v. Pazera*) that involved allegations that a youth had been repeatedly beaten and raped, the mother's claim in federal court was dismissed because the child had failed to file a grievance within the time limit of two business days as prescribed by the facility policy.[25]

It is this author's contention that embracing juvenile inmates within the purview of PLRA was an especially inappropriate and unjustifiable step because the amount of litigation brought on behalf of juveniles was hitherto minimal. (As of 1998, fewer than a dozen reported opinions directly involved challenges to conditions in juvenile detention centers.[26])

According to Jessica Feierman of the Juvenile Law Center:

Juveniles do not file frivolous lawsuits. Indeed, there was no legislative history when the Act was passed to suggest that children file frivolous lawsuits. Even before the PLRA was enacted, juveniles engaged in very little inmate litigation. . . . More importantly, a preexisting mechanism protects the courts from a flood of frivolous litigation by incarcerated youth: persons under age 18 cannot file civil lawsuits on their own. Federal Rule 17(c) requires that a guardian, "next friend" or guardian *ad litem* represent a minor in any civil lawsuit. . . . Such an adult will not proceed with a frivolous lawsuit—the Federal Rules of Civil Procedure provide for sanctions against lawyers who file frivolous suits, and our experience is clear that parents do not bring suits on their children's behalf without going to lawyers first.[27]

Several significant lawsuits involving juvenile facilities are mentioned later in this chapter—and none involve trivial or frivolous complaints.

The PLRA also limits the ability of the federal court to appoint special masters and allows them to be appointed only during the remedial phase of the action. Their involvement is restricted to conducting hearings and preparing proposed findings of fact. Moreover, the special masters are prohibited from any ex parte communications. Consequently, because all contact with any party must take place in a formal hearing on the record and with all parties represented, the special masters no longer can attempt through individual negotiation and persuasion to facilitate settlement or cooperative working among the parties to the case.

The PLRA severely limits the monetary compensation that may be paid to attorneys and special masters. Compensation of the special master is no longer to be paid by the defendants and must now be paid out of judicial funds. Some lawyers refuse to touch prisoner litigation because of the cost of experts, limits on fee recovery under the PLRA, and unsympathetic juries.

Because the PLRA did not prohibit receiverships, it may be that receivers will be appointed in situations where special masters may have been used in the past. The court still can appoint experts who may be able to perform some of the functions that masters typically have done. In simple terms, the difference is this: a receiver has direct executive authority and acts in place of the agency administrator. Special masters monitor the compliance activities of other parties, lack direct executive authority, and must rely on the federal court to order changes when they discover problems in compliance with court orders. Unlike the monitor and special master, the receiver completely displaces the defendants. The receiver makes both large and small decisions, spends the agency's funds, and controls hiring and firing decisions.[28]

These and other PLRA provisions have had a decidedly chilling effect on prisoner litigation. Essentially, access to the courts is severely restricted, initial liability is harder to demonstrate, and broad relief is more difficult to obtain.

Urgent Need for Reform of the PLRA

The PLRA was a "backdoor" legislative amendment to an appropriations bill and might not have achieved successful passage had its terms been subjected to appropriate deliberation and public airing. In fact, this sweeping bill was the subject of a single legislative hearing before the House Committee on the Judiciary, Subcommittee on Crime, and was accorded extremely limited debate. Margo Schlanger and Giovanna Shay[29] point out that, because of its hurried and sloppy drafting, within its first 10 years it required six decisions by the U.S. Supreme Court to resolve conflicting interpretations or challenges by federal appellate courts.[30]

The Commission on Safety and Abuse in America's Prisons included this recommendation in its 2006 report:

Several misguided provisions of the Prison Litigation Reform Act enacted in 1996 must be changed so that the federal courts can deliver justice to individual prisoners who are victims of rape, excessive use of force, and gross medical neglect, and compel reform in facilities where prisoners and staff are in danger.[31]

In January 2007, the Supreme Court [*Jones v. Bock*, 127 S. Ct. 910 (2007)] ruled that the U.S. Sixth Circuit Court of Appeals was overly zealous in the way it was applying the PLRA. Although the PLRA was designed to weed out frivolous lawsuits by prisoners, the Sixth Circuit had been tossing out such cases unless prisoners demonstrated in their complaints that they had exhausted all ways of resolving their grievances short of going to court. Thus, lawsuits were being dismissed if each defendant named in the lawsuit had not also been named in the original griev-ance that the prisoner had filed with prison officials. The court found this to be an excessive burden for the prisoners, and although the prisoners must exhaust adminis-trative remedies before going to court, it is up to the government to raise that issue as a potential defense, not for prisoners to demonstrate in the complaint. Writing for the Court, Chief Justice Roberts stated that we "now concede that these rules are not required by the PLRA, and that crafting and imposing them exceeds the proper limits on the judicial role."

In a recent Maryland case, a prisoner alleged assault by two officers and reported the incident to an internal investigative unit that found against one of the officers. The inmate then sued in federal court, and the officer was found liable. However, the other officer raised as an affirmative defense that the plaintiff had not exhausted all administrative remedies, and the case was dismissed. The inmate appealed, claiming that the internal investigation process was a substitute for other adminis-trative remedies. The appellate court found in favor of the inmate, stating that " 'spe-cial circumstances' can excuse a failure to comply with administrative procedural requirements, particularly when the inmate reasonably, even though mistakenly, believed he had sufficiently exhausted his remedies." The U.S. Supreme Court unan-imously (eight to zero) overturned the appellate court (*Ross v. Blake*) in June 2016, ruling that "[t]he PLRA speaks in unambiguous terms, providing that '[n]o action shall be brought' absent exhaustion of available administrative remedies. § 1997e(a). Aside from one significant qualifier—that administrative remedies must indeed be 'available'—the text suggests no limits on an inmate's obligation to exhaust. That mandatory language means a court may not excuse a failure to exhaust, even to take 'special circumstances' into account."[32]

As Justice Elena Kagan stated, in her opinion deciding *Ross v. Blake*, "Manda-tory exhaustion statutes like the PLRA establish mandatory exhaustion regimes, foreclosing judicial discretion." Thus exhaustion is mandatory, regardless of any "special circumstances." In view of this decision, it is now clearly evident that legis-lative action will be required to correct this excessive impediment to access to the courts by prisoners and to ensure that their right to judicial review will be safeguarded.

Although the PLRA achieved its two explicit principal objectives—limiting the number of frivolous prisoner lawsuits and addressing intrusive consent decrees governing prison conditions—as Schlanger and Shea assert, "it has become clear that the PLRA is undermining the rule of law in America's prisons."[33]

If the intent of the PLRA was not to impede legitimate lawsuits that allege serious cases affecting life-threatening deliberate indifference by authorities, sexual assaults, religious discrimination, and retaliation against use of free speech rights, then we would certainly expect to see a noticeable increase in the percentage of successful inmate-initiated lawsuits along with a reduction in the overall number of lawsuits. Indeed, the latter result is clear and obvious. The number of prisoner-initiated fed-eral lawsuits dropped by nearly 60 percent from 26 cases per thousand in 1995 to just 11 per thousand in 2005. However, the proportion of successful lawsuits also declined. Many more cases are dismissed, and fewer settle. What is occurring is that constitutionally meritorious cases are now faced with new and often insurmountable obstacles. One major impediment is the requirement that there be physical injury for an inmate to recover damages. Mental or emotional injury suffered while in custody is no longer a sufficient reason. Even cases of sexual assault, coerced sodomy, and rape are being dismissed as not constituting physical injury. In one case of an inmate suing because his face had been burned, the court dismissed charges on grounds that the burns had healed and there were no lasting effects (*Brown v. Simmons*).[34] A second reason is the requirement [42 U.S.C. §1997e(a) (2007)] that "no action shall be brought with respect to prison conditions under section 1983 of this title, or any other Federal law, by a prisoner confined in any jail, prison, or other correctional facility until such administrative remedies as are available are exhausted."

Schlanger and Shay ask, "What if the administrative remedies are very difficult to access? If the deadlines are very short, for example, or the number of administrative appeals required is very large? Or if the requisite form is repeatedly unavailable, or the prisoner fears retaliation for use of the grievance system? . . . What if the grievance system seems not to cover the complaint the prisoner seeks to make? Or if he is unable to fill out a grievance because he is in the hospital?"[35]

To bring the importance and urgency of radical PLRA reform to the attention of legislators, a concerted and sustained effort will be required on the part of thoughtful correctional personnel and correctional health care personnel, including their professional associations.

As a result, the PLRA offers a perverse incentive for correctional administrators to create even higher procedural hurdles in their grievance processes. After all, the more onerous the grievance rules, the less likely a prisoner will successfully sue. It is reasonable to expect a governmental agency to want to avoid lawsuits and adverse judgments. Thus, the PLRA's exhaustion provision effectively and arbitrarily places constitutional violations beyond the purview of the courts. While prisoners should be required to present their grievances and claims to authorities for review and redress prior to court filing, there needs to be a reasonable limit or suitable alternatives.

Since 1996, legal services programs that receive federal funding have been prohibited from representing prisoners. Such programs used to assist prisoners in bringing meritorious suits regarding truly egregious practices, and they also advised prisoners when there was no basis for bringing a suit. This is the most effective way to prevent frivolous lawsuits.[36]

The Prison Abuse Remedies Act has been brought repeatedly before the U.S. House of Representatives, thus far without success.[37] It calls, inter alia, for amendment of the PLRA by eliminating the requirement of a prior showing of physical injury, providing for a 90-day stay of nonfrivolous claims to allow prison officials to consider such claims through the administrative process, excluding application of the PLRA to prisoners under age 18, expanding the discretionary authority of judges in awarding relief in actions involving prison conditions, and revising the requirements for assessing filing fees and costs against prisoners in such actions. Each of these recommendations was included in a policy approved by the American Bar Association's House of Delegates in February 2007.[38]

To bring the importance and urgency of radical PLRA reform to the attention of legislators, a concerted and sustained effort will be required on the part of thoughtful correctional personnel and correctional health care personnel, including their professional associations.

MISCELLANEOUS LEGAL ISSUES

Adequacy of Funding

Courts have taken the position that cost should not be a factor in determining what is "adequate" health care for prisoners. The principle that a limited budget will not justify insufficient care has been clearly acknowledged by numerous courts. For example:

- The position of (then) Judge Harry Blackmun in *Jackson v. Bishop* [404 F. 2d 571, 8th Cir. (1968)] is representative: "Humane considerations and constitutional requirements are not, in this day, to be measured or limited by dollar considerations. . . ."
- "Lack of funds for facilities cannot justify an unconstitutional lack of competent medical care or treatment of inmates" [*Anderson v. City of Atlanta*, 778 F. 2d 678 (1985)].
- "Inadequate resources can never be an adequate justification for depriving any person of his constitutional rights" (*Hamilton v. Love*). Similar statements are found in *Gates v. Collier*, *Moore v. Morgan*, and *Battle v. Anderson* (1977).[39]
- "Humane considerations and constitutional requirements are not, in this day, to be measured or limited by dollar considerations" [*Ozecki v. Gaugham*, 459 F. 2d 6, 8, 1st. Cir. (1972)].
- "Where state institutions have been operating under unconstitutional conditions and practices, the defense of fund shortage(s) and the inability of the district court to order appropriations by the state legislature, have been rejected by the federal courts" [*Smith v. Sullivan*, 553 F. 2d 373 (1977)].

Thus, where the need for health care reaches constitutional proportions, these courts would require that it be provided regardless of cost.

Persons with Disabilities

Section 504 of the Rehabilitation Act of 1973 [29 U.S.C. §794(a)] established a policy requiring public entities that receive federal funding to operate without discrimination on the basis of disability. Thus, this law applies to the Federal Bureau of Prisons and to any state prisons or local jails that receive federal funds. In 1990, the Americans with Disabilities Act (ADA) was passed by Congress, and its sponsor, Senator Tom Harkin (D-IA), hailed it as an "emancipation proclamation for all persons with disabilities." It is certainly the most extensive civil rights legislation since the Civil Rights Act of 1964. Its stated purpose is to provide "a clear and comprehensive mandate for the elimination of discrimination against individuals with disabilities."[40] An important point to note is that, whereas Section 504 applies only to facilities that have some federal funding, the ADA applies to all public facilities. Its Title II (42 U.S.C. §12132) is the section that is relevant to correctional facilities: "[N]o qualified individual with a disability shall, by reason of such disability, be excluded from participation in or be denied the benefits of the services, programs, or activities of a public entity, or be subjected to discrimination by any such entity." Note that courts have repeatedly held that the ADA and the Rehabilitation Act are generally construed to impose the same requirements. Because the language of the acts is substantially the same, they apply the same analysis to both.

This language initially held great promise for physically and mentally disabled prisoners. Their plight includes problems with mobility, activities of daily living, hearing, eyesight, mental and intellectual disability, and access to such areas as law libraries, visiting areas, yards, laundry facilities, dining halls, vocational training, recreational facilities, bathing and restroom facilities, medical clinics, classrooms, and religious services. Mentally ill inmates often face a range of discriminatory practices, including punishment for conduct they cannot control that may result in solitary confinement for months or years at a time. Prisoners are almost totally dependent on the institution for their care. The handicapped who cannot even take care of their own personal needs are deprived indeed. Few prisons made accommodations sufficient to enable handicapped persons to participate in institutional employment or in rehabilitation programs (including sex-offender rehabilitation, substance-abuse rehabilitation, anger management, and life-skills training), even when such programs were mandated as a condition for parole or release.

The preamble to the federal regulations for Title II of the ADA states: "A public entity is not, however, required to provide attendant care, or assistance in toileting, eating, or dressing to individuals with disabilities, except in special circumstances, such as where the individual is an inmate of a custodial or correctional institution" [28 CFR subpart B, §35.130 (b)(8)].

The Title II Technical Assistance Manual of the Department of Justice specifically lists "jails and prisons" as types of facilities that, if constructed or altered after the effective date of the ADA (January 26, 1992), must be designed and constructed so that they are readily accessible to and usable by individuals with disabilities.[41] Five percent of residential units in jails and prisons, reformatories, and other detention or correctional facilities must be accessible.

"[N]o qualified individual with a disability shall, by reason of such disability, be excluded from participation in or be denied the benefits of the services, programs, or activities of a public entity, or be subjected to discrimination by any such entity."
—Title II of the Americans for Disability Act of 1990

When the ADA was enacted, however, many states adopted a defensive posture based on the Eleventh Amendment and states' rights vis-à vis federalism and also on the need for penological necessities to trump legislative mandates. They argued that operation of prisons is a "core state function" [*Torcasio v. Murray*, 57 F. 3d. 1340, 4th Cir. (1995)] and that the states' sovereign immunity cannot be abrogated without the unmistakably clear intent of Congress.

Three Supreme Court decisions are instructive.

1. *Pennsylvania Department of Corrections v. Yeskey* (524 U.S. 206 [1998]). In this case, the Supreme Court held that Title II prohibits state prisons as "public entities" from discriminating against inmates who are "qualified individuals with a disability." The unanimous Court said that the ADA's "language unmistakably includes State prisons and prisoners within its coverage" and that Congress stated clearly that the states will not be immune under the Eleventh Amendment for violations of the ADA. The Court, however, explicitly refrained, on grounds that this issue had not been addressed by the lower courts, from ruling on whether the application of the ADA to state prisons is a constitutional exercise of congressional power.

2. *Tennessee v. Lane* (541 U.S. 509 [2004]). Both Lane and Jones, paraplegics who use wheelchairs for mobility, claimed that they were denied access to the state court system and its services by reason of their disabilities. Lane alleged that he was compelled to appear to answer a set of criminal charges on the second floor of a county courthouse that had no elevator. At his first appearance, he crawled up two flights of stairs to get to the courtroom. When Lane returned to the courthouse for a hearing, he refused to crawl again or to be carried by officers to the courtroom, and he consequently was arrested and jailed for failure to appear. Jones, a certified court reporter, alleged that she has not been able to gain access to several county courthouses, and thus lost both work and an opportunity to participate in the judicial process. They sought damages and equitable relief. Ultimately, the Supreme Court in 2004 ruled that Title II, as it applies to cases implicating the fundamental right of access to the courts, constitutes a valid exercise of the authority of Congress to enforce the guarantees of the Fourteenth Amendment. However, the Supreme Court refused to consider Title II's application beyond the issue of access to the courts.

3. *Goodman v. Georgia* (*United States v. Georgia et al.*), 126 S. Ct. 877, 882 (2006). Goodman, a paraplegic, required a wheel chair for mobility. Housed more than 23 hours each day in a cell that is only 12 feet by 3 feet, he could not turn his wheelchair. He claimed that the prison failed to make toilet and bathing facilities accessible to him, denied him medical care such as catheters, treatment for bedsores, and access to mental health

counselors, and also excluded him from programs and activities because of his disability. The district court rejected his claims on grounds of state sovereign immunity. The appellate court agreed that the Eleventh Amendment precludes suits against states for money damages under the ADA, but the Supreme Court ruled that ADA applies in the prison context, and that insofar as ADA claims involve conduct that violates the Fourteenth Amendment, states do not have sovereign immunity. In its unanimous decision, Justice Antonin Scalia wrote: "No one doubts that §5 grants Congress the power to enforce the provisions of the [Fourteenth] Amendment by creating private remedies for actual violations of those provisions. This includes the power to abrogate state sovereign immunity by authorizing private suits for damages against the states."

In other words, the *Goodman* Court held in 2006 that "insofar as Title II creates a private cause of action for damages against the States for conduct that *actually* violates the Fourteenth Amendment, Title II validly abrogates state sovereign immunity."

The Supreme Court declined, however, to decide the extent to which sovereign immunity is vitiated for nonconstitutional Title II claims because the lower courts had not yet determined whether the claims in that case asserted independently viable constitutional claims or purely statutory ones. On remand, the Court instructed that the lower courts must determine "on a claim-by-claim basis (1) which aspects of the State's alleged conduct violated Title II; (2) to what extent such misconduct also violated the Fourteenth Amendment; and (3) insofar as such misconduct violated Title II but did not violate the Fourteenth Amendment, whether Congress's purported abrogation of sovereign immunity as to that class of conduct is nevertheless valid."

Meanwhile, some district courts have ruled in favor of states' rights, denying prisoners access to the benefits and safeguards of ADA. *Spencer v. Earley*, 278 Fed. Appx. 254, 261 (4th Cir. 2008) is one such example. Alongside these states' rights issues, however, another formidable set of impediments is imposed by the PLRA, making it extremely difficult for prisoners to succeed in ADA suits:

1. Indigent prisoners are no longer excused from paying a filing fee in federal court. For some, this can pose a major obstacle.
2. Prisoners must exhaust all available administrative remedies before filing suit in federal court.
3. Prisoners may not bring a federal civil action for a mental or emotional injury unless they make a showing of concomitant physical injury. This effectively precludes claims like denial of meaningful access of a blind inmate to any law library, recreation, education, job assignment, or other program.
4. Prospective (injunctive) relief is prohibited unless the court explicitly finds that such relief is narrowly drawn, extends no further than necessary to correct the violation of the federal right, and is the least intrusive means necessary to correct the violation of the federal right. Moreover, such relief may be terminated after two years unless the court finds there is a "current and ongoing violation" of federal law.

5. The hourly rate for attorneys, even in successful suits, is limited to 150 percent of the rate paid to court-appointed attorneys in criminal cases in that district. And in damage cases, attorneys' fees are limited to 150 percent of the amount of the judgment.

The U.S. Department of Justice has entered amicus curiae briefs on behalf of plaintiffs in several of these cases to plead the constitutionality of ADA's applicability to state facilities and programs. The department has also been helpful in other ways. It is empowered to intervene by bringing suit against a governmental agency such as a prison or jail only if their efforts at persuasion or mediation have proved unsuccessful. An impressive list of successful informal settlements[42] of problems experienced by prisoners with disabilities attests to the fairness and decency of prison officials. However, the heart-rending stories in this report of disabled prisoners whose cases were denied access to the courts because of the PLRA seem, to this author at least, to cry out persuasively for a just resolution.

Paul Evans concludes that Title II prohibits the exclusion of qualified individuals from access to the courts solely by reason of their disability and requires that "reasonable modifications" be made to public services. In the prison context, the flexibility of this requirement leaves room for necessary security measures. He says:

While the Supreme Court held in *Goodman* that Title II is valid in instances when its protections overlap with the Constitution, Title II should also be valid in its entire application to prevent unconstitutional conduct. . . . [In that case,] Title II would relieve an inmate of the burden of showing a particular mental state on the part of a prison official that he would have to show when proving "deliberate indifference" under the provisions of the cruel and unusual punishments clause of the Eighth Amendment. . . . The fact that inmates with disabilities often suffer unduly in prison is unjust. The punishment of an inmate with a disability and of an average inmate for the same crime should be the same; and Title II could go a long way toward rectifying the present inequity.[43]

Robert Greifinger[44] estimates that, if we were to take seriously a rehabilitative purpose for imprisonment in practice, it would not be unrealistic to expect that a third of all prisoners would qualify for reasonable accommodation and thus would not be excluded from participation in educational or training programs as a result of their disability. With the rising percentage of elderly persons in prison, the number of inmates with disabilities will inevitably increase.

In its amicus curiae "Memorandum of Law,"[45] the Department of Justice stated: "Neither the ADA nor section 504 require a fundamental alteration in the way prisons operate; indeed, the unique features of any state program, including prisons, must be taken into account in determining what the statutes require in a particular situation. Put simply, neither statute calls for an abrogation of common sense." For example, the regulations make it clear that "prisons must make only 'reasonable' modifications to their policies, practices, and procedures, when those modifications are necessary to avoid discrimination" [28 CFR §35.130(b)(7)] and that "covered entities such as prisons are never required to take any action that would result in a fundamental alteration in the nature of the programs they provide or that would pose undue financial and administrative burdens" [28 CFR §35.130(a)(3)]. Moreover, the statutes do not "mandate that prisons create particular programs or activities for prisoners or provide 'special treatment' for inmates with disabilities. They simply require the state to provide inmates with disabilities with as equal an opportunity as that provided to inmates without disabilities to participate in, and benefit from, the programs, activities, and services of the state prison system—whatever they happen to be."

> With the rising percentage of elderly persons in prison, the number of inmates with disabilities will inevitably increase.

When legitimate requests of prisoners are precluded by clear penological requirements or because of excessive cost, there should be a concerted effort to find and implement reasonable accommodations so as to provide due relief from unnecessary pain or deprivation. ACA standards explicitly "prohibit discrimination on the basis of disability in the provision of services, programs, and activities administered for program beneficiaries and participants,"[46] require that "programs and services [be] accessible to inmates with disabilities who reside in the facility,"[47] and insist on "staff and offender access to an appropriately trained and qualified individual who is educated in the problems and challenges faced by offenders with physical and/or mental impairments, programs designed to educate and assist disabled offenders, and all legal requirements for the protection of offenders with disabilities."[48]

Adequate Documentation

A system that has relevant patient information within its possession, but does not use it, can be held liable if this information could have prevented adverse outcomes. An obvious example is the suicide of a person whose unsuccessful attempt at self-harm during a previous stay at the same jail was documented in the medical record, but because that record had not been retrieved from storage upon his or her return to the system, it was not taken into account in planning the patient's care and supervision. Although it is undoubtedly costly and burdensome to retrieve old records, the issue of heightened liability remains. Here the virtues of a computerized record program are evident.

Another concern is when care providers, often of different disciplines, do not read one another's relevant notes or when such notes cannot be easily or accurately read because of poor handwriting or because they are not filed in the same chart.

Health Insurance Portability and Accountability Act

The Health Insurance Portability and Accountability Act (HIPAA) was enacted in 1996. Many correctional facilities have been ignoring its requirements on grounds that it was not applicable to them. This reasoning is understandable because the regulations originally exempted inmates' health information. However, the Department of Health and Human Services (DHHS) later revised its regulations, stating that "individually identifiable health information about inmates is protected health information under the final rule." Consequently, it is important for each correctional facility to evaluate whether and to what extent it is required to comply.

According to attorney Deanna Johnson, now that DHHS classifies correctional institutions as health care providers, the remaining question is whether a particular institution electronically transmits health information for any of the specific transactions regulated by DHHS. The three types of electronic transactions "that could apply are (1) transmission of encounter information for the purpose of reporting health care, (2) requests for the review of health care in order to secure an authorization for the health care and (3) payment of health care claims from a private/public health plan."[49] Accordingly, sending patient information electronically to request approval for a nonformulary medication or for a nonstandard medical, surgical, or diagnostic procedure would make the correctional facility a "covered entity under HIPAA." Similarly, electronic transmission of health information in order to conduct oversight activities like quality control or audits would have the same result. Another example would be any facility that takes advantage of Medicaid reimbursement for the care of hospitalized inmates because this will involve coverage by public insurance and the type of electronic communication addressed by the law.

In addition to what is otherwise already required, complying with HIPAA means that patients must be notified about their privacy rights and how their information can be used, specific privacy procedures must be implemented, employees must be trained to understand the privacy procedures, and an individual must be designated as responsible for seeing that the privacy procedures are adopted and followed. Consequently, correctional facilities should obtain competent advice from legal counsel and from health record professionals to ensure they are in full compliance with the law.

HIPAA does allow some exceptions regarding inmates, such as permitting disclosure of an inmate's health information to those having custody, if this is necessary for providing care and for the health and safety of the inmate or others.

Special Problems of Juveniles

The chief source of constitutional protection for detained juveniles is the Fourteenth Amendment, which guarantees due process.[50] The Eighth Amendment guarantees for adult prisoners are somewhat less applicable because they are based on freedom from "cruel and unusual punishment," while these youths are being confined for rehabilitation, for the most part, rather than for punishment. According to Austin et al.,

Youth detained in adult facilities under criminal court jurisdiction have the right to humane treatment, mental health and medical care, education, due process protection, and access to their families and the courts. These rights extend also to children who are confined in juvenile detention centers, training schools, adult jails and prisons, and other secure institutions. These rights emanate from the U.S. Constitution and federal laws, including the Juvenile Justice and Delinquency Prevention Act,[51] from state constitutions and laws, and from court interpretations of these laws.[52]

Many states have laws that require children to be placed in the least-restrictive environment consistent with public safety needs or that prohibit the detention of children under juvenile court jurisdiction in adult facilities.[53]

Of note, relatively few lawsuits have been brought by or on behalf of incarcerated juveniles. The Prisoner Litigation Reform Act,[54] however, applies to juvenile facilities as well as to prisons and jails and severely restricts their access to the courts. See further details previously in this chapter under "Prison Litigation Reform Act of 1996."

This author believes that juveniles should be exempted from the PLRA's provisions. They do not have a history of filing frivolous lawsuits. Applying the PLRA to children not only reduces public safety at potentially great cost to society without commensurate benefits but also oppugns our ethical convictions and basic humanitarian principles. The PLRA exhaustion provision is particularly damaging to juveniles, given the fact that many of them are functionally illiterate. In one case (*Brock v. Kenton County*),[55] the child explained that he had not known that there was a grievance system, that other children in the facility did not know of the system, and that the grievance system had never been used by a child incarcerated in that facility. Nonetheless, the court dismissed his suit for failure to exhaust administrative remedies.[56]

Even more than adults, children need the assistance of an attorney. They generally do not have access to law libraries or legal materials. Indeed, they *cannot* represent themselves in court. Even when faced with a legitimate legal problem such as physical or sexual abuse by correctional officers, persons under age 18 cannot file civil lawsuits on their own. Federal Rule 17(c) requires that a guardian or guardian *ad litem* represent a minor in any civil lawsuit.[57] Thus, PLRA provisions limiting attorney's fees have a particularly chilling effect on access to the courts for young people.

SOME IMPORTANT LEGAL CASES

A selection of significant legal cases directly or indirectly affecting correctional health care is presented here in chronological order along with excerpts or commentary.

Cases Concerning Adults

- *Schloendorff v. Society of New York Hospital*[58] (1914) New York. This is perhaps the earliest judicial statement of the right of competent adults to refuse treatment—the foundation for the medicolegal doctrine of "informed consent." Justice (then Judge) Benjamin Cardozo wrote in the court's opinion: "Every human being of adult years and sound mind has a right to determine what shall be done with his own body; and a surgeon who performs an operation without his patient's consent commits an assault for which he is liable in damages. This is true except in cases of emergency where it is necessary to operate before consent can be obtained."

- *Spicer v. Williamson*[59] (1926) North Carolina. This ruling states the common law requirement that "[it] is but just that the public be required to care for the prisoner, who cannot by reason of the deprivation of his liberty, care for himself." In fact, this case did not deal with failure to provide medical care to a prisoner but with the obligation of a county government to pay a medical specialist who had already treated a prisoner.

- *Ex parte Hull*[60] (1941) Michigan. The Supreme Court held that inmates had a right to unrestricted access to federal courts. State officials cannot enact regulations that "abridge" or "impair" an inmate's right of access to the courts. They cannot, for example, interfere with the right of inmates to file petitions in court or screen, censor, or interfere with an inmate's mailings and submissions to the courts.

- *Coffin v. Reichard*[61] (1944) Kentucky. "A prisoner retains all the rights of an ordinary citizen except those expressly, or by necessary implication, taken from him by law. While the law does take his liberty and imposes a duty of servitude and observance of discipline for his regulation and that of other prisoners, it does not deny his right to personal security against unlawful invasion."

- *Trop v. Dulles*[62] (1958) United States. "The basic concept underlying the Eighth Amendment is nothing less than the dignity of man. While the State has the power to punish, the Amendment stands to assure that this power be exercised within the limits of civilized standards. . . . The Amendment must draw its meaning from the evolving standards of decency that mark the progress of a maturing society."

- *Monroe v. Pape*[63] (1961) City of Chicago. The Court held that the old Section 1979 of the revised statutes, derived from the Ku Klux Klan Act of 1871, and which became 42 U.S.C. Section 1983, gave to individual citizens a viable remedy in the federal courts for deprivation of federally protected rights by persons acting under color of law. Also, exhaustion of judicial remedies is not a prerequisite for Section 1983 action.

- *Robinson v. California*[64] (1962) California. The Court's ruling established that the cruel and unusual punishment clause of the Eighth Amendment applies to the states in appropriate cases by reason of the due process clause of the Fourteenth Amendment.

- *Jackson v. Bishop*[65] (1968) Arkansas. The court stated: "We have no difficulty in reaching the conclusion that the use of the strap in the penitentiaries of Arkansas is punishment which, in this last third of the 20th century, runs afoul of the Eighth Amendment; that the strap's use, irrespective of any precautionary conditions which may be imposed, offends contemporary concepts of decency and human dignity and precepts of civilization which we profess to possess; and that it also violates those standards of good conscience and fundamental fairness enumerated by this court."

152   Humane Health Care for Prisoners

- *Holt v. Sarver*[66] (1971) Arkansas. The court ruled that inmates may challenge not merely individual practices but also the totality of a prison's conditions as unconstitutional.
- *Bivens v. Six Unknown Agents of the Federal Bureau of Narcotics*[67] (1971) United States. This case provides a mechanism that serves as a parallel to 42 U.S.C. §1983 suits when federal officials are sued. The Court based its action on the premise that "where legal rights have been invaded, and a federal statute provides for a general right to sue for such invasion, federal courts may use any available remedy to make good the wrong done." This reasoning reflects the principle "Where there is a right, there is a remedy," as in the old Latin maxim *Ubi jus, ibi remedium.*
- *Procunier v. Martinez*[68] (1974) California. "A prisoner is not stripped of constitutional rights at the prison gate, but rather he retains all the rights of an ordinary citizen except those expressly or by necessary implication taken from him by the law."
- *Wolff v. McDonnell*[69] (1974) Nebraska. The Court held that prisoners are not wholly stripped of constitutional protections and that they are entitled to certain minimal due process requirements consonant with the unique institutional environment.
- *Newman v. Alabama*[70] (1974) Alabama. Federal District Judge Frank Johnson found deplorable conditions in the prison medical system and other conditions of confinement. He declared the entire Alabama prison system to be unconstitutional and issued sweeping orders designed to improve conditions. As just a single example, it was found that all of the medical care for 900 inmates at one prison was provided by a medical technical assistant and some inmate assistants.
- *Gates v. Collier*[71] (1974) Mississippi. A landmark ruling by a U.S. federal district court in 1972 was confirmed on appeal by the Fifth Circuit in 1974. It brought an end to racial discrimination and the trusty system with its flagrant abuse of inmates at the Mississippi State Penitentiary at Parchman and dealt with inadequate medical care and inhumane conditions of housing, among other issues, finding constitutional violations. The appellate court also rejected the claim that the state lacked funds needed to comply.
- *Battle v. Anderson*[72] (1974) Oklahoma. Prisoners are not required to provide "optimal" medical care to inmates, but rather "prison officials have an affirmative duty to make available to inmates a level of medical care which is reasonably designed to meet the routine and emergency health care needs of inmates."
- *Estelle v. Gamble*[73] (1976) Texas. The Court wrote, "We therefore conclude that deliberate indifference to serious medical needs of prisoners constitutes the 'unnecessary and wanton infliction of pain,' proscribed by the Eighth Amendment."
- *Todaro v. Ward*[74] (1977) New York. According to the court, "The Eighth Amendment prohibits not only deprivations of medical care that produce physical torture and lingering death, but also less serious denials [of care] which cause or perpetuate pain. A constitutional claim is stated when prison officials intentionally deny access to medical care or interfere with prescribed treatment."
- *Rennie v. Klein*[75] (1978) New Jersey. Involuntary patients have a qualified right, absent an emergency, to refuse psychotropic drugs. On appeal, the Federal Court of Appeals for the Third Circuit[76] asserted that mental patients who are involuntarily committed to state institutions retain their constitutional right to refuse antipsychotic drugs that may have permanently disabling side effects. This constitutional right to be free from intrusive treatments may be limited only by the "least intrusive infringement" required by the inmate's

medical care needs or legitimate administrative concerns. A conscious weighing of an inmate's constitutional liberty interest is necessary in any determination of proper treatment alternatives.

- *Bell v. Wolfish*[77] (1979) New York. The Court found that it was not a violation of the Fourth Amendment to perform intrusive body searches on pretrial detainees following contact with persons from outside the institution because the possibility of their innocence does not contradict the need for a mutual accommodation between institutional needs and objectives and the provisions of the Constitution. "Simply because prison inmates retain certain constitutional rights does not mean that these rights are not subject to restrictions and limitations." This case also weakened some earlier challenges to double celling. It further rejected the idea that standards adopted by professional association (such as ACA or NCCHC) represented a proper measure of what the Constitution requires: "While the recommendations of these various groups may be instructive in certain cases, they simply do not establish the constitutional minima; rather, they establish goals recommended by the organization in question."

- *Rogers v. Okin*[78] (1979) Massachusetts. The federal court in Massachusetts enjoined hospital physicians from forcibly medicating committed mental patients, except in emergency situations presenting a substantial likelihood of physical harm to the patient or others. The court urged physicians to pursue less intrusive alternatives. On appeal, the First Circuit Court of Appeals also adopted the "least restrictive means" approach.

- *Vitek v. Jones*[79] (1980) Nebraska. According to the Court, "The stigmatizing consequences of a transfer to a mental hospital for involuntary psychiatric treatment, coupled with the subjection of the prisoner to mandatory behavior modification as a treatment for mental illness, constitute the type of deprivations of liberty that requires procedural protections."

- *Carlson v. Green*[80] (1980) Indiana. The Supreme Court allowed a federal prisoner to bring an Eighth Amendment claim, following the *Bivens* remedy, against federal government officials for deliberate indifference to medical needs.

- *Ruiz v. Estelle*[81]—(1980)—Texas—A consent decree applied the American Medical Association's Standards for Prisons in ordering comprehensive statewide improvements in medical care and mental health care. The court also ruled on the conditions of confinement and ended the brutal inmate "building tender" system.

- *Youngberg v. Romeo*[82] (1982) Pennsylvania. Absent specific legal rules or testimony from an expert that the social worker's actions did not meet professional standards, courts generally assume that a social worker has exercised sound professional discretion. This Court recognized deference to professional judgment. Also, the Court held that institutionalized retarded persons have "constitutionally protected liberty rights which require the state to provide minimally adequate training to insure their safety and freedom from restraint," based on the due process clause of the Fourteenth Amendment.

- *Dean v. Coughlin*[83] (1986) New York. The court said conditions are considered serious if they "cause pain, discomfort, or threat to good health."

- *Turner v. Safley*[84] (1987) Missouri. The Court defined basic ground rules for balancing competing claims between an inmate's constitutional right and a prison's legitimate penological interests. It provided a "Turner test" for analysis of competing interests.

- *West v. Atkins*[85] (1988) North Carolina. "A physician who is under contract with the State to provide medical services to inmates at a state prison hospital on a part-time basis acts 'under color of state law,' within the meaning of §1983, when he treats an inmate." Thus, the state cannot avoid liability by contracting out. Furthermore, the contractor also becomes liable for constitutional violations.

- *Phillips v. Michigan Department of Corrections*[86] (1990) Michigan. A suit was brought by Phillips, a transsexual inmate who was being denied estrogen treatment. The U.S. District Court found "that plaintiff suffers from a serious medical need, being deprived of treatment, whether the diagnosis is transsexualism or the gender identity disorder of adolescence or adulthood, non-transsexual type. . . . The medical testimony was clear that [these] are serious psychiatric disorders with profound emotional and physical effects." Based on the finding of deliberate indifference, the court granted a preliminary injunction and ordered the state to provide her the same standard of care she was receiving prior to her incarceration at that facility—2.5 mg per day of Premarin. This decision was affirmed by the Sixth Circuit Court of Appeals in 1991.

- *Washington v. Harper*[87] (1990) Washington. The Supreme Court made it clear that forced medication of inmates with mental disorders could be ordered only when the inmate was a danger to himself or others and when the medication is in the inmate's own best interests. Substantive due process requirements need to be met. In addition, "alternative, less intrusive means" must first be considered before resorting to the involuntary administration of psychotropic medication.

- *Wilson v. Seiter*[88] (1991) Ohio. The Court ruled that an express intent to inflict pain need not be shown, but a subjective showing of deliberate indifference is required. A plaintiff "must show a culpable state of mind on the part of prison officials."

- *Helling v. McKinney*[89] (1993) Nevada. According to the Court, "An injunction cannot be denied to inmates who plainly prove an unsafe, life-threatening condition on the ground that nothing yet has happened to them." Furthermore, "that the Eighth Amendment protects against future harm to inmates is not a novel proposition."

- *Farmer v. Brennan*[90] (1994) Indiana. For a deliberate indifference claim to succeed, the Court ruled that the defendant must know of and disregard a substantial risk, and this can be inferred from the surrounding facts where failure to respond to a clear risk is reckless. In other words, the defendant must actually draw the inference. It is not sufficient that the official "should have known." A transgender federal prisoner was housed with male inmates and was raped and beaten by her cell mate. According to the Court, if the correctional officials knew that they were exposing her to risk of serious harm and were deliberately indifferent, this would be a violation of the Eighth Amendment.

- *Madrid v. Gomez*[91] (1995) California. In this landmark challenge to total isolation and the supermax genre of prisons, the court stopped just short of declaring the supermax strategy to be unconstitutional, but it did find supermax conditions at the Pelican Bay State Prison unconstitutional for mentally ill prisoners. Supermax conditions "may well hover on the edge of what is humanly tolerable for those with normal resilience particularly when endured for extended periods of time."

- *Sandin v. Conner*[92] (1995) Hawaii. This decision marked a sharp move by the Court away from its holdings in several earlier prisoner rights cases and made it more difficult for prisoners to bring lawsuits challenging the management of prisons on constitutional grounds. For a due process claim to succeed after *Sandin*, the plaintiff must show that the nature of the deprivation imposes an "atypical and significant hardship on the inmate in relation to the ordinary incidents of prison life." Otherwise, the prisoner will not have a liberty interest in avoiding the deprivation.

- *Lewis v. Casey*[93] (1996) Arizona. In the case, the Court held that "an inmate cannot establish relevant actual injury simply by establishing that his prison's library or legal assistance program is *sub par* in some theoretical sense . . . and the inmate therefore must go one step further and demonstrate that the alleged shortcomings in the library or legal assistance program hindered his efforts to pursue a legal claim."

- *Pennsylvania Department of Corrections v. Yeskey*[94] (1998) Pennsylvania. The Supreme Court interpreted the federal statute (Americans with Disabilities Act of 1990), holding that its protections applied also to inmates.

- *Sell v. United States*[95] (2003) Federal Bureau of Prisons. The Supreme Court imposed stringent limitations on the right of a lower court to order forcible administration of antipsychotic medications to a criminal defendant who had been found incompetent to stand trial for the sole purpose of rendering him competent and thus able to be tried.

- *Stouffer v. Reid*[96] (2010) Maryland. The highest court in Maryland reviewed the case of a prisoner who was refusing hemodialysis, a life-sustaining treatment for his end-stage renal disease. The court found that "an inmate, by virtue of his incarceration, is not divested of his right to disagree with his medical providers" and ruled that "absent evidence that Reid is a direct threat to the safety and well-being of others or that he is protesting any prison policies or attempting to manipulate an official, we agree with the Court of Special Appeals that the State has not shown a valid penological interest in compelling Reid to submit to dialysis."

- *Minneci v. Pollard*[97] (2012) California. In January 2012, the U.S. Supreme Court held that a *Bivens* action cannot be brought against a private prison's personnel to raise Eighth Amendment violations. Pollard had sought damages from employees of the Wackenhut Corrections Corporation, which housed federal inmates at its private facility. The Court declined to imply a remedy to bring constitutional claims under *Bivens* against Wackenhut's employees on the grounds that state tort law provides an adequate alternative for damages (namely, claims for negligence or medical negligence). As a result, inmates at privately operated federal prisons are unable to sue under federal law when their constitutional rights are violated, although they can bring a tort claim that would not be available in federal facilities.

- *Coleman v. Brown/Schwarzenegger/Wilson*[98] (initially filed 1990) California. This case raised constitutional issues of prisoner mental health care and was consolidated with *Plata v. Brown* in 2007 to become *Brown v. Plata* (2011).

- *Plata v. Brown/Schwarzenegger*[99] (initially filed 2001) California. This case raised constitutional issues of prisoner medical care. The case was consolidated with *Coleman v. Brown* in 2007 to become *Brown v. Plata* (2011).

- *Brown v. Plata*[100] (2011) California. In this landmark case, the Supreme Court ordered a substantial reduction of prison overcrowding to enable relief of unconstitutional medical and mental health care. The case is discussed at length in this chapter under "A New Challenge—The Impact of Mass Incarceration."

- *Ross v. Blake*[101] (2016) Maryland. In this case, the Supreme Court ruled unanimously that a court may not excuse failure of a prisoner to exhaust all available administrative remedies, even under "special circumstances," because that would be contrary to the text and history of the language of the PLRA.

Cases Concerning Juveniles

- *Lollis v. New York State Department of Social Services.*[102](1970) New York. A 14-year-old status offender who got into a fight with another girl was placed in isolation in a six-by-nine foot room for 24 hours a day for two weeks with no recreational facilities or reading material. The court found this isolation to be cruel and unusual punishment and thus unconstitutional.

- *Nelson v. Heyne*[103] (1974) Indiana. The Seventh Circuit Federal Court of Appeals held that the misuse of tranquilizing drugs in an Indiana juvenile institution constituted cruel and unusual punishment. These drugs were being administered solely for the purpose of controlling excited inmate behavior. (The drugs Sparine and Thorazine were administered by a nurse on recommendation of the custodial staff under standing orders by the physician. Neither before nor after injections were the juveniles examined by medically competent staff to determine their tolerances.) The court also found that the severe disciplinary beatings with a paddle constituted cruel and unusual punishment.

- *Morgan v. Sproat*[104] (1977) Mississippi. This case was filed in Mississippi in 1975 on behalf of confined children, with final judgment occurring in 1977. The U.S. attorney general subsequently initiated an investigation in 2002 of two training schools, stating that the conditions were shocking and that the state had made little or no progress since 1977. More than 20 years later, children were allegedly still being maced, hog-tied, and shackled to poles; suicidal teens were being stripped and confined in isolation rooms without toilets, light, or ventilation for days on end; and even staff members were too frightened of retaliation to report incidents of child abuse.[105] The Southern Poverty Law Center and the Mississippi Center for Justice joined forces to take over as class counsel in *Morgan*. The court held that where "the purpose of incarcerating juveniles in a state training school is treatment and rehabilitation, due process requires that the conditions and programs at the school must be reasonably related to that purpose."

- *D.B. v. Tewksbury*[106] (1982) Oregon. The court ruled that juvenile institutions in Oregon have a constitutional duty to protect from harm children they detain.

- *Morales v. Turman*[107] (1987) Texas. The suit was filed in 1971 on behalf of a class of minors incarcerated in institutions for delinquent juveniles operated by the Texas Youth Council (later the Texas Youth Commission in 1983 and the Texas Juvenile Justice Department in December 2011). Fourteen-year-old Alicia Morales was being held at the request of her father because she disobeyed his order to work and turn her earnings over to him. She hired an attorney and filed a federal suit. She and many other confined juveniles had had no court hearing or attorney before being sent to the Texas Youth Commission. Plaintiffs sought to establish a constitutional right to treatment of incarcerated juveniles. The case attracted national attention. After years of negotiations and court proceedings rising to the U.S. Supreme Court in 1977, a settlement agreement was reached in 1984 and a monitoring committee finished its work in 1988. Its terms remain in effect because the class action plaintiffs included all youth who would be committed to the Texas Youth Commission in the future. The court of appeals rejected the plaintiff's assertion of a constitutional right to treatment for incarcerated juveniles, but the *Morales* case established the first national standards for juvenile justice and corrections and prompted many changes in Texas, including prohibition of corporal punishment, extended periods of isolation, and all forms of inhumane treatment. The case required establishment of an effective grievance system and minimum staff qualification and training requirements.[108]

- *Gary H. v. Hegstrom*[109] (1987) Oregon. This case concerned the management of Oregon's MacLaren Facility for adolescent wards of the juvenile court. The Ninth Circuit Court of Appeals applied some helpful reasoning. The appellate court agreed with the findings of fact and the finding of unconstitutional conditions by the district court but disagreed with the imposition of a highly detailed remedial order based on Eighth Amendment violations. The appellate court acknowledged the district court's findings of many violations of proper health care, sanitation, and decency in the segregation unit, which included, inter alia, failure to evaluate students' health as they are admitted to the segregation unit; lack of a sick-call system that ensures that each segregated student with a health problem is identified; administration by untrained staff members of psychotropic, stimulant, and tranquilizing medication to some students; no adequate system for evaluating students and no physician available for medical emergencies; an almost nonexistent monitoring system to detect side effects of the medications given; provision of little or no mental health treatment; failure to provide mental health care to many students after they had engaged in self-mutilation; the practice of using lockup instead of providing treatment; and long delays in obtaining any treatment (for example, a student who intentionally cut himself had to wait for a month to see a psychiatrist). However, the appellate opinion stated that the more protective Fourteenth Amendment due process clause—which implicitly incorporates the cruel and unusual punishments clause standards as a constitutional minimum—is the appropriate standard for reviewing conditions at an institution that is noncriminal and nonpenal as with these juvenile facilities.

- *Alexander S. v. Boyd*[110] (1995). South Carolina. In this class action suit, a district court found that plaintiffs "have proved that certain conditions of confinement" in the institution "violate their constitutional and statutory rights" and ordered the state to create and implement a comprehensive remedial plan.

- *S.D. v. Parish of Orleans, LA*[111] (2001) Louisiana. S.D., a 17-year-old youth with a history of delinquent behavior, filed a lawsuit alleging that he had been assaulted at least three times, twice by guards, suffering serious injuries both times, including a broken jaw, and that he had spent approximately two months in isolation. Juvenile justice experts from the U.S. Department of Justice found that the conditions at the Tallulah Correctional Center for Youth and Louisiana's three other juvenile prisons were "life-threatening and dangerous" to the children confined therein. In the first 20 days of August 1996, the Department of Justice found that 28 Tallulah children were sent to the hospital for evaluation or treatment of serious injuries, including fractures or suspected fractures and serious lacerations in need of suturing. In 1997, the Department of Justice threatened to file suit if Louisiana did not take adequate remedial measures to protect children from harm in these institutions. When negotiations between the state and the Department of Justice failed in November 1998, for the first time ever the Department of Justice sued a state because of the conditions at its juvenile prisons.[112] The court found in 2001 that the injury sustained when plaintiff's jaw was broken violated his federal and state constitutional rights because the injury bore no relation to the purposes of his detention. (This reference is to the due process rights guaranteed by the Louisiana constitution, which in some respects exceed those guaranteed by the Fourteenth Amendment to the U.S. Constitution.)[113] Plaintiff was entitled to a safe environment.[114]

- *Jackson v. Fort Stanton Hospital and Training School* and *Jackson v. Los Lunas Hospital and Training School*[115] (first filed in 1987) New Mexico. The case(s) first found serious violations of the Rehabilitation Act involving people with severe developmental disabilities who were subjected to discrimination and unnecessary segregation. A remedial action plan was negotiated and ordered. Contempt motions were filed in both 1996 and 2004 because many identified deficiencies had not been corrected. Still unresolved in 2016, this lawsuit has radically changed the way New Mexico treats its developmentally disabled. The institution was closed and care was shifted to intimate, community-based programs that allow disabled people to interact with the public and to programs that pay family members to care for them. An extensive ongoing monitoring program[116] reports significant progress in numerous areas.

- *A.M. v. Luzerne County Juvenile Detention Center*[117](2004) Pennsylvania. The court ruled that this Pennsylvania facility is obliged to protect the welfare of children in its custody. It found sufficient evidence that the facility was deliberately indifferent to substantial risk of harm to a 13-year-old boy with mental illness who was placed in the general population, where he was repeatedly assaulted by fellow residents.

- *K.L.W. v. James.*[118](2005) Mississippi. In this case, a settlement agreement was reached to guarantee that incarcerated children in Mississippi will have meaningful access to the court system. The case was brought on behalf of K.L.W., a developmentally disabled 14-year-old who had been assaulted by a security guard at the Columbia Training School. When the mother attempted to arrange a meeting with her son and an attorney, the superintendent told her to get a court order and hung up on her. Under the settlement, the state is required to tell children that they have a constitutional right to ask for help from a lawyer, help children make legal requests, ensure that the requests are delivered, and abandon its policy of requiring a court order before allowing a lawyer to respond to a child in trouble.

- *Minix v. Pazera*[119](2005) Indiana. This case was dismissed in federal court because the child had failed to file a grievance within the two business days' time limit required by the juvenile facility policy. The plaintiff claimed that he had been beaten and suffered sexual assaults and that facility staff was aware of the abuse but failed to prevent it. Shortly thereafter, the Civil Rights Division of the U.S. Department of Justice concluded its investigation of the South Bend Juvenile Facility, where the plaintiff had been detained, and reported that staff there failed to adequately protect the juveniles in its care from harm and that the grievance system was "dysfunctional" and "contribute[d] to the State's failure to ensure a reasonably safe environment." Ultimately, after he was released from the facility, the plaintiff in *Minix* amended his suit, thereby overcoming the barrier posed by failing to have exhausted all administrative remedies as required by the PLRA because it was now viewed as a new suit to which the PLRA did not apply. The federal district court then heard his claims, although in the end it dismissed the case inter alia because the plaintiff failed to provide clear proof that officials had knowledge of the assaults.

- *J.A. et al. v. Barbour et al.*[120] (2007) Mississippi. The suit was filed on behalf of mentally ill teenaged girls living at the Columbia Training School in Mississippi who were shackled for between eight days to one month for 12 hours each day, physically and sexually abused, and provided with inadequate mental health treatment. Seven months after the suit was filed, state officials announced they would close the training school. The plaintiffs inadvertently failed to respond to a motion for relief, and the court entered an order granting the request to dismiss. After the case failed to settle, the court dismissed the case with prejudice in 2010.

STRATEGIES TO AVOID LITIGATION

A Checklist of Risk-Prone Areas

Although one can always be sued, there are ways that a correctional health care program can reduce the likelihood of lawsuits and minimize the prospect of losing the case if sued. The following is a suggested checklist of 25 areas that often lead to problems and litigation if ignored or neglected. This checklist may be thoughtfully adapted to specific situations and experiences, with items added or subtracted as appropriate.

- [ ] 1. **Implement a good health care program**, giving careful attention to every important issue, especially intake health screening and follow-up, chronic disease management with fail-safe follow-up, unimpeded access to a good sick-call program with prompt referral of acute conditions for follow-up, proper identification and surveillance of the suicide prone, timely kite response and follow-up, and a reasonable and fair grievance system that is taken seriously.
- [ ] 2. **Employ an adequate number of qualified staff**. Staff members should be fully qualified by community standards. Provide them adequate in-service training. Assign support staff for the medical service providers. Be sure they are trained to know what they should and should not do. In addition, set up an effective fail-safe physician and nurse on-call arrangement.
- [ ] 3. **Insist on proper and legible documentation with due confidentiality safeguards**. Health records are best integrated rather than fragmented by discipline. The record may be electronic, paper, or a combination of both. Be sure the medical record adequately explains what the clinical staff did or did not do on behalf of each patient. Documentation of the physician's rationale is important. Factual errors, omissions, illegible entries, unresolved contradictions, and questionable alterations are potential problem areas. Be sure the records and all information derived from the delivery of care are held confidentially. Follow applicable HIPAA requirements.
- [ ] 4. **Pay attention to thorough history taking** and be sure that relevant medical information is solicited and documented, such as allergies, drug use, family history, and prior medical problems. Undue delays in diagnosing problems can often be traced to an incomplete history.
- [ ] 5. **Establish a pattern of thorough diagnostic procedures appropriate to each situation**. To safeguard against overlooking significant test results, policy should prohibit filing such items unless and until the doctor has initialed them as evidence that they have been reviewed. Claims in which filed, unreviewed reports result in a delayed diagnosis or treatment and contribute to a patient's injury are rarely defensible—and always costly.

☐ 6. **Require the regular use of approved physician practice clinical guidelines and nurse protocols**. These help achieve consistency among providers and ensure current standard of practice.

☐ 7. **Ensure consistent follow-up**. Meticulous attention by clerical and nursing staff is essential to prevent patients from being inadvertently lost to follow-up, which can lead to episodic care. When a medical service provider fails to enter into the progress note a "return to clinic" date or "no follow-up needed," policy should require that nursing or clerical staff either ascertain and document the doctor's intent or reschedule the patient within a reasonable default period. It is acceptable for a physician to elect to observe and monitor rather than refer the patient to a specialist or to order diagnostic studies, but in each such case the physician should (1) document the reasons for deferring action and (2) revisit the problem on subsequent visits, documenting a course of action or noting that the problem has been resolved.

☐ 8. **Obtain informed consent**. For routine care, implicit or verbal consent is usually sufficient. Explicit, formal written consent applies to all invasive or risky procedures such as surgery, dental extractions, and psychotropic medications. Do not rely on a generic consent obtained at time of admission. Where minors are concerned, consent should be obtained from parents, guardians, or the institution head consistent with state law and community practice.

☐ 9. **Be sure that refusals are informed**. Patients have the right to decline hospitalization, referral to other doctors, immunizations, or any recommended treatment. Let the communication be directly between patient and doctor or patient and nurse so that there is no misunderstanding. A corrections officer should not be the recipient of a refusal. When the patient declines, the provider is obliged to explain the possible or likely consequences of the patient's choice, which should be noted in the medical record. When the risks of nontreatment are great, the explanation should also be documented by a confirming letter to the patient.

☐ 10. **Avoid miscommunication among health professionals**. Keep track of referrals, question delays in receiving reports, and document telephone conversations with colleagues and patients in which important information is given or received. All health professionals need to function as a team, and communication breakdowns can result in serious problems for patients.

☐ 11. **Insist on strict procedures and accountability for medication administration**. Take care that patients on chronic medications obtain refills promptly. Careless charting and incomplete documentation of prescriptions and refills are common factors in facilitating claims. Use a medication control record to track medications and reduce the risk of overlooking drug interactions or patient-dosing errors. Providers should be aware of all medications currently prescribed by other caregivers.

In the community, the physician is not responsible for ensuring a patient takes a prescription to the pharmacy or goes to the pharmacy each month to obtain a refill. But in the correctional setting, the patient is totally dependent on the system to provide the medications. It may be acceptable to place some responsibility on patients receiving "keep-on-person" (KOP) medications (of which a prisoner is allowed to keep a small supply for daily use without having to have each dose administered by a nurse) to send a kite when the medications need to be refilled. But there is no excuse for not providing the medications once the refill request has been submitted. It would be irresponsible to impose such burdens on a patient who receives nurse-administered medications.

☐ 12. **Make patient education a priority**. Without adequate information, patients may inadvertently fail to cooperate or comply with their treatment plans. Oral education may be inadequate and easily forgotten or confused by patients. It is common practice in the community to provide written information about diseases or conditions, drugs prescribed, self-care, and follow-up and to document that this information was duly dispensed. Conversely, if there is reason to believe that the patient is not fully literate, be sure to read and explain the information to the patient and answer any questions.

In a correctional system, this area is of particular import, given the well-known fact that persons entering jail, prison, or a juvenile facility are typically persons who have not received adequate or accurate health information. Every clinical contact with a prisoner affords an opportunity for relevant and meaningful patient education to occur.

☐ 13. **Encourage a therapeutic alliance.** Patients are less likely to sue a doctor with whom they have a trusting relationship. Fostering a good doctor–patient relationship is important in the community—and even more so in corrections. The patient has not freely chosen the provider and the care is taking place in a context that may be adversarial. Moreover, a sound therapeutic alliance is conducive to effective healing. Hence, the importance of treating patients respectfully. Courtesy, respect, and a caring attitude are essential. It is important to listen to the patient and not rush through patient encounters.

☐ 14. **Be sure that all corrections officers are trained** in what they need to know about medical and mental health matters, including recognition of the signs and symptoms of illness and knowledge of the proper referral procedure. Particularly those officers who will work in medical and mental health areas should receive regular ongoing training pertinent to their role.

☐ 15. **Minimize or avoid the use of segregated housing for the mentally ill**. The conditions of isolation and deprivation of normal stimuli can be severely harmful to mental health and yet fail to reduce violent behavior. Professional treatment in a suitable therapeutic environment is not only more humane but also better management. Frequent and proper rounding of persons in segregation is essential and should include a bilateral albeit brief exchange of relevant communication.

☐ 16. **Avoid co-payment programs**. If this is not an option and a co-pay system is required, monitor it closely and ensure it does not deny legitimate access, especially to chronic, infectious, or mentally ill patients. Not everyone who appears at sick call needs an extensive work-up, but take enough time to be sure.

☐ 17. **Do not allow medical or mental health staff to participate, even remotely, in nonethical activities or in punitive correctional measures.** Initial and periodic training of staff in the principles of professional ethics and their practical application is essential.

☐ 18. **Instruct all staff to report suspected abuse promptly**. This critical area is discussed in Chapter 2, "Areas of Significant Ethical Role Conflict," under "Reporting Abuses by Staff." There should be a policy of zero tolerance for any abusive behavior.

☐ 19. **Have a good program for quality-improvement monitoring** and program evaluation. This, if done well with broad participation among staff, can help prevent errors and improve procedures

☐ 20. **Seek and obtain accreditation**. It helps to invite an objective outside observer, and affords another set of eyes to discover problematic and risk-prone areas early.

☐ 21. **Take care to have a caring staff.** Encourage caring attributes. Let patients know that their legitimate health needs are important to the staff. Staff attitudes toward patients are critically important, and these should always be respectful, caring, and attentive. Referring to them as *patients* rather than *inmates* is helpful. It is too easy for staff to slip into attitudes that Dr. Robert Greifinger terms *cynical*, such as "They all lie," "She is just drug-seeking," "He just wants to get out of the jail," and "What does he want, a Cadillac?"[121] This is counterproductive and leads to inadvertent lapses in quality of care such as undue delays, failure to follow policies, departure from scope of practice, failure to document, and neglected continuity and coordination of care.

☐ 22. **Accord due medical autonomy** to health care professionals who attend patients. Do not hesitate to challenge any infringement of the authority or ability of health care providers to treat their patients.

☐ 23. **All health care staff should serve as patient advocates**. Take the initiative to be proactive on behalf of your patients, making their health and well-being your highest concern.

☐ 24. **Don't try to hide problems** if you detect a gap or a deficiency. A cover-up can be more serious than the crime. Recognize the problem and get on with trying to solve it. Enlist interdisciplinary cooperation. Get supervisors involved. Think about systemic repair, not ad hoc Band-Aids. Do not blame the staff, but fix the problem. When you see problems that require fixing, report them promptly to the proper supervisor and document the report.

☐ 25. **Make grievance procedures as simple and uncomplicated as possible**. If you are the recipient of a lawsuit or a grievance—even if the complaint goes nowhere because it is deficient on technical grounds—look carefully at the merits of the complaint and set about to fix the problem. Give inmates a ready means to raise concerns and challenge perceived mistreatment or neglect. Not every grievance is meritorious, and some are inartfully written, but it may be a legitimate cry for help. Whenever feasible, conduct at least a brief meeting with the grievant to clarify your understanding of the real issue being raised, overlooking minor technical deficiencies in the format or wording or timing of the written document. A grievance system is not a game to see who will win. Rather, it is a mechanism for sensing problematic areas before they become serious or widespread.

Don't Fight the Courts

Though it may seem counterintuitive, a correctional agency need not always adopt a strategy of implacable resistance to each and every lawsuit filed against it. Certainly some lawsuits are frivolous and inappropriate and should be strongly resisted from the outset. But if the evidence suggests that the plaintiff's case may have merit and that the treatment or conditions of confinement of prisoners are indeed seriously inadequate or inhumane, then the agency will likely cut its losses and emerge with a better outcome by admitting fault and promptly developing a suitable plan of correction.

Such a plan of correction should specify what needs to be done, a reasonable calendar for its accomplishment, and identification of needed resources (funds, personnel, space, equipment, supplies). Sometimes what is needed is simply a change of policy or procedure. At other times, staff training is necessary. It may require an effort to coordinate the roles of multiple agencies or units in carrying out the plan of correction.

This approach would suggest an honest, straightforward examination of the evidence—perhaps accompanied by the agency's own independent investigation and involvement of an outside consultant. Face facts and do not deny the evidence or make excuses. If a wrong was done, a responsible agency will acknowledge the error, fix the problem, and move on.

This strategy, however, is rarely adopted in the real world where politics, pride, and ambition occupy such prominent positions. Managers and directors do not like to admit errors. Politicians fear reprisal at the ballot boxes if they acknowledge mistakes or if they accede, without kicking and screaming, to arrangements that might cost taxpayers money.

IMPACT OF THE COURTS

As indicated previously in this chapter, many of correctional health care's needed reforms have come about through access by prisoners to the courts for relief. "No serious student of American correctional history can deny that litigation has provided the impetus for reforms of medical practice in prisons and jails,"[122] says Vincent Nathan, who has had extensive experience as a court monitor and special master. He also identified the principal effects that court involvement has achieved in correctional facilities: "Judicial intervention over the past three decades has had an enormously positive impact on the operation of correctional institutions in the United States, and on the conditions in which prisoners live and staff work."[123] The most tangible impact has been on environmental conditions and elimination of widespread environmental hazards. The courts have also ameliorated horrendous crowding in some facilities, improved the control of unnecessary and excessive force, and enhanced the delivery of medical and mental health care to prisoners. The courts have brought about improvements in disciplinary procedures, helped integrate women and minorities into the ranks of professional and line staff, made strides in food services, and encouraged preventive maintenance.

Nathan regards two other results of judicial intervention to be of enduring importance. First, it has had a significant impact on the thinking and mindset of correctional administrators and midlevel and line staff so that the goal of humane and constructive treatment of prisoners is now more widely recognized and carried out in practice. An example is the extent to which many correctional systems are refusing to take advantage of the recent opportunities that more conservative court decisions have given them to reduce services or relax due process protections (as in *Sandin v. Conner*[124] or *Lewis v. Casey*[125]). Despite these rulings and the impediments to gaining access to the courts resulting from the PLRA, it is encouraging to note how few prisons are rushing to eliminate due process safeguards for assignment to disciplinary segregation or are closing their law libraries. Most prisons still offer far more than the minimum of one hour per day, five days a week of physical exercise and recreation that courts have defined as constitutionally sufficient (for example, *Watts v. Ramos*).[126] Second, according to Nathan, "correctional litigation has brought a measure of newly found self-respect to many prisoners. They know that they are no longer entirely outside the scope of legal protection—mere castaways from society about whom the laws have nothing to say or do. . . . They are no longer anyone's slaves."[127]

Nevertheless, PLRA's reactionary attempt to correct perceived excesses in prisoner litigation has seriously weakened the courts' salutary impetus and support for good correctional medicine and has notably impeded judicial inquiries into tragic violations of justice and humanity.

On the other hand, perhaps the need to depend on judicial relief could be obviated by certain offsetting strides that have been made in recent years, among them, efforts to professionalize correctional health care. Professional associations such as the National Commission on Correctional Health Care, the Academy of Correctional Health Professionals, the American Correctional Health Services Association, the American College of Correctional Physicians, and the Health Professional Interest Section of the American Correctional Association have been organized to address the pressing issues of health care in corrections. Professional codes of ethics and published position statements also lay out the responsibilities of caregivers involved in the system. The quality of physicians, nurses, health care administrators, and other health care staff serving many prisons, jails, and juvenile correctional facilities has improved notably over the past few decades. Excellent professional certification programs sponsored by the Academy of Correctional Health Professionals and the American Correctional Association assess initial competence by examination and require evidence of ongoing proficiency for continued certification. As quality and professionalism of staff have improved, there has been increasing utilization of quality assurance activities intended to monitor the safe and effective practice of medicine in corrections.

Also important is the growth of professionalism in the correctional industry. Correctional officers no longer see themselves as "guards" but as members of a profession to whom society has entrusted the care and custody of persons required by law to serve time in correctional institutions. They have their code of ethics and their standards to observe. By and large, correctional officers across the nation live up to these professional standards. And correctional physicians, nurses, psychologists, and other health professionals have also developed and promulgated codes of ethics for their members to follow. In an important clarification issued by the American Correctional Association, "The term 'guard' evokes a stereotypical and negative image that does not recognize their professionalism. The duties of corrections personnel, whose primary responsibility is custody and control, also include direct or indirect support of habilitative or rehabilitative programs that require advanced or specialized training."[128] Both the ACA and the American Jail Association also publish and sponsor excellent professional journals and offer the benefits of regional and national training conferences for correctional professionals.

Accreditation programs under the auspices of the NCCHC and the ACA will certainly continue to lead the way by signaling the essential characteristics of a humane and acceptable correctional health care program and effectively promoting their adoption. These programs also contribute significantly to the betterment of conditions of confinement in our country. Unfortunately, however, participation is voluntary and only a small fraction of prisons, jails, and juvenile facilities currently avail themselves of the benefits and safeguards of accreditation. Furthermore, neither the ACA nor the NCCHC, including their accreditation programs, is independently subsidized; instead, the bulk of their funding for conferences, programs, accreditation, and administration is derived from corporate sponsorship within the correctional or correctional-medical industry and from fees paid by facilities requesting accreditation. Consequently, it is at least conceivable that the accrediting agencies themselves could feel pressure to compromise if strict application of the standards might result in the loss of paying customers (that is, facilities seeking accreditation).

Only time will tell whether and to what extent the substantial and needed improvements made during the last four decades will survive. Strong and purposeful leadership by correctional officials outside the health field—especially commissioners and directors of corrections, wardens, and jail administrators—is highly critical in this regard. Their principled and unwavering commitment to ensure that inmates have prompt access to necessary health care services and their uncompromising insistence on quality of care that meets community standards of professional practice could go far to safeguard the progress that has been already achieved.

It is reasonable, therefore, to ask whether we can now rely on the forces of professionalism, self-monitoring, and accreditation to carry us forward in meeting our ethical and legal obligations. Can we do so without the intervention of the courts to require jails, prisons, and juvenile correctional facilities to maintain humane conditions of confinement? Sadly, we conclude that we cannot. Countervailing forces are only too evident. Witness the general public outcry against "coddling criminals" and the demand for "law and order." Politicians win no votes by expressing support for prison reform. Some legislators and their constituents espouse harsher conditions of confinement and hold that prisoners are deserving of every bad thing that happens to them. The PLRA provides that prisoners must exhaust all administrative remedies before they are eligible to bring a suit in law, and these provisions have been carried to their most extreme interpretations.

Restaurants, hotels, and the airlines, just like most other business enterprises, operate in a context in which market competition affords an incentive to strive for quality. Owners (proprietors) are motivated to be better than their competition in order to attract business and earn a profit. Even so, as experience has amply demonstrated, strictly enforced government regulation of each of these industries is essential to ensure safety, sanitary conditions, and environmental protection. The reason is that, without regulation, businesses are motivated to focus their efforts mainly on what is obvious to the public (their customers), such as amenities, courtesies, and outward display. The situation in correctional facilities stands in marked contrast. There is no built-in incentive either to provide amenities and attractive accommodations or to ensure safe and sanitary facilities and effective programs because their "customers" are not free to take their business elsewhere.

Inspired or enabled by the PLRA, some correctional agencies have taken purposeful steps to increase the number of complex administrative steps and shorten the filing time available to inmates in the hope they can remain immune to scrutiny by the courts as long as they are able to show that a prisoner's fumbling attempt to file a grievance was deficient on technical grounds. Some jurisdictions have allowed only two to five days after an event takes place for a valid grievance to be filed. Some make the requisite forms for the grievance difficult to obtain, or they may even require that the inmate request the grievance application from the very officer who is the target of the grievance. In juvenile facilities, the situation is even worse because the young inmates are too immature to comprehend the nature of their situation or understand the vague and complicated administrative procedures required of them to file a valid lawsuit petition. As the consent decrees were gradually terminated and court-imposed supervision ended, many states have visibly tended to slip back into their old ways.

William Collins, an experienced correctional attorney, said,

Looking at the changes in American prisons and jails over the past third of the twentieth century, one development produced more positive change across the country than any other: judicial oversight of the operation of prisons and jails. . . . More than any other trend, the federal courts have forced accountability on those persons and institutions whose responsibility it is to hold offenders accountable.[129]

Collins goes on to say: "Surely, one might argue public pressure would have put an end to these sorts of barbaric practices. But would it? Would the public have even been aware of these practices? Recent examples of public attitudes toward offenders show that today the public cares little about what happens to offenders and assumes offenders deserve whatever they get, as long as it is not good." But at least corrections can be trusted to police itself through accreditation and professionalism, can it not? Reported events such as "the 'counterfeit' internal investigation system, the tolerated staff brutality, the code of silence and the naked inmates in small cages come not from 1965 but from the early part of this decade [referring to the heinous conditions and practices brought to light in *Madrid v. Gomez* (1995) about the Pelican Bay prison complex in California].[130] Public pressure did not bring these practices . . . to light. Modern professional practices did not prevent these problems from developing virtually simultaneously with the opening of the institution. Litigation brought these problems to the light of day."[131]

It is reasonable to ask whether we can now rely on the forces of professionalism, self-monitoring, and accreditation to carry us forward in meeting our ethical and legal obligations. Can we do so without the intervention of the courts to require jails, prisons, and juvenile correctional facilities to maintain humane conditions of confinement? Sadly, we conclude that we cannot. Countervailing forces are only too evident.

What, then, is to be done? Experience teaches us that self-monitoring, although important, has its limitations. Organizations such as correctional systems possess their own internal supervisory and quality-assurance mechanisms. However, the operational goals of the agencies may themselves become self-serving and not well aligned with broader societal goals. There is also a risk that these internal monitors may tend to cover up mistakes or simply fail to notice them. For all these reasons, external reviews with no vested interests are beneficial. Accreditation can play a role, but its effectiveness is somewhat blunted by the factors already mentioned: it is voluntary and can be co-opted because the auditors work under tight time constraints.

Perhaps the situation is aptly described in the words of Juvenal, the ancient Roman satirical poet: *Sed quis custodiet ipsos custodes?* (But who will watch the watchmen?).[132] An objective outside perspective is needed, especially in total institutions such as prisons where the well-being and lives of so many prisoners is at stake. Correctional and health care administrators can and should be expected to behave honorably as their professional organizations encourage them to do, but they are being constantly squeezed by lawmakers and the public who criticize every expenditure and loudly clamor for harsher measures. In view of all this, the logic of requiring ample and ready access to the courts and effective judicial oversight is persuasive.

A New Challenge—The Impact of Mass Incarceration

Over the past few years, a new and important chapter in the history of court involvement in prison health care has been playing out as the U.S. Supreme Court deliberated and issued its response to *Brown v. Plata* [563 U.S. 493 (2011)]. This followed a lengthy litigation saga regarding inadequate health care services in the California Department of Corrections and Rehabilitation (CDCR). *Coleman v. Schwarzenegger* [912 F. Supp. 1282 (1995)] was a class action suit brought in federal court in 1990 that alleged serious deficiencies in prisoners' mental health care. *Plata v. Schwarzenegger* (Docket no. 3:01-cn-01351-TEH, N.D. Cal), another class action suit, was filed in 2001 and alleged unconstitutionally inadequate medical services. Ultimately, these class action cases were combined into *Brown v. Plata.*

After years of impasse, the *Coleman* court appointed a special master in 1995. In *Plata,* the court appointed a receiver in 2005 because, as the court found, implementation of the remedial plan had not been completed in a single prison by 2005. Plaintiffs in both cases filed motions to convene a special three-judge court, as required by the PLRA, to rule on a remedial order to reduce the California prison census. On August 4, 2009, this three-judge court unanimously held that a reduction in the California prison population was essential to allow provision of constitutional levels of medical and mental health care and ordered that the state of California reduce its overpopulation from 195 percent of rated capacity to 137.5 percent within two years and required the state to submit a plan for how it would accomplish this. It was left to the state to determine whether it would construct more prisons, transfer prisoners to other states, make greater use of parole, release certain classes of prisoners, increase use of good-time provisions, or modify the sentencing criteria. California initiated some steps toward reducing the census but appealed the decision to the U.S. Supreme Court, where hearings were held on November 30, 2010.[133] The central question before the court was whether a court order requiring California to reduce its prison population to remedy unconstitutional conditions in its correctional facilities violates the Prisoner Litigation Reform Act, which restricts the ability of federal judges to affect the capacity and conditions of prisons and jails beyond what is required by federal law and further limits a judge to order the "least intrusive [remedy] necessary to correct the violation of the Federal right."[134]

The California state prison system is the nation's largest. The three-judge court had concluded that "a primary reason" for the inadequacy of health care services is the severe crowding of California's 33 state prisons. As summarized in the *Harvard Law Review*, "Considering the testimony of seven expert witnesses, the court found that overcrowding led to a variety of impediments to the adequate provision of health care, including poor reception and treatment areas, an inability to house inmates by mental health classification, a lack of beds for mentally ill patients, an inability to recruit medical and mental health staff, poor medical records management, and poor suicide prevention care."[135] Among other findings, experts determined that an average of one unnecessary death per week was occurring in California prisons. Evidence was also submitted of unqualified health care providers and inadequate and unsuitable space for the provision of health care services.

In fact, even California's state inspector general, David R. Shaw, found significant problems in 17 prisons reviewed, stating that:

First, nearly all prisons were ineffective at ensuring that inmates receive their medications. Sixteen of the 17 institutions either failed to timely administer, provide, or deliver medications or failed to document that they had done so. The 17 prisons' average score of 59 percent in medication management was significantly below the minimum score for moderate adherence. . . .

The second recurring problem among the 17 prisons was poor access to medical providers and services. Prisons were generally ineffective at ensuring that inmates are seen or provided services for routine, urgent, and emergency medical needs according to timelines set by CDCR policy. Effective prison medical care depends on inmates' timely access to providers and services. No prisons met the 75 percent minimum score for moderate adherence on access to providers and services, while seven prisons scored 60 percent or less. . . .

Prisons scored particularly poorly in four component areas: preventive services, inmate hunger strikes, access to health care information, and specialty services. The average score for preventive services was only 37 percent, and we found alarmingly low scores in tuberculosis treatment. . . . Prisons also scored a very poor 60 percent average in specialty services; we found prisons not granting inmates timely access and not providing prompt follow-up related to those services.[136]

In its decision on May 23, 2011, a narrow majority of the Supreme Court ruled that CDRC needed to make massive reductions in its prison census. They affirmed the following: "Courts may not allow constitutional violations to continue simply because a remedy would involve intrusion into the realm of prison administration." The opinion also said that prison overcrowding in California "creates a certain and unacceptable risk of continuing violations of the rights of sick and mentally ill prisoners, with the result that many more will die or needlessly suffer. The Constitution does not permit this wrong." Moreover, "Just as a prisoner may starve if not fed, he or she may suffer or die if not provided adequate medical care. A prison that deprives prisoners of basic sustenance, including adequate medical care, is incompatible with the concept of human dignity and has no place in civilized society."

There were, however, strong objections. Justice Antonin Scalia, joined by Justice Clarence Thomas, sternly admonished the majority for affirming "what is perhaps the most radical injunction issued by a court in our Nation's history: an order requiring California to release the staggering number of 46,000 convicted criminals." Justice Samuel Alito filed a separate dissenting opinion, joined by Chief Justice John Roberts, in which he wrote that the "Constitution does not give federal judges the authority to run state penal systems."[137]

In the years following this landmark decision, California attempted to modify the decision or have it removed and made little progress in meeting the target reduction. The three-judge panel, instead of modifying the order, granted a two-year extension. California's prison census had hit a peak of 162,804 on November 1, 2006, and was at 143,565 on May 25, 2011, two days after the *Brown v. Plata* ruling. On January 20, 2016, it reached 112,792, which was 136.5% of capacity.[138]

As noted, the Court in *Brown v. Plata* allowed defendants discretion on how to relieve the overcrowding. California released some prisoners but transferred many more to local jails or to prisons in other states. Time will tell whether this may have compounded the problem by fragmenting the mass incarceration into multiple jails where it is more difficult to monitor and in facilities that were not designed for long-term incarceration.[139]

Had this all-important *Plata* ruling been otherwise, many thoughtful persons feared a serious erosion of the notable gains in prison health care achieved over the preceding 35 years. Yet Parsons warns, "Due to the fragility of the majority in *Brown* and the fact that the decisions of the Rehnquist Court and the PLRA echo Scalia's and Alito's concerns about the ruling, the arguments cannot be taken lightly and may prevail in future decisions."[140]

What the ACA's Public Correctional Policy on Conditions of Confinement has concluded is worth mentioning: "To support safe, secure and constitutionally acceptable conditions, agencies should . . . [e]stablish and maintain a safe and humane population limit for each facility and housing unit therein based upon recognized professional standards."[141] The challenge, of course, is to define and quantify as precisely as possible the operational requirements of "a safe and humane population limit."

CONCLUSION: LOOKING TOWARD THE FUTURE

Much has changed since the day that prisoners were deemed to be slaves of the state and to have lost all their civil rights. The concept of "civil death" is now all but abrogated. Since the 1960s, the courts have continued to struggle to define the extent of prisoner rights.

Johnson v. California [543 U.S. 499 (2005)] challenged the unwritten policy of the California Department of Corrections and Rehabilitation, which racially segregated prisoners for as many as 60 days in double-occupancy cells each time they entered a new correctional facility. The stated reason for this practice was to prevent violence caused by racial gangs. The Court said the Fourteenth Amendment ban on racial segregation outweighed the prison system's claim for deference because it is possible to address prison security concerns through individualized consideration without using racial segregation.

The *Harvard Law Review* commented on the *Johnson v. California* decision (which insisted on the application of *strict scrutiny* to the policy of racial segregation of prisoners, thereby requiring California to demonstrate that its policy was narrowly tailored to serve a compelling state interest). After acknowledging the standard objection that courts do not know much about the real dangers and risks involved in the operation of prisons and therefore should not meddle in their management, the article pointed out that prisons are no more unknown to judges than are other public institutions, such as universities and the police, which are frequently subject to strict scrutiny. In other words, the argument that there is a singular gap in expertise between prison administrators and courts is not persuasive. Perhaps, rather, the true reason some courts have taken this stand is an unspoken belief that prisoners have forfeited their rights by committing crimes and that the extreme and oppressive conditions of incarceration represent a just punishment. As the *Harvard Law Review* suggests, the real question may well be "Why do prisoners lose full constitutional protection at all?"

The Court should return to the fundamental question of why prisoners have a subordinate constitutional status in the first place. . . . The key question . . . is why prisoners lose full constitutional protection at all. Historically, the normative justification for stripping prisoners of constitutional protection was that they had committed crimes. . . . One may question whether a punitive purpose still motivates some who would limit prisoners' claims to constitutional protection. . . . No matter how heinous their crimes, a rule that would deprive prisoners of equal protection would only serve to punish "society as a whole."[142]

Some additional signs of hope are on the horizon. A shift in U.S. public opinion concerning the overuse of incarceration is encouraging. Topics of discussion include revising harsh and determinate sentencing practices, modifying parole guidelines, and repealing draconian and ineffective drug laws. There is growing awareness that the high rates of incarceration and the disproportionate representation of African Americans, Hispanics, other minorities, and the poor are direct results of factors like the war on drugs, institutionalized racism in our society, and profit-induced pressures brought by the corporate prison industry. Certainly, a driving force in this focus of interest is the economic reality of the surging cost of prisons and jails in the face of a sluggish economy and the devastating impacts this has had in depleting funds needed for schools, infrastructure, health, and other public priorities. Moreover, people do not like being reminded that we have, by far, the highest rate of incarceration anywhere in the world. Also of significant importance are recent symbolic events—especially the visit of President Barack Obama to a federal prison in Oklahoma in 2015 and the visit shortly thereafter by Pope Francis to a Philadelphia prison. These events called widespread attention to the reality and excesses of incarceration in our country. President Obama announced criminal justice reform as a high priority. "Reformation of our broken system of criminal justice is long overdue not only for humanitarian reasons, but also for our national economic health."[143]

Reflecting this shift in public perception, there was little strident clamor for "law and order" from the 2016 presidential candidates, and a few of the candidates repeatedly spoke out for revision or repeal of the drug laws, reform of sentencing practices, elimination of private prisons, and the urgent need to downsize the prison system and correct the disproportionate racial and ethnic composition of inmate populations. Given the outcome of the 2016 elections, however, it remains to be seen what trends will emerge. Nevertheless, the *Plata* decision highlighted the plight of persons incarcerated in grossly overcrowded conditions and, as a result of all these influences, there appears to be some convergence of energy toward constructive action in this arena. As a nation and a people, we are much better than this, and it will be to our credit that we take decisive action to reverse these unfortunate trends. We should be reminded that what *Plata* revealed about California is by no means limited to that state alone, and these travesties—including overcrowding, racial and ethnic disparities, and extreme isolation—must be detected and addressed wherever they exist. The courts are uniquely able to bring the light of day to bear on the hidden world of corrections. We are a society of law, and we do ourselves a great disservice when we systematically deny justice and dignity to any of our members, for (as both John Locke [1689] and William Pitt [1770] proclaimed) "Wherever law ends, tyranny begins." Finally, Fyodor Dostoevsky's admonition again rings clear: "The degree of civilization in a society can be judged by entering its prisons."

Chapter 5

How Much Health Care Is Appropriate and Necessary?*

A COMPLEX ISSUE

Whenever a correctional system denies prisoners access to necessary and adequate health care, it perpetuates a collective crime against the prisoners that is equally as wrong and abhorrent as their heinous crimes against society.

Occasionally someone asks how much health care a prisoner is entitled to receive. This is a difficult question. In truth, we do not even have a satisfactory method for defining how much health care a person in free society should receive. As our society is structured today, the answer often depends on the patient's ability to pay, either personally or through insurance. Government programs provide a safety net of sorts for some, as do charity and uncompensated care. Insurance and government third-party payers have their own criteria, benefit packages, and mechanisms for prior approval and utilization review of procedures and services. The extensive national debate that culminated in the Patient Protection and Affordable Care

---

* This chapter has been extensively revised by the author from the version that appeared in the predecessor to this volume [Kenneth L. Faiver, *Health Care Management Issues in Corrections* (Lanham, MD: American Correctional Association, 1997) in the chapter entitled "Defining Appropriate and Necessary Health Care," 69–82]. The current chapter contains a reformulation of some key elements of the previous model for decision making. This prior version was itself adapted with permission from an article that was published in the *Journal of Correctional Health Care* [B. Jaye Anno, Kenneth L. Faiver, and Jay K. Harness, "A Preliminary Model for Determining Limits for Health Care Services" 3(1) (Spring 1996), 67–84]. An even earlier version of this material, "Setting the Standard for Correctional Health Care Services," written by Kenneth L. Faiver (MLIR, MPH) in collaboration with Jay K. Harness (MD, FACS) and B. Jaye Anno (PhD, CCHP-A) was first delivered by Dr. Harness at the Fourth World Congress on Prison Health Care in London, England, in August 1988.

Act of 2010 addressed some of these underlying questions in an effort to render health care services more accessible to all Americans.

Given the exploding medical and pharmaceutical technologies and the ever-spiraling costs of health care, the United States may be approaching a time when explicit rationing of health care services will be necessary, at least for the highest-cost procedures. Some other countries with nationalized health coverage programs are already effectively doing so through decisions of public health authorities.

> Whenever a correctional system denies prisoners access to necessary and adequate health care, it perpetuates a collective crime against the prisoners that is equally as wrong and abhorrent as their heinous crimes against society.

Even in the United States, rationing of health care services is already common. It is clearly implicit in the prior authorization mechanisms used by health maintenance organizations and health insurance companies and is operative by way of the economic ability of self-payers to purchase their care. Moreover, we use explicit rationing as our system of allocating scarce human organs for transplantation such as kidneys, livers, hearts, lungs, and corneas. In selecting recipients for vital human organs, hard choices are made that effectively determine who shall live and who shall die.

When it comes to how much we are willing to spend on the health care of an individual prisoner, are there any upper limits? Undoubtedly there are, just as there ultimately must be in the larger society. But we need to decide which societal values we wish to safeguard in this process. If we ever reach the point when these explicit criteria need to be established, there will be long and arduous debate and many points of view will be expressed. In the end, American citizens should and will demand clear and transparent criteria that, above all, demonstrate fairness, ethics, and due regard for human dignity.

Using medically sound prognostic criteria seems best for now: eligibility should be based on how much net benefit can be expected at the margin from the procedure relative to its cost and given the available alternatives. Care should be taken to prevent, insofar as possible, bias and prejudice from inequitably tilting the balance. Use of medical criteria is far preferable to the torturous approach of biased and self-righteous judgment that would characterize the creation and use of a "social worth" model. Such an approach is based on the premise that some persons, because they are deemed able to make a greater contribution to society, are therefore of greater value than others—a premise that runs counter to the self-evident truth announced by our founders in the Declaration of Independence that "all men are created equal."

Established standards for correctional health care primarily emphasize structural and process issues involved in the delivery of care. In a few instances, they attempt to address outcomes of care, but none specifically define the quality of care that must be provided nor the extent of care that is required. Perhaps a closer approach may be found in the clinical practice guidelines now available to correctional health providers for many chronic diseases. Although courts have given a few hints, they also have not directly dealt with the question of how much health care is necessary—nor are they likely to do so.

> The "social worth" model of allocating scarce health care resources is based on the premise that some persons, because they are deemed able to make a greater contribution to society, are therefore of greater value than others—a premise that runs counter to the self-evident truth announced by our founders in the Declaration of Independence that "all men are created equal."

The issue is complex because so many variables are involved. How badly is the care needed? How quickly is it needed? What will happen if it is not provided? How much does it cost? How long has the patient had this condition? How painful is the condition, and can the treatment be expected to alleviate the pain? What loss of function is associated with the condition, and can the treatment be expected to improve function? How risky is the procedure? How did the illness or injury happen? How long will the patient remain in the correctional system? What other treatments are available and how effective are they? How much does the patient want the care? What evidence has the patient shown that she or he will cooperate in the treatment process? Is the intervention likely to bring significant improvement? How old is the patient? Is it a prison, a jail, a juvenile facility, or an immigration detention center? What concomitant medical condition does the patient have? Is the treatment a well-accepted procedure, or is it new and experimental? How long, complicated, costly, and risky will be the recovery? What are the enduring side effects? Many of these questions are relevant in each case and must be explicitly or implicitly addressed.

If it is difficult to make such decisions for members of a free society, then how might we expect prisoners to fare in the process? Fortunately, we have some basis for optimism. The U.S. Supreme Court held that deliberate indifference to the serious medical needs of prisoners violates the Constitution. Numerous courts in recent years have enforced decisions that require access to health care for prisoners. The ethics of the medical profession require the physician to place the well-being and health of the patient first and beyond any and all other considerations. The call to fairness of the American people harkens back to the principle that we are all essentially equal no matter what our station in life. The Constitution prohibits deprivation of the rights of any person without due process. Criminal trial courts, in depriving convicted persons of their liberty, do not intend to diminish their access to proper health care. Such is not a component of their punishment.

Some persons have staunchly maintained that a correctional system is not obliged to restore or repair health problems of a person if these existed before incarceration but only to prevent, insofar as possible, any deterioration of health. According to this view, inmates should leave prison no sicker than they arrived except for the unavoidable and natural effects of aging.

These issues merit serious consideration precisely because denial of health care is not included in the punishment decreed by society. Jails, on the one hand, are short-term facilities and thus usually not held responsible for more than maintaining patients at their current levels of health, including stabilization and treatment of emergencies, relief of pain, avoidance of loss of limb or function, and prevention and treatment of injuries and infections. Prison systems, on the other hand, do much more. They must invest in the restoration of preexisting conditions when this can be expected to extend life, improve (or prevent loss of) function, relieve pain, or significantly affect quality of life. Juvenile facilities, in addition, must take into account the developmental needs of young persons and may have an even greater obligation to restore function to the extent possible, taking into consideration the expected length of stay in the correctional system. This topic is discussed further in this chapter under "Preexisting Conditions."

Because resources are limited, priorities must be set. In a sense, the first priority service for any correctional system is intake health screening. Actually, this is a prerequisite for service. By learning what health problems enter through the front door, a correctional system can know what services will be required, who will need them, and how urgently. The obvious next priority is to give appropriate and timely follow-up care to the health problems detected at intake and to those that subsequently arise.

This chapter will not provide precise or definitive answers that quantify the extent of medical interventions to which prisoners are entitled. Instead, it will attempt to define the issues and present explicit criteria for decision makers to consider in determining whether a particular health service should be provided in a specific case. It will offer a model for thinking about the complex set of variables involved in decisions of this nature.

Practitioner Guidelines

Clinical guidelines do not precisely specify how much care should be rendered. Rather, they offer an evidence-based and acceptable process of care. As their name suggests, practitioner guidelines are neither standards nor mandates. Although their proper use and application depend on competent exercise of clinical expertise and judgment, they do represent what is currently held to be a proper clinical response to a given set of symptoms and problems.

Clinical guidelines are useful for several reasons. First, the practice of medicine is complex and new advances are continually being made, so no single provider can ever be fully conversant with the best practice for all treatment situations. Second, especially in the practice of institutional medicine, there is value in maintaining some reasonable consistency of practice among providers so that patients with similar conditions are treated in essentially the same manner. Practice guidelines are designed for the purpose of ensuring good quality of care while avoiding treatment modalities that are unnecessarily costly. In this regard, Dr. Robert Greifinger writes:

Correctional health care programs should use evidence-based treatments. Too few correctional health care programs use nationally accepted guidelines for the diagnosis and treatment of chronic disease and mental illness. Diabetes, hypertension, coronary artery disease, hyperlipidemia, and asthma are examples of diseases for which a consensus agrees that there are clear, cost-effective methods for reducing morbidity and mortality. There is no good reason not to implement these methods. Without them there is excess morbidity, mortality, and cost. Why shouldn't correctional clinicians follow nationally accepted methods for diagnosing and treating the most prevalent conditions behind bars, especially when they are cost-effective for society?[1]

While practitioner guidelines are based on the best available current evidence at the time they are published, they are not always perfect. They are not derived from randomized clinical outcome studies as much as from clinical judgments and expert opinions of reputable practitioners. Nor can they anticipate all possible situations. They do contain helpful suggestions and recommendations. For example, guidelines for treatment of diabetes specify that regular monitoring of glycemic control by HbA1c is required. Failure to do this or to have periodic funduscopic retinal examinations or regular podiatric examinations would suggest unacceptable care of diabetic patients, whether in prisons or in the free world. Consequently, when practitioners deviate from published practitioner guidelines, they need to document in the patient record the reasoning that led them to choose another path unless the rationale is otherwise obvious from the record.

Clinical guidelines can be obtained from learned professional associations of physicians specializing in various areas of medicine. Examples include the American Diabetic Association; the National Heart, Lung and Blood Institute; the American College of Physicians; and the American Academy of Pediatrics. Another excellent source of clinical practice guidelines that may be particularly useful for jails and prisons is the set developed by the Federal Bureau of Prisons.[2] These cover a wide range of topics. Doctors working in corrections may confidently use these as guidelines but not as substitutes for their own professional judgment and skill.

Another source of helpful clinical guidelines from a recognized panel of authorities can be found in the recommendations of the U.S. Preventive Services Task Force that was convened by the U.S. Public Health Service. Rather than offering systematic guidance on the overall treatment of specific conditions, they deal with particular questions that arise in the course of treatment. These recommendations are organized by topic for ready access on the Web site. In its own words, the task force "was convened to rigorously evaluate clinical research in order to assess the merits of preventive measures, including screening tests, counseling, immunizations, and preventive medications. The topics in these lists include all recommendations: active, inactive, and in progress."[3] The work of the task force is widely recognized as "the gold standard" for preventive care strategies, and it has been charged by the Patient Protection and Affordable Care Act of 2010 to make annual reports to the Congress regarding preventive care.

An essential standard of the National Commission on Correctional Health Care requires that for chronic diseases the responsible physician establish clinical protocols consistent with national clinical practice guidelines, and the standard further requires that the medical record document the use of these guidelines by the clinicians.[4]

Universal Principles

Adequate health care services are essential for all elements of society in all parts of the world. These services are equally important to the inmates of jails, prisons, and juvenile facilities and must be provided to at least the extent that is commensurate with contemporary community norms. Receiving health care is as fundamental as obtaining food, clothing, and shelter. Denial of health care should never be justified as part of an inmate's punishment.

The reference here is to *contemporary* norms because the standards of professional practice evolve over time, as well as to *community* norms because they may differ somewhat from place to place. The standards depend on technological and scientific advances; on the ability to process, disseminate, and use information; and on the availability of skilled practitioners and other resources. Some aspects of the professional standards of practice are influenced by cultural factors and sensibilities. Economic factors also can shape the standards, a process much in evidence today as third-party payers apply the principles of managed care and as incentive shifting occurs in the medical marketplace. How much society can afford to pay is not irrelevant, especially in view of new and costly technology.

Given the universal requirement for health care, certain basic standards and norms related to those services must apply equally in and out of correctional facilities. These primarily have to do with the fundamental ethical principles[5] of *beneficence* and *autonomy*.

> Denial of health care should never be justified as part of an inmate's punishment.

As used here, the term *beneficence* includes its positive aspect (the norm of providing a benefit) and its double-negative aspect, which is sometimes called *nonmaleficence* (the norm of avoiding causation of harm). This norm of *beneficence* requires the medical system to intervene to do some good for the patient and does not allow it to cause intentional harm. Thus, the medical system will provide the specific services that correspond to the contemporary community standard of professional practice. It will do so in a manner (type, quantity, and intensity) that is consistent with the needs, wishes, and condition of the patient and in a manner (quality) that is also in keeping with the standard of practice. Because it will do no harm to the patient, the medical intervention will respect the patient's *dignity* (causing no unnecessary embarrassment or humiliation and acknowledging the value and intrinsic worth of the person), respect the patient's *privacy* (safeguarding the confidentiality of the patient's medical record and condition), honor the patient's *liberty* (choosing the least-restrictive mode of management), and ensure the patient's *safety* (achieving a safe and sanitary treatment setting to avoid undue risk of infection or other harm and selecting those intervention modalities that offer the best *net benefit* (that is, a balance of overall benefit with the risk of unintended harm or injury) to the patient.

The norm of *autonomy* respects the decision-making capabilities of the patient. A medical procedure will be performed only if the patient gives informed consent. Therefore, the patient is entitled to full and truthful information about the condition, diagnosis, treatment plan, and prognosis in plain and understandable language, and he or she has a right to participate in determining treatment decisions. Autonomy likewise recognizes the right of a competent person to refuse any unwanted and therefore unlawful touching of his or her person. This is challenged in the noncorrectional setting only if there is question about the patient's ability to make a competent decision, and not merely because someone in authority may not happen to agree with that decision. For overriding public health or safety reasons, involuntary treatment of an incompetent person or quarantine of a competent but unwilling person requires due process, usually a court order. These rules are no different for prisoners.

The failure of care professionals to meet an acceptable contemporary standard constitutes negligence and malpractice. No convincing ethical or legal argument can be made that would justify denying to inmates of a correctional institution a level of health care that is equivalent to the contemporary standard and practice of the community.

Prisoners are entitled to the same contemporary standard of medical, dental, surgical, psychiatric, and nursing care, inclusive of diagnostic, preventive, rehabilitative, and palliative strategies, as are persons in the free world. For example, management of diabetes would be essentially the same, whether or not the patient was incarcerated. In the United States and in most industrialized countries, a "contemporary standard" for the management of diabetes and its known complications and sequelae has evolved. This is also true of most medical, dental, and psychiatric maladies. The failure of care professionals to meet an acceptable contemporary standard constitutes negligence and malpractice. No convincing ethical or legal argument can be made that would justify denying to inmates of a correctional institution a level of health care that is equivalent to the contemporary standard and practice of the community.

Prisoners also must be deemed to have the same fundamental rights as any free world patient. This includes respect for the person's dignity as a human being, as well as the right to receive care in a safe, sanitary, and clean environment with an adequate amount of space and in an area that is sufficiently equipped to allow the delivery of contemporary quality of care. Qualifications and credentials of the providers must meet the same licensing and certification standards that society holds to be required in the community. Contemporary health care cannot be provided in a substandard setting with inadequate space or equipment, unqualified providers, or excessive time constraints. A reaffirmation of the universal health care issues just discussed is essential to ensuring that inmates receive adequate and dignified care.

CONCEPTUAL FRAMEWORK FOR DECISION ANALYSIS

Resources available for providing health care in correctional settings are limited. In a free market economy, scarce resources are allocated according to the price consumers are willing to pay. An insurance mechanism that affords benefits to enrollees may be available to offset the out-of-pocket costs to consumers. Some governments provide health care to all their citizens on an entitlement basis through a national health service. In the United States, many who cannot afford private health services and do not have insurance are aided through a complex system of Medicaid, welfare, and other social assistance programs.

Prisoners are recognized as having a right to receive health care, their entitlement resting on a common law theory that the warder is responsible for the life, safety, and well-being of the ward. In the United States, there also is a constitutional obligation to provide health care to prisoners who are deprived of the opportunity to seek care on their own. To be "deliberately indifferent" to their serious medical needs has been declared a violation of the Eighth and Fourteenth Amendments to the Constitution, in view of the right to be free of cruel and unusual punishment and the right to due process [*Estelle v. Gamble*, 429 U.S. 97 (1976)].

Not every request a prisoner makes for a specific health service must be granted. How much care should be provided, as a matter of good public policy, is the subject of this chapter. The principles and recommendations described here are not always founded in law or enforceable by a court. They do represent, however, what is becoming recognized as the proper level of care by many qualified expert groups, agencies, and individuals—namely, care that generally is deemed important or necessary in the free community. In addition, the quality of whatever care is provided must also be in keeping with contemporary standards of professional practice.

Rather than attempt to construct an exhaustive list of procedures and treatments to which prisoners are entitled under specified circumstances, it may be more helpful to develop a conceptual framework for considering factors that influence the selection of services to be provided. This framework begins by describing a spectrum of services that ranges from those that ought to be provided to those that may appropriately be denied. In between these extremes are diagnostic and therapeutic procedures that arguably should be provided to prisoners or whose acceptability depends on one or more relevant circumstances. For example, almost no one would withhold emergency first aid or obstetrical care, but few believe that prisoners are entitled to cosmetic hair transplants or face-lifts at public expense. Thus, it is clear that not every medical procedure that is technologically possible or commonly performed in free society is obligatory for prisoners. Moreover, the Supreme Court determined that the Constitution prohibits "deliberate indifference to the serious medical needs" of prisoners. Thus, unnecessary care, or care that promises only trivial health benefit, is not required.

Dr. Dean P. Rieger offers some criteria for determining seriousness:

- Will the condition if untreated cause loss of life or limb, or make it significantly more likely?
- Does the condition cause or lead to significant pain or other suffering?
- Does the condition cause or lead to significant negative impact on activities of daily living (as defined by our nursing professionals)?[6]

Disagreement, however, may vary on different levels about whether a prisoner should be afforded open-heart surgery, a kidney transplant, gender change surgery, an artificial limb, or a hearing aid. Such disagreement is reasonable when it concerns a clinical appraisal of the patient's condition and prognosis with and without the procedure so that the issue is a comparison of the benefit with the cost. But it would be unacceptable to hold that a person qua prisoner ought to be treated differently from others.

After describing characteristics of the spectrum of care and providing a few illustrations, a model will be presented for the decision-making process. The model attempts to cope with the multiple factors that can or should influence the outcome, sometimes independently and sometimes in combination, in each specific case.

The conceptual framework presented here may be useful to individual clinical practitioners, to ethical advisors, and especially to utilization review committees in organizing and weighing the multiple variables that necessarily factor into the decision process. In most large correctional systems, there is need for a highly structured, multidisciplinary utilization review process that will proactively review all nonurgent clinical decisions involving costly or unusual procedures. The intent is to avoid unnecessary health expenditures and achieve consistency and fairness. There are evidence-based resources, textbooks, and software applications that can assist correctional systems in reaching these decisions. The success of such a system, however, in terms of protecting the patients' access to necessary care is critically dependent on the effective advocacy efforts of primary care providers on behalf of their patients.

A pharmaceutical formulary serves as a similarly helpful guide for practitioners, requiring them to utilize first-line remedies unless there are sound clinical reasons to deviate such as allergies, a history of poor response to the first-line medication, or another contraindication. The content of the formulary should be predicated on considerations of efficacy, patient safety, and cost-effectiveness.

A coalition of national organizations representing health care professionals, government officials, and business leaders formed a working group to develop a set of principles specifying the essential features of a sound drug formulary system. Their definition of a *drug formulary* is "a continually updated list of medications and related information, representing the clinical judgement of physicians, pharmacists and other experts in the diagnosis and/or treatment of disease and promotion of health." Their recommendations for a formulary program are also appropriate for every correctional system:

- Enable individual patient needs to be met with nonformulary drug products when demonstrated to be clinically justified by the physician or other prescriber.
- Institute an efficient process for the timely procurement of nonformulary drug products and impose minimal administrative burdens.
- Provide access to a formal appeal process if a request for a nonformulary drug is denied.
- Include policies that state that practitioners should not be penalized for prescribing nonformulary drug products that are medically necessary.[7]

International Implications

This book may well be read by practitioners and correctional authorities in countries outside the United States where decidedly different customs and cultures prevail. Most of what is said here should still apply, but it is relevant to consider what is meant throughout this book by the phrase "contemporary standards of community practice." These standards are evolving and depend in part on the introduction of technological advances and new scientific knowledge. The prevailing community standards are also related to the affluence of a society in terms of being able to afford the latest and the best. In some Third World countries, only rudimentary medical practice and basic hygiene are available for the majority of citizens. Then the level of care required in a prison system may be no higher than that which is generally available to the free citizens. By the same token, however, it must not be less.

Adequate health care services are essential for all elements of society, no matter where people live, yet we find great discrepancies in what is available in the general free world community across countries or regions just as we do across economic and social strata. Because health care is still widely held to be a good or service that money can buy, not everyone defines it as a basic human right. Still, decent people are not comfortable seeing extreme examples of want or lack of the basic necessities of life—including health care—among any group or class of people or any set of individuals. There is a basic norm, an entitlement to receive medical care that transcends the economics of buying and selling. Some countries have addressed this by adopting social programs that include a form of universal health insurance. Each of these plans or approaches, however, still needs to face the question: given available resources and the recognized unmet need, how do we decide to allocate these limited resources so as to accomplish the greatest good?

Consider the issue of local community standards (what level of health services free citizens commonly receive) being relevant to the standard of care for prisoners in that society. As we rapidly become a global economy both in principle and in reality, we find we are less comfortable with this situation. The extreme examples of lack of basic health care for incarcerated persons (and of free citizens) in some locales cannot be condoned. Some generous physicians and other health professionals are actively involved in their own small way to address these inequities and freely give of their skills and time and resources to provide health care services to prisoners in Third World countries as often as they are able. Physicians, nurses, and others are doing commendable work in Caribbean, African, and other resource-poor regions with programs like Health through Walls, an organization founded and directed by Dr. John P. May,[8] just as Doctors Without Borders (Médecins Sans Frontières) and similar organizations try to mitigate extreme lack of health care services among free citizens of these societies.

In summary, although geographic variances can influence the application of this model, the thought process should remain substantially the same.

A SPECTRUM OF CARE MODEL

Visualize a spectrum or range of health care interventions plotted with two axes. The horizontal axis represents the necessity or *need* for the intervention. As will be seen, this is a complex variable essentially comprising the net expected benefit to health, function, life expectancy, and relief from pain conditioned by factors such as urgency, desire, chronicity, and availability of alternatives. The vertical axis represents *cost* of the procedure and its associated aftercare. The higher the cost and the lower the need, the more likely the procedures will move toward rarely or never approved, and the lower the cost and the higher the need, the more likely a procedure will tend to be usually or always approved.

At one end are those interventions to which an inmate is *always* entitled. These are where need is high relative to cost. An example would be emergency treatment to save a life or limb or to alleviate severe pain. Giving first aid to a burn victim, setting a broken limb, and cleansing and dressing a wound also illustrate interventions of this type. Other examples might be treatment of acute and severe psychiatric illness; an emergency appendectomy or gall bladder surgery; medication for chronic conditions such as high blood pressure, diabetes, asthma, or epilepsy; treatment of infectious disease; and emergency dental care to relieve pain. These are represented in the lowest zone labeled "always" in Figure 5.1.

Figure 5.1
Spectrum of care model: Likelihood of approval for medical care decisions.

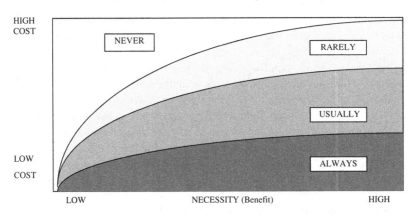

LIKELIHOOD OF APPROVAL FOR MEDICAL CARE DECISIONS:

Effect of *Cost* versus *Necessity* of Care

Those items *usually* recognized as services to which prisoners are entitled might include psychological counseling, group therapy, basic prosthetic limbs and orthotic devices, dental fillings, hernia repair, orthopedic surgery, physical therapy, renal dialysis, a pacemaker, a CT scan or magnetic resonance imaging (MRI) for certain indications, cataract surgery, completion of transsexual surgery, preventive interventions and immunizations, replacement of missing front teeth, and removal of a gang tattoo. Many medications are also in this category, including antiretroviral therapy for HIV and antiviral treatment for hepatitis C (HCV). When these services can safely be deferred for a time, the expected length of incarceration becomes particularly relevant to the decision process. For those who face a short stay, a somewhat greater need or urgency is required, relative to cost, to justify the intervention. These services are depicted in Figure 5.1 in the area labeled "usually."

Medical procedures that safely can be deferred for a time are sometimes called "elective procedures," meaning that they are not urgent. Another common but quite different understanding of the term "elective" is "of doubtful necessity" or "optional." To avoid any confusion and because this chapter is about the determination of medical *necessity* rather than *urgency*, the term "elective" will be avoided. If the term does arise in deliberations or policies regarding what services to provide, its meaning should be carefully clarified to prevent miscommunication.

A third group comprises procedures that are *rarely* approved for prisoners, or at least are subject to much greater scrutiny and review. These include extremely expensive procedures as well as those of doubtful necessity. Examples are bone-marrow and other major organ transplants,[9] certain plastic and reconstructive surgeries, and possibly initiation of transsexual surgery. In view of the high cost, the need (and expected benefit) of these procedures must be recognized as being especially great to justify their approval, as illustrated in the area labeled "rarely."

Finally, there has been close to universal consensus that prisoners are *never* entitled to certain procedures at public expense. Examples might include purely cosmetic or luxury treatments or expensive alternatives to conventional treatment—such as gold crowns or dental implants. These are in the upper portion of the chart in the area labeled "never."

The preceding examples are not intended to be normative but to illustrate the process and applicability of the model. Further, the boundaries are not rigid. There remains room for debate and clarification in specific instances, but the proposed paradigm may serve as a useful format to aid the discussion. Any procedure or treatment, for example, may cross boundaries as it shifts along the axes of need and cost.

The case of treatment for persistent gender incongruence can illustrate how these boundaries can be crossed and how some procedures can migrate from one category to another over time in light of developing understanding of diseases and evolving social norms. For example, *completion* of transsexual surgery, which had been assigned to the "rarely" category in an earlier edition of this chapter, is now viewed as belonging to "usual." Similar reasoning places the *continuation* of hormonal therapy for transsexual patients in the "always" category unless medically contraindicated. Finally, the real medical rationale for not placing the *initiation* of transsexual surgery into the "usually" segment of the benefit package has more to do with its lack of urgency and the difficulty of predicting success of the initial procedures. Hence, we have tentatively classified it as "rarely," where several other factors can be assessed to determine the relative necessity of the procedure for any given individual. Those, on the other hand, who believe this procedure to be unnecessary would prefer to assign it to the "never" category. However, this is an evolving area in that the severity of pain and suffering from gender dysphoria is becoming more widely recognized, and the technology for successful and safe treatment is advancing.[10] When there is a recognized medical necessity for transsexual surgery, based on community standards, the "rarely" category is clearly inappropriate.

At least theoretically, some level of need is so trivial as not to be required, no matter how low its cost. Likewise, some interventions may cost so much that they would not be provided, however great the need. Hence, the idealized curves in Figure 5.1 begin at zero, rise, and then gradually decrease in slope over their relevant range.

The graphic representation illustrates a somewhat oversimplified formulation of the relationship of necessity and cost to the decision to provide health care. The lower the necessity (benefit) or the higher the cost, the greater the ease of denying the service. The lower the cost or the greater the necessity (benefit), the more difficult it should be to deny the procedure. Necessity of the procedure is intended to represent a function of the net benefit that the procedure would bring to the patient. Hence, the terms *necessity* and *benefit* are largely interchangeable in this context. There are times when net benefit to others is also relevant, as when considering the treatment of an infectious condition or the treatment of mental illness.

Cost is usually measured in or translated into dollars. For example, the cost to a correctional agency for medical transport and for guarding a patient at a community hospital is just as real an expenditure as the hospital bill or the doctor's bill. Other less tangible costs also can be incorporated into this model, at least conceptually, such as the cost of potential harm to society from the escape of a violent prisoner during a hospital stay. As medical advances continue and new medications or the increased use of laparoscopic, laser, microscopic, and robotic surgical techniques renders the need for a lengthy hospital stay less frequent, these developments can possibly shift the outcome of the cost–benefit equation.

> The graphic representation illustrates a somewhat oversimplified formulation of the relationship of necessity and cost to the decision to provide health care. The lower the necessity (benefit) or the higher the cost, the greater the ease of denying the service. The lower the cost or the greater the necessity (benefit), the more difficult it should be to deny the procedure.

Some people will object to a model that allows an explicit trade-off between cost and need on grounds that human life cannot be valued in dollars. Others might object from the standpoint that several courts have ruled that a state is not excused from providing required care to a prisoner simply because it would be too costly.[11] The response to the first objection is that all of us make the cost-versus-need trade-off each day, often implicitly. A smoker decides to risk eventual cancer for the current enjoyment of tobacco. An insurance company covers certain benefits and not others. A society quickly would go bankrupt if it were bound to spend unlimited amounts—say, millions of dollars per each death averted—on behalf of each of its citizens. In answer to the second objection, the court rulings in these instances were far down the scale of costliness from the level envisioned here as an outer boundary.

The question can be phrased using different terms. How much should be spent at the margin to achieve various levels of benefit? For example, one might willingly pay a large sum to extend a life by 20 healthy years, but how much would the same person (or society) be willing to pay if the expected benefit were only an additional year, one week, or just one day? Or what if the quality of life during that extended period of life were severely diminished? Again, it needs to be emphasized that the application of this concept must be essentially the same whether or not the patient is a prisoner.

From Whose Perspective?

Where costs are high, a greater expectation of benefit is required to justify the proposed intervention. But from whose perspective should costs and benefits be considered? Among the possibilities are the perspectives of the individual patient, the attending provider or health care delivery system, fellow prisoners, and society in general.

From the *point of view of the individual patient*, the desired benefit may be cure or improvement in health as far as is technically achievable, no matter what the cost. In contrast, in free society, there comes a point at which most people reach a balance between the marginal benefit to be gained from additional units of treatment and the marginal cost (or price) of that treatment. At some point, a patient, who must bear all or a significant portion of the cost of the treatment finds that the additional care "is simply not worth it."

This trade-off is relevant to inmates because nonmonetary costs also temper the demand for health services. For prisoners, just as for free world patients with full health benefit coverage through an insurance plan, the time spent, the expense of travel, and the inconvenience incurred in seeking and receiving care are real costs. Treatment itself can bring its own pains, discomforts, adverse side effects, and risks. There are times when people object to the "probing" or "guessing" of doctors and prefer more conservative or "natural" remedies or even no treatment at all. People can resent the assault on their privacy and the negative consequences that certain types of diagnostic and treatment procedures involve. These disincentives to seek care are operative among inmates as well, serving effectively to curb a theoretically limitless desire to avail themselves of every possible treatment option.

In correctional facilities, a countervailing secondary gain may be associated with the receipt of health services because of the opportunity for social contact with inmates, nurses, and others—or for an excursion outside of a confined living unit. This perceived "nonhealth care" benefit is greatest in facilities that severely curtail movement and social interaction.

From the *perspective of the provider or the correctional health care agency*, the desired objectives may be to accomplish maximum good for the patient and also to protect oneself and the agency from risk of lawsuit for denial of necessary care. Thus, whether out of benevolence or the defensive practice of medicine, there may be a tendency to overtreat. On the other hand, the health care providers in a jail or prison usually are given a limited budget and therefore have an incentive to be cost conscious. These predetermined budgetary limitations need not be regarded as absolute. In meritorious cases of extraordinary need, the health care provider (correctional agency) may seek a supplemental appropriation or other adjustment from the funding authority. Sometimes they may need to reduce other nonnecessary expenses so as to enable provision of required care.

In attempting to use available dollars to provide essential services to the greatest number of prisoners, health systems necessarily engage in some rationing of care. Beyond this, the contracting of health care services by state and county governments to private for-profit corporations adds a new element of concern that appropriate care could be denied in order to increase profits.

In some circumstances, one must consider the *perspective of fellow prisoners* to the extent that their well-being may be affected by the outcome. Perhaps the clearest example is in the case of a contagious disease, where prompt and effective treatment, even though costly, would be judged worthwhile if it reduces the risk of other prisoners contracting the disease. In addition, the case of contagious disease has a bearing on the costs to the correctional agency, to the well-being of security staff, and even to the general public because interruption of the chain of disease transmission can yield a real public health benefit. The behavior of a seriously mentally ill patient can have a disruptive impact on other prisoners housed in the same area.

There is also the *societal perspective*. In part, it comprises the summed perspective of all of its members, even if these are not always consciously expressed or in full agreement. It also calculates the overarching good of society, although this might be in conflict with the summed good of individuals, a point well illustrated by the paradox of the commons: what is best for all in general may be less than the sum of what each would want individually. Society necessarily considers trade-offs involving tax increases or foregone social improvements in this context. But society also regards it as a good for each member of society to achieve and maintain a high level of physical and mental well-being.

The paradox of the commons just noted refers to the practice in times past for farmers to graze their cattle in the commons, a publicly owned plot of grassy land near the center of the village. Although each farmer would desire to bring additional animals to graze on this free land, each realized that overgrazing would soon render the land worthless to everyone. Consequently, a form of mutually agreed rationing had to occur, whereby each one would choose to bring a limited number of cows, thus ensuring, out of a fundamentally selfish motive, the perpetuity of this benefit for all.

A recent example is the prospect of achieving societal benefit from eradicating the risk of exposure to hepatitis C. This severe disease is largely concentrated among incarcerated persons, where the prevalence is nearly 10 times that of the free world population. (People used to acquire HCV infection through blood transfusions. Since the implementation of new safeguards for the U.S. blood supply in 1992, the principal avenue for HCV transmission is sharing contaminated needles by users of injectable illegal drugs and hence the concentration of HCV among prisoners.)

Recent pharmaceutical advances have made available new direct-acting oral medications that are simple and safe, have relatively few side effects, and have a remarkable 90 percent cure rate for this disease (compared to less than 40 percent, coupled with complex treatment regimens and very high risk for serious side effects for the older treatment regimens). But these new medications are extremely costly—more than $1,000 per pill. Typical treatment requires one pill per day for 12 weeks or at least $84,000 for the medications alone for a single course of treatment and as much as $153,000 for patients who require additional medications.

In the community, insurance companies have imposed restrictive reimbursement policies in view of the high cost of treatment. "In response, the Centers for Medicare and Medicaid Services notified state programs that limitations on drug coverage should not deny access to clinically appropriate antiviral therapy for beneficiaries with chronic HCV infection."[12] This same principle should apply as well to prisoners.

The costs for prisons and jails to identify and treat all HCV-infected persons in their facilities would be staggering, but the benefit to society would be even greater in eliminating sources of infection. The solution will require adoption of a national public health strategy to supplement correctional budgets and fund this effort. With planning and coordination, a public health strategy can stop HCV transmission and ultimately eliminate HCV as a threat.

This approach illustrates a clear example of how society is not well served if the rights and basic needs of prisoners are ignored. It is sound public policy to accord prisoners the type of health care that is consistent with contemporary standards of professional practice in the free community.

The decision-making process described in this chapter is considered primarily from the point of view of society, which recognizes the importance of strategies that foster good public policy and takes into account society's evaluation of the need facing each individual patient. Fundamental to this approach is the belief that society is not well served if the rights and the basic needs of prisoners are ignored. It is sound public policy to accord prisoners the type of health care that is consistent with contemporary standards of professional practice in the free community. Obviously, different solutions could emerge if the benefits and costs from another perspective were incorporated into this model. A prisoner may desire a personal benefit that society rejects in its larger and less personal view.

As stated previously, we are dealing with an evolving process. Community standards do change over time. A procedure that was once regarded as not necessary, too risky, or excessively costly may later become an accepted practice with improved technology. Thus, the examples of medical care decisions given in this chapter should be regarded as a reflection of the times in which the book was written. As always, one should look at contemporary standards of care.

FACTORS THAT SHOULD NOT INFLUENCE A DECISION TO TREAT

In determining whether a prisoner should receive a particular form of treatment, certain factors should be seen as completely irrelevant to the decision process. These include such matters as gender, race, ethnic origin, sexual orientation, nature of the crime, behavior in prison, contributory behavior, profession, social standing, celebrity status, and preexisting conditions.

Gender, Race, Ethnicity, or Sexual Orientation

It should be obvious that gender, race, ethnic origin, and sexual orientation or identity ought not to be counted at all in determining whether to treat a prisoner. To do so would be unjust discrimination and a violation of the individual's civil rights based on membership in any class.

There may, however, be some disagreement concerning other factors, such as the nature of the crime; the inmate's behavior while in prison; any incidents of self-harm; social standing, profession, or educational attainment; celebrity status; and preexisting conditions.

Nature of Crime or Behavior in Prison

In keeping with the norm of beneficence,[13] which requires the medical practitioner to intervene only for the purpose of accomplishing some good for the patient, the denial of medical care never should be used or even appear to be used as punishment, as was previously stated. Incarceration itself is the punishment imposed by law. The patient's behavior in prison—even hostile, deceitful, abusive, reprehensible, or threatening—should not be considered in making a decision to approve or deny a needed therapeutic procedure. One does not "earn" an entitlement to health care, nor does one become unworthy of medical treatment because of bad behavior. The correctional agency should never withhold or threaten to withhold health care services as a punishment for rule violations or as a deterrent to improper behavior by prisoners. Accordingly, the model prisoner in the honor housing block and the troublemaker in disciplinary segregation should be assessed equally as candidates for a needed medical intervention. For this reason, it is perhaps best when the medical decision maker is unaware of the criminal or behavioral history of the patient.

> One does not "earn" an entitlement to health care, nor does one become unworthy of medical treatment because of bad behavior. The correctional agency should never withhold or threaten to withhold health care services as a punishment for rule violations or as a deterrent to improper behavior by prisoners.

Self-Harm or Contributory Behavior

Some people suggest that the correctional system may appropriately withhold treatment to persons who have brought on themselves their own illness or injury. Thus, the ravages of alcohol or substance abuse, sexual promiscuity, tobacco, or self-mutilating behavior might be given a lower priority for treatment than would an illness for which the patient is entirely without blame. This moralistic and self-righteous line of reasoning is deficient on at least two counts. First, because it is not the practice in the community to determine whether the patient is at fault before providing or paying for treatment, it has no place in the prison. Second, true culpability is not so easily determined in many cases because all of the relevant and possibly mitigating circumstances cannot be known. For example, the tendency to engage in acts of self-harm may be a consequence of mental illness.

Contributory behavior may be relevant in some situations, but only in the sense that willful and protracted failure to comply with treatment or the continued use of tobacco, alcohol, or drugs, for example, would diminish the likelihood of a successful outcome of the treatment intervention. This effect, however, would already be accounted for in the model by way of the expected benefit from treatment. This may also be the case with organ transplants.

Self-inflicted injuries sometimes are managed with a conservative therapy until the propensity for repetition of the injury is reduced. This is a narrow but appropriate exception to the position stated here. For example, an inmate who frequently swallows foreign objects may be examined and then closely observed for any signs of an impending problem rather than be rushed to the emergency room each time for an endoscopic or surgical procedure. Furthermore, these cases often suggest that treatment be coupled with counseling and relevant life-skills education. They should not be handled punitively.

Celebrity Status, Notoriety, Social Class, or Profession

Celebrity status or notoriety poses a somewhat thorny problem because the decision maker knows that the eye of the world—magnified and perhaps distorted through the media lens—will be watching closely. There may be political ramifications. If a costly procedure is performed, it will be labeled favoritism and an "extravagance." If denied, it will be called "inhumane." The press will scurry to discover how many other inmates have or have not received this type of care but will fail to inquire about relevant individual circumstances. A legislator may telephone the agency director demanding preferential treatment for a friend or constituent.

From both an ethical and a pragmatic standpoint, therefore, the facility should try to remain as neutral as possible about the identity or notoriety of the recipient when making these decisions. Here is where already established, clear, and objective criteria and policy will pay off—policy that has been reviewed and endorsed, if possible, by an objective community body such as the medical ethics committee at a medical school or community hospital. If this policy is followed regardless of the celebrity or social status or the profession of the patient, the allegations of partiality and discrimination will be more easily countered.

Preexisting Conditions

Some persons have advanced the general premise that correctional systems are obligated only to maintain a prisoner in as healthy a state as when he or she entered prison, after due adjustment for aging and natural deterioration, and thus have no obligation to improve health or to restore health that was lost before incarceration. The author disagrees. This position not only fails to consider whether the patient was aware of this condition or had the ability to obtain treatment in the community but also is inconsistent with community standards. As required by the Patient Protection and Affordable Care Act of 2010, third-party payers may no longer exclude coverage on the basis of preexisting conditions.

Moreover, a condition that previously existed only in subclinical or mild form and is discovered or progresses to the point of causing significant pain or disability only after incarceration should not be regarded as preexisting. Some cases may have not been treated in the community because of inability to gain effective access to health care, whether because of ignorance, lack of resources, lack of mental competence, or some other reason. (It is also unlikely that, in any practical way, decision makers could obtain accurate and reliable information of this kind.) The mere fact that the condition was or was not preexisting ought to be irrelevant to the decision to treat, just as it is in the community. If a preexisting condition is growing more severe or more painful, the situation is no different than it would be for a new illness. The goal of the physician is to restore health or function or to relieve pain, not to judge peoples' motivations.

If the unhealthy condition or disability commenced in the institution rather than prior to incarceration, a further question arises about potential liability. Just as an employer can be held responsible for treatment of a job-related injury, there should be no hesitation to provide restorative treatment for an injury sustained through no fault of the patient while incarcerated. The injury may be the result of willful or careless action by another inmate or an officer, or it may be accidental. Contributory negligence by the patient could be a mitigating factor.

FACTORS THAT MAY INFLUENCE THE DECISION TO INTERVENE

A variety of factors can affect the decision to provide a particular health benefit. Table 5.1 lists 10 factors to consider. This is an attempt to discover the net benefit of an intervention by mapping the relationship between various types of cost and how much a particular treatment procedure is needed. The first eight factors listed in the table can be viewed as dimensions of the *need* for rendering a therapeutic procedure. The latter two relate to *cost*.

Dimensions of Necessity

The goals of treatment are accounted for in the first three factors: *improvement of health, improvement of function*, and *relief of pain*. These are the principal determinants of necessity. Every treatment procedure is intended to have a beneficial impact on one or more of these factors. Necessity for a procedure, therefore, is reckoned according to the expected benefit to be derived in terms of health, function, and freedom from pain—or conversely as the net harm or loss suffered from denial of

Table 5.1
Factors to Be Considered in Making the Decision to Perform a Health Care Procedure

Dimensions of necessity		Factor	Polarity[a]	Expectation		Interaction[b]
				If procedure is not performed	*If procedure is performed*	
Goals	1	Improved Health	+	Patient will die or remain ill	Patient will survive, and health will improve	
	2	Improved Function	+	Patient will become disabled, bedridden, or incompetent	Patient will enjoy improved physical and mental function	
	3	Relief of Pain	+	Patient will experience extreme or continued pain.	Patient will be pain free or have greatly reduced pain	
				Less inclined to treat	*Favors decision to treat*	
Mediating factors	4	Adverse Side Effects	−	Serious or likely	None or unlikely	Interacts with side effects[b]
	5	Urgency	+	Stable	Rapidly deteriorating	
	6	Availability of Alternative	−	Acceptable conservative treatment option available	Alternative unavailable or has expected pessimistic outcome	
	7	Patient's Desire	+	Refusal or indifferent	Intense desire for treatment	Based on 1, 2, 3, and 4
	8	Length of Stay	+	Very short time remaining in prison	Long term or life sentence	May interact with urgency
Cost	9	Chronicity	−	Ongoing course of treatment	One procedure or shorter course	Affects cost
	10	Cost	−	High	Low	

[a] Polarity effect or direction of the influence that each factor has on the decision to treat.
[b] Potential interaction or overlap because of the side effects associated with the alternative procedure.

the intervention. Depending on the context, these first three factors can be seen as the need for a particular intervention or the net benefit of receiving the intervention.

The next five factors are secondary determinants of necessity—that is, they can contribute to or detract from the need to treat but are not themselves reasons for treatment. These are conditional factors that mediate the need for treatment. The first of these conditional factors, and the fourth dimension of necessity, is the *likelihood of adverse side effects* if the procedure is performed. Obviously, this will condition the desirability or necessity of the contemplated procedure. The fifth dimension of necessity is *urgency*. The procedure will be deemed more necessary if it is urgent—that is, if the patient's health condition is unstable and will deteriorate rapidly without treatment. The sixth dimension of necessity is the *availability of alternative treatment* methods. If a safe and promising but less costly and more conservative treatment alternative is available, then the initially contemplated approach is rendered less imperative. The seventh dimension involves the intensity of the *patient's desire* for the procedure, which can range from outright refusal to an eager desire for treatment. This, of course, can be influenced by the expected outcomes of treatment (1, 2, 3, and 4 in Table 5.1) and can itself offset the outcomes, especially by virtue of eagerness or reluctance to cooperate. The eighth dimension is the expected *duration of stay* of the patient in the correctional facility. This can interact with the urgency of the procedure so that a less urgent treatment may be more easily deferred for a short-stay patient.

Taken together, then, we can say that implementing a treatment procedure is more necessary when it is more likely to restore good health, improve or restore function, and relieve pain; when it can be accomplished without serious adverse complications; when it is urgent; when there is no acceptable alternative; when the patient strongly desires the treatment; and when the patient is likely to remain incarcerated for a long time.

Cost Factors

The final two factors relate to cost. The ninth factor is *chronicity* of the care that will be required. It makes a big difference whether only a single procedure is involved or if a lifetime of ongoing treatment will be needed. This can directly affect the cost and possibly also the patient's desire for the treatment. The 10th factor is the *cost* of the procedure.

Referring back to Figure 5.1, a procedure such as a liver transplant would perhaps be positioned in the upper-right quadrant of the chart in the sector labeled "rare." But as procedures such as liver transplants become the accepted standard of care for persons with end-stage liver disease and their successful outcomes become more frequent, it will be more difficult to deny these treatments to otherwise eligible prisoner candidates. The procedure can be lifesaving, although the costs are staggering, both for the transplant procedure itself and lifelong immunosuppressant therapy.

Organ transplants are representative of the most costly medical procedures. They are also a scarce resource. More than 30,000 lifesaving organ transplants took place in the United States in 2015, and more than 120,000 Americans were on waiting lists for lifesaving organs.[14] An estimated 22 people die every day while waiting for a vital organ. In addition, more than 40,000 corneal transplants took place in 2015.[15] For some patients, transplants constitute the only hope for survival. If the prognosis is good on all counts and no other viable option is available, the fact of prisoner status is not an acceptable reason to deny eligibility for transplant procedures.

Some people resent hearing about a prisoner who receives an organ transplant. They argue from the standpoint of cost and that organs are scarce and prisoners should not receive them as long as law-abiding citizens are in need. At first blush, this reasoning about organ scarcity appears to have merit, but it ignores the fact that some prisoners receive transplants with organs donated by relatives or friends. In some circumstances, kidney transplants for long-term inmates with end-stage renal failure is a cost-effective alternative when compared to lifelong hemodialysis treatment, especially when a family donor is available. More important, however, this country has not taken the position that preferential treatment on organ supply should go to celebrities or "important" people or that prisoners represent a class of people unworthy of an organ donation. This would exemplify the "social worth" or "social value" theory mentioned previously in this chapter under "A Complex Issue." Under this approach in the selection process, the implied reasoning would be that because society underwrites much of the cost of the transplants, organs should go on a priority basis to persons who have the greatest potential to return benefit to society.

Instead, we have chosen in the United States to use a combination approach of "best tissue match" and "first-come, first-served," giving priority to urgency and to persons under age 18. Some programs use a lottery approach, adding points for blood-type matching, length of time on waiting list, degree of urgency, and patient proximity to the transplant center. The patient with the highest points receives the available organ.

This issue has a special relevance because of the large number of prisoners who have been infected with hepatitis C, some of whom will develop cirrhosis and liver failure. For them, a liver transplant can be a lifesaving intervention.

Description of Factors to Be Considered in the Decision to Treat

This model is mostly relevant to decisions about so-called big ticket items—medical, surgical, and diagnostic procedures with the highest costs—because few people would even question the need for prisoners to receive a good medical diagnosis and treatment for an infection or injury or for chronic conditions such as diabetes, hypertension, asthma, epilepsy, or psychosis. But most people might require greater scrutiny and prior authorization for referral to a specialist, hospitalization, an MRI, or major surgery. As such, the model described here is not expressly intended for routine primary care procedures, although the reasoning process would be similar.

Improvement in Health, Improvement in Function, or Relief of Pain

Improved health, improved function, and *relief of pain* together represent the essential purposes for which a medical procedure would be undertaken. They are the principal reasons why any treatment would be deemed necessary. Therefore, they will be discussed here together, subsumed under the rubric of *medical necessity.*

Necessity can be evaluated on an ordinal scale. At one extreme, the intervention may be a life-or-death matter that assumes the highest importance. It could be an appendectomy, gall bladder surgery, cardiac catheterization, or surgical excision of a malignant tumor. Without surgery, the patient is likely to die. It might be eye surgery to preserve sight for a person whose other eye cannot be restored. A total hip or knee replacement may be required for an elderly patient to have any hope of not becoming wheelchair bound. A full panoply of palliative medicine may be required for a cancer patient experiencing extreme pain.

At the next level, the intervention may be intended to save an arm or a leg or alleviate severe pain and distress. It could be a corneal transplant or cataract surgery for a person with another sighted eye, knee surgery to relieve moderate pain and improve ambulation, or provision of a prosthetic device such as an artificial limb or a hearing aid. It might be that the newest, most costly, and sophisticated imaging technique is recommended for diagnosing a particular patient with a serious and potentially remediable condition.

At the lowest end of the scale are situations where intervention is of trivial therapeutic benefit, as would be the case with most cosmetic surgery.

A reasonable reference point or guide for determining whether a procedure is "unnecessary" may be whether and under what circumstances Medicaid covers the procedure for its beneficiaries in the state. Some may argue that even these criteria are too limited and restrictive. However, they can serve as a starting point for referencing the applicable community standard.

Probability of a Successful Outcome with Few Adverse Side Effects

Like any third-party payer such as a health insurance carrier or health maintenance organization, a correctional agency is usually more willing to cover treatments that have a high likelihood of achieving the desired successful outcome than those that will probably not succeed or will leave the patient with serious adverse consequences even though they may be successful. To recognize this factor, the expectation of an overall successful outcome after considering all of the risks and potential adverse side effects might be rated as excellent, good, guarded, or poor. As an example, a bone marrow transplant for a leukemia patient with 50-percent probability of a five-year survival is much more defensible than the same costly procedure for a person whose likelihood of even a one-year survival is estimated by experts to be between 5 and 10 percent.

An expensive course of chemotherapy or radiation therapy for a cancer patient is justifiable only if the patient is able and willing to tolerate the side effects of treatment and if it holds a good chance of retarding spread of the cancer and giving the patient a commensurate increase in expected quality of life. All else being equal, the therapy ought not to be denied merely because the patient is a prisoner.

Urgency

An emergent or urgent procedure, in contrast to one that is deferrable, by definition cannot be delayed without risk of incurring additional harm to the patient or reducing the likelihood of a successful outcome. In itself, urgency does not address the necessity or importance of the procedure. For example, a patient may experience moderate pain, such as that from a thrombosed hemorrhoid, that could be alleviated quickly through surgical treatment or that would remit after some days either spontaneously or with conservative treatment. In such a case, the surgical procedure would be described as urgent although low in terms of necessity because life, limb, or function are not at risk, severe and long-term pain is not involved, or there are acceptable alternatives.

Availability of an Acceptable Alternative

If an alternative of more conservative therapy is available and this is considered to be acceptable practice, then it may be chosen by the patient and the physician. Its availability reduces the need to select a more expensive form of treatment. Examples might be continued hemodialysis rather than a renal transplant or wearing a truss instead of undergoing surgical repair of a hernia.

Patient's Desire for Treatment

Just as a competent patient's right to refuse treatment should be respected, so also the intensity of the patient's desire to receive treatment can be a relevant factor for the decision maker. One patient, considering the advantages and risks of a given intervention, may eagerly desire to receive the treatment. Another patient may consent yet remain substantially indifferent.

As another instance of potential interaction among these various factors, the likelihood of successful outcome may well be influenced by the patient's desire for the treatment. The eager patient is likely to cooperate fully with the treatment plan. Cooperation and compliance with the prescribed treatment plan can significantly alter the outcome of treatment, as can an optimistic and hopeful attitude on the part of the patient and a trusting relationship with the physician.

Expected Remaining Duration of Incarceration

The urgency factor described above is particularly relevant for jails, where many inmates are incarcerated for only a few days or weeks. If the expected length of stay is short, a procedure of low necessity or of low urgency might be legitimately deferred until the prisoner is able to obtain care in the free world at no cost to the correctional system. Many restorative dental procedures fall in this category and often need not be performed in a short-term jail setting if the patient can easily wait until his or her release back into the community. This is why it is justifiable for most jails to provide only emergency dental care to patients who will be released in a matter of days or weeks or a few months. But this factor interacts with the urgency of need so that even a short-term jail is required to provide life-sustaining surgery for a patient in urgent need.

Chronicity of Care

The intervention may be a single, one-time episode for an acute condition, after which the patient is expected to resume normal good health. At the other extreme, the condition may be chronic and require lifelong care. This factor can become important in two ways. First, if the prisoner arrives with a chronic illness currently under treatment, it would be difficult for the prison or jail to deny continuation of the treatment except when medically contraindicated because of other complications. An example might be an HIV-seropositive patient receiving antiretroviral therapy or a cancer patient undergoing radiation therapy or a psychiatric patient who is responding well to a treatment regimen with expensive psychotropic medication. Second, the correctional decision maker may be considering whether to initiate a long and costly course of treatment. Here the choice may not be so simple.

The whole cost and course of treatment often cannot be reasonably anticipated at the beginning. Decisions are therefore made one stage at a time. Complications and relapses lead to more expenditures and new decisions. Each of these must be made on the basis of revised prognosis and estimated future costs without looking retrospectively at the costs already incurred. Sometimes, it is reasonable to commence a medically conservative form of treatment and progress to more costly treatment modalities only if and as indicated.

Some procedures should not be started on a patient about to be released to the community except when there is reason to be confident that the patient has the will and the resources to continue it. An example is chemoprophylaxis to prevent tuberculosis infection from progressing to an active disease. Once started, this treatment must be faithfully continued and closely monitored for six to nine months. A Pap smear is not appropriate for a woman about to leave the jail in a day or two because she will not be there when the results become available and proper treatment can be prescribed. The same might be said about initiating treatment for hepatitis C unless competent follow-up can be ensured.

Cost of the Intervention

The cost of the intervention is appropriately taken into consideration when approving or disapproving a procedure. Given that the intervention is desirable on medical or therapeutic grounds, the overall benefits must be commensurate with the cost incurred as a matter of good public policy.

Costs can be described in a variety of ways. Often estimated dollar cost may be the most direct scale to use so that a $150,000 course of treatment is recognized as more costly than a $2,000 procedure, but precise estimation is not required. For purpose of this analysis, relative cost is sufficient, and a simple seven-step scale is offered: (1) exceedingly high, (2) very high, (3) high, (4) moderate, (5) low, (6) very low, and (7) trivial. The administrator also should consider whether the cost of the intervention will be offset by direct savings—for example, if a hepatitis B vaccination were determined to be cost-effective considering direct medical care and legal costs that might eventually be avoided, or if a renal transplant were deemed less costly in the long run than many years of hemodialysis for a person serving a life sentence.

Avoid Confounding the Variables

In applying this method of analysis, we should avoid counting the same factor under multiple headings. Doing so inadvertently could assign undue weight to that factor. Where the factors themselves can easily overlap, a statement to this effect has been provided. For example, *expected functional improvement* may already be recognized in *few side effects* or in *relief from pain* or in *patient's desire for treatment*. In this example, functional impairment may be the essential element of what is being measured in all four variables, and it then should be counted only once. However, if the factor *few side effects* is measuring ability to survive a surgical procedure or avoidance of infection, it could be measuring something other than restoration of function. Similarly, if extreme pain is largely the cause of the functional disability, *relief from pain* may be capturing the essence of the *restoration of function*.

Some factors are not explicitly included in the model because they would almost always duplicate matters already incorporated in one or more of the factors already discussed and would thus skew the analysis. These include a patient's history of compliance, comorbidity, treatment delays, age and general health, and quality of life.

History of Compliance with Treatment

The patient's prior *history of compliance* with prescribed treatment sometimes can serve as a predictor of future compliance and should be considered in evaluating the probability of a *successful outcome*.

Comorbidity

Existence of a *comorbid condition* could also be a factor that reduces the probability of a *successful treatment outcome*.

Treatment Delays

The potential effects of *delay of treatment* on the eventual *outcome* are also important, but these are explicitly accounted for in the context of *urgency*.

Age and General Health of Patient

All else being equal, it is often reasonable to predict more *favorable outcomes* for a younger patient than for an elderly one. Similarly, expected *outcome* and *useful functioning* are more likely to be improved in the case of a patient who is otherwise generally healthy than for one who suffers from multiple serious or degenerative maladies. Therefore, while the *age and general health* of the patient are each clearly relevant to the decision maker, they are easily confounded with other factors that essentially represent the same factor, and the calculus should carefully identify the correct variable of interest to avoid double counting.

Quality of Life

Whether the intervention will appreciably improve or possibly detract from the *quality of life* for the patient is a most important consideration. However, this also may be redundant with other factors explicitly included in the model such as *functional improvement, improved health, freedom from pain, fewer side effects,* or *patient's desire.* Therefore, it should be employed cautiously, if at all, as a discrete factor in the analysis.

CONCLUSION

This preliminary model for decision making is offered as an aid in weighing the appropriate criteria for approval or disapproval of a particular health care service in a specific case. Ultimately, it may be possible to assign numerical values to the salient factors to improve the usefulness of the model. It should be stressed that this is still a highly preliminary formulation. The input of correctional health colleagues and others, especially physicians and medical ethicists, is needed to refine the model and improve its utility. In the same way that national standards for correctional health care evolved through a deliberative and inclusive process, so consensus is also needed in deciding how much health care is enough.

Correctional health care professionals are recognizing the importance of seeking a consensus policy on medical necessity.[16] Although each jurisdiction could attempt to reach its own definition, it may be difficult to defend and explain the differences. Why, for example, does one correctional jurisdiction "always" treat a deviated septum or an elective hernia while this is "never" done in a nearby state?

Dr. Armond H. Start[17] proposed a structured process for gathering and organizing information before making a decision. At some point it would involve the completion of a form in the presence of the patient. His questionnaire, reproduced below, comprises a set of questions to assist the decision maker in approving significant but expensive technical diagnostic studies or ordering costly but nonurgent procedures.

Once completed, the primary care physician would send the form to the medical director of the health care system or to the utilization review committee. If the medical director or utilization review committee renders a negative decision, both the patient and primary care provider should have an opportunity to express in writing to the decision maker why they perceive the denial to be wrong. Many issues covered in the form are related directly to the factors proposed in our model so that it can be a complementary and useful instrument.

Evaluation for Approval of a Major Medical Procedure
(As Suggested by Armond H. Start, MD[18])

1. What medical evaluation has been done previously to solve or define this problem?
2. How long has the problem existed?
3. Did the problem exist prior to incarceration?
4. What was done about the problem? (i.e., previous efforts made by the patient or other care providers to take care of the problem)
5. Did the problem begin or occur while incarcerated?
6. How long before the patient's release from custody?
7. What is the degree of disability is associated with the problem?
8. Can housing or work supervisors validate the degree of disability?
9. How long has the patient cooperated in the primary management of the problem?
10. Why do you believe the patient will cooperate in a therapeutic alliance—if this problem is addressed?
11. What are the chances for long-term therapeutic success if the problem is treated?[19]

Conceptualizing Mental Illness as a Chronic Condition*

MENTAL ILLNESS SHOULD BE TREATED, NOT PUNISHED

Correctional officials used to have a saying: "Most prisoners are bad, but some are sad and a few are mad." In their view, this meant most prisoners were truly obnoxious characters—bad actors—but some were depressed and possibly suicidal, and a few were so obviously mentally ill as to require professional mental health treatment.

Because jails and prisons are structured to deal with bad actors, there is a tendency to see most sick or deviant behavior as bad behavior. Some correctional staff strongly resist the therapeutic approach because it appears to be "coddling" prisoners. In such an environment, it is easy for medical professionals to capitulate to the ever-present pressures of their surroundings. Professional and medical standards and ethical principles can be eroded. This is dysfunctional for the institution, and the skill of the psychiatrist or psychologist is not being put to its best use.

The "bad, sad, and mad" paradigm really does not work. Life is just not this simple. The fifth and latest version of the *Diagnostic and Statistical Manual of Mental Disorders* (DSM-5)[1]—the major reference manual for mental health

---

* This chapter is adapted and expanded from a 1998 article written by Robert S. Ort and Kenneth L. Faiver titled "Mental Illness as a Chronic Condition: Coping with Chronic Mental Patients in a Correctional Setting," *Corrections Compendium* 23(5) (May 1998), 1–6. A similar paper was presented by the same authors at the National Commission on Correctional Health Care Conference in San Antonio, TX on November 10, 1997, titled "Recognizing Mental Illness as a Chronic Condition."

professionals—catalogs and defines every conceivable mental disorder. Its pages contain many more diagnostic categories than "bad, sad, and mad."

This manual also describes the factors and criteria that mental health professionals must consider before reaching a diagnosis and preparing a long-term treatment plan. This is a considerable change from DSM-IV-TR, its predecessor. For example, mental retardation is now called intellectual disability, and there is a strong focus on assessment of cognitive capacity as well as adaptive functioning, the latter being the determinant of severity rather than the IQ score. Gender dysphoria (new in DSM-5) emphasizes "gender incongruence" rather than "cross-gender identification," and is not classified as a sexual dysfunction or a paraphilia. Substance abuse and dependence are no longer separate diagnoses, as in DSM-IV-TR, but it is now substance use disorder. Criteria for personality disorders have not changed from DSM-IV-TR, but DSM-5 does include an alternative approach to the diagnosis of personality disorder that has been referred for further study.[2]

Under previous editions of the DSM, each psychiatric diagnosis was organized into five aspects or dimensions (axes).[3] However, the multiaxial system was discontinued in DSM-5. This change "suggests that there is no differentiation between medical conditions and mental health disorders" and reinforces "an assumption that mental disorders are rooted in biological causes."[4]

Unfortunately, even in light of what we now know about mental illness, some within the world of corrections still think it cute or clever to characterize their populations as "bad, sad, or mad." This is not only misleading but also trivializing, and it distracts from the severity of the problem.

> Now that sheriffs, jail administrators, and prison wardens are responsible for operating facilities that house large numbers of mentally ill individuals, some of the traditional methods of managing incarcerated persons may be outmoded. A more effective and humane management of mentally ill patients requires a radically different approach.

For reasons discussed later in this chapter, far more mentally ill persons in the United States are housed today in correctional institutions than in community mental health facilities. This is inappropriate and brings tragic consequences because jails and prisons are completely unsuited to the task of effective treatment and humane management of these persons. The mentally ill should be housed in places of treatment, not punishment. Dr. Ahmed Okasha, president of the World Psychiatric Association, made this point emphatically. His admonition deserves careful attention:

The presence of mental patients in prisons does not only deprive them of their right to proper treatment and care, but also leads to possible maltreatment and stigmatization. It is an ethical obligation to stop both. The [United Nations] resolution[5] on the human rights of mental patients requires that they should be treated in adequate facilities, preserving their dignity. The *Madrid Declaration* states that mental patients should be treated by the least restrictive methods. Incarcerating mental patients is a violation of both.[6]

Our society generally disapproves of punishing mentally ill people for behavior that results from impaired understanding and control. But it happens all the time. Too few community resources are available to permit an adequate and timely response to concerns raised about the behaviors of mentally ill people, many of whom are also homeless or on drugs. Police find themselves with insufficient alternatives in these circumstances, so the mentally ill are arrested and held in jail on a variety of charges. The unfortunate consequences are well known.

Now that sheriffs, jail administrators, and prison wardens are responsible for operating facilities that house large numbers of mentally ill individuals, some of the traditional methods of managing incarcerated persons may be outmoded. A more effective and humane management of mentally ill patients requires a radically different approach.

What psychologist Dr. Lisa Boesky[7] said about residents of juvenile justice facilities is also true of adults in prisons and jails. Although mental illness does not excuse negative behavior and offenders should be held accountable for their behavior, whether or not they suffer from a mental health disorder, they should also receive appropriate mental health treatment. At one end of the spectrum are persons described as "antisocial" or "sociopathic," who know exactly what they are doing when they commit crimes and do them anyway. On the other end of the spectrum are those who are seriously mentally ill, may experience psychotic thinking and may have even been psychotic at the time they committed their crimes, or may have substantial cognitive deficits that result in their having little understanding of the behavior expected of them. Such severely mentally ill persons typically do not belong in the justice system, and they require intensive services from the mental health system.

SOCIETY'S FAILURE—DEINSTITUTIONALIZATION

In 1780, John Howard, a renowned British prison reformer, wrote about how the bridewells were crowded and offensive because so many of the rooms that were designed for prisoners were now occupied by lunatics. He went on to report:

I must here add, that in some few gaols are confined idiots and lunatics. These serve for sport to idle visitants. . . . The insane, where they are not kept separate, disturb and terrify other prisoners. No care is taken of them, although it is probable that by medicines, and proper regimen, some of them might be restored to their senses, and to usefulness in life.[8]

In the first part of the 19th century, jails and almshouses in the United States were also becoming repositories of the mentally ill. Beginning in the 1840s, Dorothea Dix, Horace Mann, Louis Dwight, and others labored long and hard to change this situation and advocated the establishment of public psychiatric hospitals. By 1880, more than 75 such hospitals were in existence, and less than 1 percent of inmates in jails and prisons were reported to have serious mental illness.[9]

From about 1880 until the end of World War II, states were viewed as meeting their ethical and moral obligations if they provided hospital care to patients with acute mental illness and humane custodial care to those with chronic mental illness. However, the 1930s and 1940s brought periodic disclosures in the news media describing deplorable conditions in these hospitals, including physical neglect, sexual abuse, and inhumane treatment. The resulting outcries set the stage for deinstitutionalization. After World War II, a sustained attack on the legitimacy of mental hospitalization emerged.

"The [United Nations] resolution on the human rights of mental patients requires that [the mentally ill] should be treated in adequate facilities, preserving their dignity. The *Madrid Declaration* states that mental patients should be treated by the least restrictive methods. Incarcerating mental patients is a violation of both."
    —Dr. Ahmed Okasha, President of the World Psychiatric Association

---

A brief historical review can help us understand this major social change. The following chronology summarizes key events in this history. After World War II, the practice of psychiatry underwent a major change. The vast majority of psychiatrists were no longer based in state and county mental hospitals. They had gone into private practice in cities and suburbs. As a consequence, the profession was not prepared to defend state hospital systems. At the same time, the largest cost item in state budgets was the maintenance of state mental hospitals. Ten years later, Thorazine was introduced on a widespread basis as an effective pharmacological treatment for psychosis. In 1961, the Joint Commission on Mental Illness and Health recommended that "no new mental hospitals be built and that mental hospitals of more than a thousand beds be gradually converted to centers for the long-term care of patients with chronic disease, including mental illness." The Kennedy administration initiated its "bold new approach" to the treatment of the mentally ill in 1963 with the promise of 2,000 community mental health centers to enable a shift from costly institutional care to what was touted as more cost-effective and more humane care in the community. Around 1978 during the Carter administration, there was a resurgence of support for continued deinstitutionalization, along with incorporation of the principle that patients with severe mental illness should be treated in the least restrictive setting. Most states have now discharged all but a scant few patients from their remaining mental institutions. In 1999, the Supreme Court ruled in *Olmstead v. L.C. and E.W.* that unjustified isolation of individuals with disabilities in institutions is a violation of the Americans with Disabilities

Act when these patients could be served equally as well or even more effectively in community-based settings.[10]

Key Dates of Deinstitutionalization

1945—Shift of psychiatrists from state hospitals to private practice
1945—High cost of operating state mental hospitals
1955—Introduction of Thorazine
1961—Joint Commission discourages expansion of state mental hospitals
1963—Kennedy's "bold new approach": community mental health
1978—Principle of "least restrictive environment"
1998—Near total deinstitutionalization
1999—*Olmstead* decision

To appreciate the full thrust of this deinstitutionalization, we must have a clear understanding of its definition. This process has two components: (1) the transfer of hospitalized persons from their institutional environments to the community and (2) the prevention of hospitalization for those people who might be considered potential candidates for hospital care.

Deinstitutionalization was not effectively opposed by the most prestigious organization representing psychiatrists—the American Psychiatric Association. At the same time, state legislators were supportive and viewed the process as a cost-shifting program. Meanwhile, federal legislators saw it as a cost-effective strategy to provide more humane care in the community. Perhaps most important, it was especially popular with the public. Meanwhile, Thorazine was being described as an effective antipsychotic medication that restored psychotic patients to a state of normalcy. This myth has largely persisted and contributed to widespread misunderstanding of the true nature of mental illness.

Throughout this time, media continued to publish horror stories about conditions in state mental hospitals while praising pilot community mental health center programs as examples of successful deinstitutionalization. Health planners, psychiatrists, mental health workers, and other interested parties promoted the deinstitutionalization movement. Two presidents provided personal support. Patient rights groups and lawyers viewed it as a civil rights issue. Thus, deinstitutionalization became a recognizable social movement with far-reaching consequences.

However, deinstitutionalization closed the option of institutional care to many persons who in reality require a structured setting, and it was accomplished without deploying adequate community resources to serve the needs of former hospital patients. Community mental health centers tended to focus their attention on the more benign forms of mental disorder for which their staffs were better prepared by training. As a result, the successful treatment of patients with minor mental disorders created excessively optimistic expectations for the treatment of more serious forms of mental illness.

The U.S. psychiatric hospital census dropped from 558,992 in 1955 to fewer than 50,000 in 2000 to 2003.[11] In this same interval—when the number of community psychiatric beds dropped by more than 90 percent—the population of the United States increased by some 124 million persons from 166 million to 290 million.[12] Most of those who were deinstitutionalized were seriously mentally ill. Some had mental retardation. Nearly 60 percent suffered from schizophrenia, and another 15 percent or so were diagnosed with manic–depressive illness and severe depression. Another 10 to 15 percent were diagnosed with organic brain diseases.[13]

Looked at another way, the per capita bed population in 1955, the peak year of psychiatric hospitalization in the United States, was more than 300 beds per 100,000 people. This is more than 20 times the ratio in 2010, according to a report by the Treatment Advocacy Center. Furthermore, nationwide in 2010, approximately one-third of all public psychiatric beds were occupied by forensic patients—either persons awaiting trial or sex offenders being held after completion of their prison sentences because they were deemed too dangerous to release. Today, public psychiatric beds are still being eliminated, and the ratio of beds per population continues to decline.[14] This is summarized in Table 6.1.

According to E. Fuller Torrey,

[I]t seems reasonable to establish a range 40 to 60 psychiatric beds per 100,000 population as a minimum standard currently needed for reasonable psychiatric care in the [United States] in light of the realities of the present funding system. . . . Currently, there are about 35,000 state psychiatric beds available, or about 11 beds per 100,000 population.

Torrey offers his caveat regarding realities of the present funding system "because we actually do not know how many psychiatric beds would be needed if we were not constrained by Medicaid and other federal regulations."[15]

Table 6.1
Number of Psychiatric Beds in United States, Selected Years

Year	Beds	Per 100,000
1955	558,992	300
2005	50,509	17
2010	43,313	14
2016	35,100	11

Source: E. Fuller Torrey, Doris A. Fuller, Jeffrey Geller, Carla Jacobs, and Kristina Ragosta, *No Room at the Inn: Trends and Consequences of Closing Public Psychiatric Hospitals, 2005–2010.* The Treatment Advocacy Center (July 19, 2012); E. Fuller Torrey, "A Dearth of Psychiatric Beds, *Psychiatric Times* (February 15, 2016).

Budget cuts in mental health funding continue to be widespread, with devastating effects on the ability of communities to meet the mental health needs of their residents. For instance, it was reported that $1.6 billion was cut from state non-Medicaid mental health spending between 2009 and 2011.[16]

The Consequences

Since 1978, deinstitutionalization has been promoted on the principle that severe mental illness should be treated in the least restrictive setting. For many of those who need help, this laudable goal has been at least partially realized. But for a substantial minority, it is a dismal failure, as evidenced by the people who are unable to adapt to living with their families, in group homes, or in flophouses. They include many of the people who now sleep in doorways, under bridges, in cardboard boxes, or—as we know all too well—in our prison and jail cells. The promised community resources did not become available to the extent needed.

All too frequently these mentally ill people come into contact with the criminal justice system. This phenomenon has been called "criminalization of the mentally ill." Suppose a homeless mentally ill patient who had been sleeping under a bridge decides on a cold and rainy night to take shelter in a deserted house. Neighbors complain, and police arrest him with a charge of trespassing—a misdemeanor. While he is in jail, a custody officer expects him to comply with the rules. When he does not, the officer becomes frustrated and verbally assertive. The inmate strikes out. Now he is accused of assaulting an officer—a felony—and faces lengthy prison time.

Scope of the Problem—Prevalence

Deinstitutionalization was not the only factor leading to the greatly increased number of mentally ill persons in corrections. Another factor was the so called "Hinkley effect." During the 1970s, society developed a greater acceptance and understanding of the nature of mental illness, and this was reflected in the criminal justice system. The "not guilty by reason of insanity" defense was used with increasing frequency, and it became common to impose probation or simply not prosecute defendants if they agreed to seek treatment voluntarily.

All that changed, however, after the highly publicized and horrific crimes committed by persons commonly believed to be mentally ill, including Charles Manson, Richard Speck, Lynette "Squeaky" Fromme, and, especially, John Hinkley (who attempted to assassinate President Ronald Reagan in 1981). As a result, protection of society, not the treatment of mentally ill patients, became the first priority. States began to enact "guilty but mentally ill" statutes. Other states passed laws making the defense plea of not guilty by reason of insanity more difficult.[17]

When persons with mental disorders are arrested, most often it is because they have been a nuisance, not because they are dangerous. Linda A. Teplin,[18] who studied the Cook County Jail for the National Institute for Mental Health, says that jails have become the unintended major intake centers for all kinds of health, welfare, and social problem cases in disguise. Too frequently, mental patients are passed along to the criminal justice system because community treatment and support programs cannot or will not handle their needs. Consequently, arrest is now the method commonly employed by police to manage the mentally ill. Even though mentally ill suspects are no more likely to commit serious crimes than are those without mental illness, studies have demonstrated that their arrest rate is significantly higher.

The jail is now the poor person's mental health facility. Although the mental health system can say "no" to a patient, the criminal justice system cannot.[19] Dollars saved through mental health program cutbacks may represent no savings at all if they are offset by higher expenditures in the criminal justice system.

Dr. Terry Kupers assigns the following reasons for the expanding prevalence of mental illness in correctional settings: the shortcomings of public mental health systems, the tendency for post-Hinckley criminal courts to give less weight to psychiatric testimony, harsher policies toward drug offenders including those with dual diagnoses, and the growing tendency for local governments to incarcerate homeless people for a variety of minor crimes.[20]

At midyear 2005, more than half (56 percent of state prisoners, 45 percent of federal prisoners, and 64 percent of jail inmates) of all prison and jail inmates in the United States had mental health problems. An estimated 15 percent of state prisoners and 24 percent of jail inmates reported symptoms that meet the criteria for a psychotic disorder. Some 74 percent of state prisoners and 76 percent of local jail inmates who had mental health problems met the criteria for substance dependence or abuse.[21]

Jail officials in Wayne County, Michigan, which includes Detroit, reported that nearly 17 percent of jail inmates were taking psychotropic medications.[22] Mental health problems were defined by two measures: a recent history or current symptoms of a mental health problem. The prevalence of mental illness has been estimated to be at least two to four times higher in correctional facilities than in the general free world population. These patients require treatment.

Relative to an estimated lifetime prevalence of 3.1 percent in the general population, the percentage of inmates reporting a history of psychotic symptoms during the previous 12 months is 10.2 in federal prisons, 15.4 in state prisons, and 23.9 in local jails. The prevalence (percentage) of inmates who reported experiencing symptoms of mental health disorders (major depressive disorder, manic disorder, or psychotic disorder, sometimes in combination) in the previous 12 months was 39.8 in federal prisons, 49.2 in state prisons, and 60.5 in local jails.[23] In the words of Bureau of Justice statisticians James and Glaze, "At midyear 2005 more than half of all prison and jail inmates had a mental health problem." These numbers are probably an underestimate because it is well known there are cases of undiagnosed mental illness in correctional settings. A large number of inmates have also suffered closed head injuries with resultant neurological deficits. As Jane Haddad pointed out, it is also a fact that the chronically mentally ill who enter correctional systems tend to serve more time than other persons facing similar charges, in some cases because of their limited ability to develop acceptable parole plans.[24] Most

Table 6.2
Estimated Prevalence of Selected Mental Disorders among Inmates of U.S. Jails and Prisons

| Disorder | Estimated Prevalence | | | |
| | Range among Jail Inmates | | Range among Prison Inmates | |
	Low (%)	High (%)	Low (%)	High (%)
Major Depression	7.9	15.2	13.1	18.6
PTSD	4.0	8.3	6.2	11.7
Anxiety Disorder	14.1	20.0	22.0	30.1

Source: Bonita M. Veysey and Gisela Bichler Robertson, "Prevalence Estimates of Psychiatric Disorders in Correctional Settings," in National Commission on Correctional Health Care, *Health Status of Soon-To-Be-Released Inmates* 2 (April 2002), 57–80.

mentally ill persons entering prison today have not been convicted of violent crimes.

Analysis performed on prevalence data of mental illness among the United States population—appropriately weighted for socioeconomic status, substance-use characteristics, race, age, and gender of persons recently released from correctional institutions—has permitted a projection of estimated or expected prevalence of various mental disorders in inmate populations.[25] Table 6.2 shows these estimates.

The numbers of inmates suffering from developmental disabilities and other forms of intellectual disability is difficult to know. Miles Santamour[26] has suggested it may be between 4 percent and 9 percent. Most of these are not profoundly retarded. Many disabilities and deficits probably go unrecognized. People with impaired cognitive skills are subject to being preyed on and misled. They are not clever enough to assess situations adequately and can be unduly influenced. Some have even confessed to crimes they did not commit because they believed they should be cooperative and agree with the officers interrogating them.

The jail is now the poor person's mental health facility. The mental health system can say "no" to a patient, but the criminal justice system cannot. Dollars saved through mental health program cutbacks may represent no savings at all if they are offset by higher expenditures in the criminal justice system.

We have looked at how we arrived at the point where large numbers of mentally ill persons are in our prisons and jails. Now we must address some of the significant issues being faced daily by correctional administrators and corrections officers as a result of the growing number of mentally disordered persons in penal institutions. The current chapter will explain some of the unfortunate results of failing to conceptualize mental illness as a chronic condition.

JAIL AND PRISON ENVIRONMENTS ARE COUNTERTHERAPEUTIC

Life in a correctional setting can be profoundly stressful. Environmental factors such as noise, crowded conditions, confined space, and too little sunshine play a part, as do fears, real and imagined, of assault or injury from other inmates and officers. Taunts and threats from fellow prisoners can be terrifying. This is particularly so for first-time arrestees. Young, weak, and physically attractive persons are targets of sexual abuse. Prison and jail environments are particularly hard on persons who have previously been subjected to physical or sexual abuse or to other traumatic stress because there are so many stark reminders of these terrifying events at every turn. Especially vulnerable are persons with histories of schizophrenia, depression, anxiety disorder, and posttraumatic stress disorder (PTSD). Any of these persons may quickly experience psychological decompensation when confronting the powerful stressors of life in jail and prison.

E. Fuller Torrey, a psychiatrist, eloquently described the plight of a mentally disordered person in a correctional institution:

Being in jail or prison when your brain is working normally is, at best, an unpleasant experience. Being in jail or prison when your brain is playing tricks on you is often brutal.

One reason for this is that jails and prisons are created for people who have broken laws. These institutions have rigid rules, both explicit and implicit, and a major purpose of incarceration is to teach inmates how to follow such rules. The system assumes that everybody can understand the rules and punishes anyone who breaks or ignores these structures. Because of illogical thinking, delusions, or auditory hallucinations, many of the mentally ill cannot comprehend the rules of jails and prisons and this has predictable, and sometimes tragic, consequences.[27]

The deliberate indifference standard has been applied by courts for failure to meet, not just the serious medical needs of prisoners, but also their serious mental health needs. This definition is found in *Tillery v. Owens*: a "serious mental illness" is one "that has caused significant disruption in an inmate's everyday life and which prevents his functioning in the general population without disturbing or endangering others or himself."[28]

The health records of mentally ill persons in correctional facilities typically contain copious notes from psychiatrists, psychologists, social workers, and nurses who address appropriate topics such as mental status, suicidal ideation, response to medication, and current symptoms. Rarely, however, do they document a patient's history of mental illness and his or her prior treatment experience. A history of repeated hospitalizations, crisis events, or relapses cogently argues against a diagnosis of malingering.

"Being in jail or prison when your brain is working normally is, at best, an unpleasant experience. Being in jail or prison when your brain is playing tricks on you is often brutal."

—E. Fuller Torrey, MD

Even less often does the health record document that even a cursory inquiry took place concerning adjustment to current surroundings or important events occurring in patients' lives—such as trials, sentencing, the prospect of prison, appeals, interactions with fellow prisoners, visitors (or lack thereof), family illness or death, unfaithfulness or abandonment by spouse or significant other, or well-being of children. Perhaps the available time for each therapeutic contact is too brief, but these can be significant and even momentous concerns for confined persons, even for those without major mental illness. Consistent failure to explore these aspects of patients' lives suggests that mental health staff may already regard the antitherapeutic environment of a prison or jail as an unchangeable reality. In abdicating the role of change agent, a mental health professional becomes less effective therapeutically. It is inexcusable for therapists to ignore major stress factors affecting their patients because the presence of such factors can suggest specific treatment modifications.

The author vividly recalls, during a visit to a large county jail, meeting a man— not yet 20 years old—who was being held in an observation cell because of suicidal tendencies. I asked to have him brought out so I could talk with him. I asked the obvious question, "Why do you want to hurt yourself?" He answered, "I just got back from court. I got my sentence today: double life for two homicides. I'll never see daylight again. What is there to live for?" This young man was the same age as my son at the time.

Confinement itself is highly stressful. A jail or prison is not a comforting, reassuring, or stabilizing environment—even in the best of circumstances. An environment favorable to treatment may be described as comforting, reassuring, stabilizing, safe, nurturing, relaxing, moderate, and familiar, as seen in the following list. This set of descriptors clearly does not resemble the typical correctional institution.

It is inexcusable for therapists to ignore major stress factors affecting their patients because the presence of such factors can suggest specific treatment modifications.

Characteristics of an Environment Favorable to Treatment

- Comforting: not annoying or troubling
- Reassuring: not intimidating
- Stabilizing: not destabilizing or disorienting
- Safe: not dangerous (or perceived as such)
- Nurturing: not draining and taxing
- Relaxing: not exhausting
- Moderate: not extreme or harsh
- Familiar: not strange or unknown

Instead, the prisoner is exposed to loud and frequent noises. He or she must associate with predatory and dangerous people. Voices are rarely gentle. Inmates live in constant fear and uncertainty, not knowing whom to trust. The environment is strange and unfamiliar. Punishment and disciplinary sanctions are almost a way of life. Little opportunity is afforded to exercise meaningful control over one's life. In addition, jail inmates may experience considerable anxiety over their trial and sentencing, over the competence and diligence of their attorneys, and over recent separations from loved ones. The following lists these negative environmental aspects.

Negative Aspects of the Correctional Environment

- Excessive noise
- Predatory types
- Fear
- Uncertainty
- Unpleasant, untrustworthy companions
- Strange, unfamiliar environment
- Threat of disciplinary sanctions for rule violation
- Loss of control over one's life
- Trial and sentencing anxiety
- Loss of and separation from loved ones

Second only to medication, the environment (milieu) in which a person lives is the single most powerful factor influencing the course of chronic mental illness, the efficacy of treatment interventions, and the patient's response to external stimuli. The nature of this environment has a direct bearing on how quickly a patient will decompensate, how severe an episode will become, and how stable the patient will be. A beneficial change in the efficacy of treatment interventions may result from a nurturing and supportive environment that encourages compliance with medication, while the benefits of treatment can be eroded or negated by stressful surroundings. Finally, even though a person may respond appropriately to stressful stimuli faced one at a time, it may be impossible to cope when the whole environment is stressful.

Crowding exacerbates the stresses of institutional life and compounds the problems endemic to prisons and jails, including poor living conditions, lack of meaningful work, inter-inmate violence, sexual exploitation, and weakening of one's usual affectional ties.[29]

Second only to medication, the environment (milieu) in which a person lives is the single most powerful factor influencing the course of chronic mental illness, the efficacy of treatment interventions, and the patient's response to external stimuli.

Admittedly, the correctional environment may be an improvement over what some mentally ill persons experienced outside in the free world. At the least they have food, clothing, and shelter, access to medical and dental care, some mental health treatment, a safe haven from enemies, and counseling and rehabilitative programming. Thus, these persons may be regarded as relatively better off in the typical correctional setting—but only because of the extremely deprived and hostile environments from which they come.

Besides medication and a therapeutic milieu, psychosocial interventions and therapies can be helpful in alleviating symptoms and assisting a patient in coping with such situations.

MENTAL ILLNESS: A CHRONIC CONDITION THAT WAXES AND WANES

The preceding discussion of deinstitutionalization makes it clear that jails and prisons in the United States have become the principal public institutions for the care of the mentally ill in our society. State mental hospitals are exceedingly rare. As a consequence, correctional facilities must establish effective treatment programs for mentally ill inmates that adequately provide for their safety, security, and humane treatment.

Two subgroups are found among the seriously mentally ill inmates. The first comprises older deinstitutionalized patients who have histories of multiple hospitalizations. These are becoming fewer in number. Those in the second and younger group, on the other hand, usually do not have a history of multiple admissions to state hospitals because there were no beds for them. Both groups of patients over time will be diagnosed as demonstrating symptoms of severe mental illness such as schizophrenia, bipolar disorder, major depression, and other psychoses.

The mental illness typically found in these patients will be chronic in nature. Unlike many physical conditions, chronic mental illness is not cured by treatment.

Pneumonia, for example, is often cured by a single dose of penicillin. A fractured forearm, properly aligned and cast, will mend in about six weeks. But with a chronic illness such as arthritis, acute symptoms (pain and stiffness of the joints) quickly return once treatment is discontinued or when the patient experiences stressful conditions such as cold, humidity, or extreme changes in barometric pressure. The illness really never goes away and must therefore be viewed as a chronic condition. Leona Bachrach described it well: "a chronic condition is characterized by a long duration of illness, which may include periods of seeming wellness interrupted by flare-ups of acute symptoms and secondary disabilities."[30] In other words, the symptoms of the illness tend to wax and wane over time for each patient rather than exhibit a steady path toward cure.

It is important to appreciate the difference between "normal" persons and those with chronic mental illness in terms of their range of adaptive behaviors. Everyone will face stress in jail or prison, but mentally ill persons are less able to cope.

A few decades ago, when much less was known about how the brain functions, speculating about the underlying causes of mental illness was easier. With advances in our knowledge about the biochemistry, neuropathways (neurons, or nerves, that connect and channel energy from one part of the brain to another), and anatomy of the brains of chronically mentally ill persons in comparison to those of "normal" persons, the field is notably more complex. There is ample evidence from application of the various imaging techniques that there are noticeable differences in brain functioning of persons with mental disorders. First, we know that the concentration of certain chemicals in "normal" brains differs from that found in the brains of chronically mentally ill patients. Second, as we know from studies of identical twins, only one of whom has mental illness, the ventricles in the brain of the schizophrenic twin are larger than those of the twin who is "normal." Third, it has been demonstrated that mentally ill people employ different portions of their brains than do "normal" people when performing the same intellectual functions, giving evidence of a physiological rationale for their less effective coping skills.

We know also that an illness such as the flu can initiate a bout of depression in chronically mentally ill patients. For patients with chronic mental illness, we know that medication is the primary treatment. We also know that the second most effective treatment for these patients is placement in a therapeutic environment. In such a setting, members of the treatment team can aid the patient by helping to establish or reestablish contact with significant others and by offering reassurance, clarification, and comfort when needed. For the most part, supportive therapy and assisting the patient in his or her executive functions should be the focus of individual therapy. (Executive functions of the brain are high-level abilities that influence more basic abilities like attention, memory, and motor skills. For this reason, they can be difficult to assess directly. Some persons may have difficulty with tasks that require divided or alternating attention. Executive functions are important for decision making and for successful adaptation and performance in real-life situations. They also enable people to inhibit inappropriate behaviors and appear to play a role in antisocial behavior.)

A patient treated with medication in a therapeutic environment often reaches a state of remission in which the more flagrant symptoms have subsided. Because of the chronic nature of mental illness, the treatment plan must address long-term care and treatment even after the patient has been stabilized on medication and no longer requires the intensive services of a hospital or other acute care setting. Although medication protects against relapse, helps to maintain stability, and assists a person with chronic mental illness in coping with life's stresses, it cannot fully protect against more extreme forms of stress, especially when combined with limited problem-solving skills or loss of social support. This helps to explain why, even with medication, about 40 percent of newly discharged schizophrenic patients in the free world tend to relapse within a year of their discharge from a hospital. In fact, psychosocial treatment is most helpful for patients who are not currently exhibiting severe psychotic symptoms and who have reached a degree of stability through faithful compliance with their medication.

Patients are best continued on their antidepressant medications for some months after full remission has occurred. The high level of recurring daily stress in prisons and jails may make normalizing of brain function longer to achieve, and medication may be needed indefinitely.[31]

The chronicity of mental illness is described by correctional psychologist Dean H. Aufderheide: "The symptom severity of mental illness, like any chronic illness such as hypertension or diabetes, will wax and wane, constantly changing in response to internal and external factors. The mental health treatment and services plan, therefore, must be individualized, reviewed and revised in response to the changing clinical needs of the mentally ill inmate."[32]

It is important to appreciate the difference between "normal" persons and those with chronic mental illness in terms of their range of adaptive behaviors. Everyone will face stress in jail or prison, but mentally ill persons are less able to cope.

Looking at chronic mental illness in these terms, relatively few mentally ill persons who are discharged from a mental health unit into the general population of a jail or prison can be expected to make an adequate adjustment. Consequently, there needs to be a carefully elaborated plan for ongoing care of a large proportion of the mentally ill population. This plan should involve housing that is specifically designed to afford relief from typical sources of stress. Correctional administrators without such a plan risk falling into the deinstitutionalization trap once again—this time within their own facilities!

Acute Stress Disorder versus PTSD

Some persons exhibit their first signs of mental illness shortly after being exposed to extreme levels of stress in a jail or prison. When a prominent and respected citizen is arrested and jailed, she or he faces the prospect of loss of prosperity and reputation and senses an overwhelming loss of control over her or his life. This can manifest itself in acute psychotic symptoms. With antipsychotic medication and a therapeutic environment, the patient recompensates—sometimes in only a few days. Because a repeat episode is not likely, the patient may be safely returned to the general population of the jail or prison.

Episodes of disabling anxiety, psychosis, depression, agitation, or mania— previously referred to as "shell shock"—have been reported in wartime. We now know that response to a severe traumatic stress can also result in the chronic mental disorder called posttraumatic stress disorder (PTSD), a disorder that is too rarely diagnosed in correctional facilities, possibly because of overly large caseloads and too little time. Yet many prisoners would qualify for such a diagnosis. As just one example, a teenaged inmate told how he watched at age four as his uncle was murdered just a few feet away from him. He reported enough symptoms to qualify for a diagnosis of PTSD. A characteristic of this disorder is that severe symptoms can later be triggered by exposure to stress that evokes painful reminders of the earlier traumatic event.

Closed Head Injury

Likewise, the diagnosis of psychiatric disorder associated with severe head trauma is often overlooked by correctional mental health staff. An appreciable number of inmates report such episodes when asked the appropriate exploratory questions, but these questions are not always asked because of time constraints or inadequate motivation on the part of the therapist. Either way, the situation is ethically indefensible. If the clinician were to pursue this line of reasoning and arrive at a connection between previous head trauma and current explosive episodes, it might lead to an appropriate treatment strategy rather than a punishing response to the patient's behavior. Through interviews with the patient, correctional officers, and family members, the therapist might learn that the young man led a normal life up to age 10 when he was hit in the head with a baseball bat, after which he was hospitalized and did not regain consciousness for four days. Subsequently, he responded inappropriately—and often violently—to frustrating circumstances. He was in constant difficulties throughout high school and eventually injured another student severely, for which he was arrested. His behavior in jail has since led to numerous disciplinary infractions for fighting. From all of this, the therapist might reasonably determine that there is a connection between the head injury and the patient's abrupt change in pattern of behavior, concluding that mental health treatment may be a more effective answer than ticketing and time spent in segregation.

Chronicity of illness fosters learning maladaptive behaviors. For example, a patient who finds the behavior of other people irritating soon learns that if he acts in a hostile and aggressive manner, those around him tend to leave him alone. But this is not a suitable adaptive behavior in a correctional setting because an officer may raise his voice to indicate that he wants compliance with the rules. If the inmate perceives this as an irritation and responds in a hostile and aggressive manner, the officer will institute punitive sanctions. Ignoring the chronic nature of the illness and treating the mentally ill patient like any other prisoner can quickly escalate an incident and disrupt a general population unit rather than maintain good order.

While the prevalence of traumatic brain injury (TBI) in the U.S. general population is around 8.5 percent, the prevalence among incarcerated persons has been estimated as ranging between 25 percent and 87 percent.[33]

Barbara Curtis, a correctional nursing director, points out that the effects of TBI "could have contributed to behavior that provoked arrest and incarceration" and often leads to substance-abuse problems and can invite disciplinary infractions during confinement. The incarcerated who suffer from TBI tend to forget where they need to be or where they should not be, have difficulty focusing on instructions, may forget the rules, and often have poor anger and impulse control. During screening, "the clinician should look for physical signs such as scars on the face or head, any physical disability like one-sided weakness and difficulty with speech or action," which can be clues to a history of brain trauma.[34]

Curtis also counsels that an individualized treatment plan should be developed for everyone with TBI. The goal of treatment, in addition to preventing further head injury, should be "to improve independent function to the best level possible" with a focus "on managing symptoms, teaching compensatory strategies, and making environmental modifications." On an inmate's release, special consideration should be given to assisting the individual in adapting to the free world, where she or he will likely be living in a much less structured environment. It will be important to establish an effective connection with supportive resources in the community that can assist with TBI as well as other mental health and substance-use issues.

SPECIAL UNITS FOR HOUSING MENTALLY ILL PATIENTS

As previously stated, even well-managed correctional environments can be inherently hostile to the mentally ill because of the characteristic noise, crowding, fear, separation from loved ones, abuse and threats from predatory inmates, lack of normal amenities, idleness, anxiety over trial and sentencing, shame, embarrassment, and loss of hope. In combination, these fears can be extremely stressful and may push a person "over the edge." An otherwise stable person can become acutely mentally ill under these circumstances. Some are readily stabilized and recompensated with medication, and others need only a brief assist from supportive therapists. But many do not get along well in the general correctional environment. Without daily encouragement, they fail to take their medications regularly. They begin to hear and respond to voices and other internal stimuli and become overly fearful and paranoid. They behave in bizarre and offensive ways. And they can be injurious to themselves or others, often without warning.

An increasing number of correctional settings have found it useful to establish inpatient units and intermediate care settings for the mentally ill who, from time to time, experience severe symptoms. Too often, however, the number of these beds is inadequate given the high percentage of mentally ill, and the units may also be notably understaffed and lacking in supportive programming and therapeutic activities. Correctional authorities and mental health professionals sometimes find it necessary to discharge the less severely ill to the general population to make room for the more severely ill. When the fragile and unstable patient is returned to the general population, the combination of environmental stressors and poor medication compliance quickly cause an increase in symptoms. The patient is then returned to the mental health unit—a game of revolving door—and experiences severe pain and distress and possibly injures him- or herself or others.

Mentally ill prisoners can easily disrupt entire housing units. Some prisoners take delight in baiting or abusing the mentally impaired. Others feel annoyed at their behavior and tend to act out in inappropriate ways. When the mentally ill are removed from the general population setting, the rest of the prison is demonstrably quieter and more manageable.

It is sensible to plan for an adequate number of sheltered living units in the correctional facility or system to accommodate all of those mentally ill inmates who require additional protection, observation, support, or assistance. Staff in these units need to be sensitive to patients' needs and trained in mental health treatment and care.

Typical Characteristics of Mentally Ill Patients by Level of Care

Some characteristics are common to persons who are appropriately classified at the various treatment levels. These treatment levels go by various names—for example, intensive care, acute care, active care, subacute care, intermediate care, structured care, residential care, and outpatient care—in decreasing order of illness severity and treatment intensity. The paradigm shown in the following list adopts the terminology of active, subacute, residential, and outpatient care. Although the margins between these levels are somewhat imprecise, the concepts themselves are sufficiently clear so that clinicians using these or similar definitions can usually agree on the category to which a patient should be assigned.

Movement of a patient from one category to another should be readily accomplished by the treatment team whenever indicated by an exacerbation or remission of symptoms and with due consideration to the patient's expressed preference.

In the community, lengths of stay in acute psychiatric hospitals have become quite short—perhaps too short. Persons tend to remain longer in community care settings (residential treatment centers). We should therefore beware of applying the community mental health guidelines to prisoners without making appropriate adjustments. For many, the stresses experienced behind bars are much more severe than those encountered in the free world. Without extra help and support, persons who could perhaps do well at home with a caring family member are simply unable to cope adequately in the jail or prison setting. Moreover, commonly accepted intervals for follow-up of chronic patients in the community assume that a given patient is known to be sufficiently stable to tolerate 30 days, 90 days, or longer periods without follow-up. Until the patient's response pattern in the correctional environment is fully observed and evaluated and the medication dosage has been adequately titrated, much more frequent contact is needed and should be ensured. Likewise, when a patient is moved from a higher to a lower intensity of care level, therapeutic contact should be frequent until the patient is stable, and only then may it be gradually decreased.

The formulation in Table 6.3 was developed in 1992 by the psychiatric and psychological staff at the Wayne County Jail in Michigan in collaboration with Dr. Robert S. Ort and the author. The objective was to reach agreement on a set of criteria for assigning patients to treatment levels. It is offered here as a sample of how the treatment staff at a facility might estimate the number of patients in need of various care levels.

PRACTICAL CONSEQUENCES OF FAILING TO RECOGNIZE THE CHRONIC NATURE OF MENTAL ILLNESS

Recognition of the chronicity of mental illness has significant policy implications. Some practices commonly seen in correctional systems can result from a misunderstanding of this concept. Examples are shown in the following list. Mental health professionals working in correctional settings have a clear ethical responsibility to speak out and raise these issues whenever, in their professional judgment, the health and well-being of patients are adversely affected.

Some Unfortunate Correctional Practices That Can Result from Misunderstanding the Chronic Nature of Mental Illness

- Premature discharge from a mental health unit into the general population
- Substitution of crisis intervention for continuity of care
- Failure to appreciate or recognize the sources of stress in the patient's daily life
- Deliberate efforts to render a treatment unit uncomfortable and unattractive
- Employment of punitive sanctions in mental health treatment units
- Failure to explore and take into account factors of impaired cognitive function or impulse control as a consequence of mental illness
- Accumulation of significant numbers of mentally ill persons in segregation
- Understaffing and underfunding of mental health programs

Patients may be returned too quickly to the general population from a mental health unit. The environment of the mental health unit is more structured, safer,

Table 6.3
Typical Characteristics of Mental Patients by Level of Care

TYPICAL CHARACTERISTICS OF PATIENTS REQUIRING *ACTIVE* CARE

Suicidal
Homicidal
Severely disturbed
Highly unstable
Agitated
Severe psychiatric or neuropsychiatric symptoms
Experiencing treatment complications
Persistent diagnostic uncertainty
Severe personal distress or psychic pain
Unable to cope with demands of everyday life in the jail
Require major assistance with activities of daily living
Require titration of various psychoactive medications
Acute psychoactive substance withdrawal
Severe or persistent self-mutilation behavior

TYPICAL CHARACTERISTICS OF PATIENTS REQUIRING *SUBACUTE* CARE

Superficial self-injurious behavior
Moderate agitation, psychotic symptoms, psychic pain, psychiatric distress
Require some assistance with activities of daily living

TYPICAL CHARACTERISTICS OF PATIENTS REQUIRING *RESIDENTIAL* CARE

Likely to decompensate in general population
Low level of psychic distress
History of chronic mental illness
No suicidal or homicidal intent
Chronic illness is stable
Illness that allows a low level of stress to initiate decompensation
Low level of current psychic distress
Unable to cope with demands of everyday life within the jail
Able to care for personal activities of daily living and grooming with minimal assistance
and encouragement
Symptoms are no longer extreme
Symptoms and behaviors frequently provoke disciplinary sanctions
Definitive diagnosis has been made
Vulnerability to victimization

TYPICAL CHARACTERISTICS OF PATIENTS REQUIRING *OUTPATIENT* CARE

No history of mental illness; single episode of psychiatric disorder
History of long remissions when kept on medication
History of dependable compliance with medication regimen
Recompensates with little or no pharmacotherapy
Behaviors are not overly offensive or provocative to other inmates

and more comforting. Staff are supportive. Disturbing and hostile stimuli are absent or minimized. Patients are encouraged to take their medication regularly. However, after transfer to the general population, they may be subjected to numerous stressful influences such as insults and threats from other inmates, unpleasant noise and sights, indignities and discomforts, and harsh or inconsiderate direction from officers. They may also receive little or no encouragement to take their medication regularly. It should be no surprise if their symptoms recur. Professional staff should not be too quick to say that a patient is sufficiently stabilized to return to the general population, although staff members are sometimes under pressure to do so when their caseloads are too high or their mental health units are too small. Although trying a person out in the general population is an acceptable course of action, a long-term assignment to a sheltered living unit should be considered if the placement is not successful. It is unacceptable to discharge a patient from a mental health unit to the general population without scheduling a follow-up visit to a mental health professional within a few days after discharge. Frequent return visits are indicated until it is clear that the patient's condition remains stable.

To discourage "malingering," some officials—even correctional mental health professionals—have recommended that mental health units not be made too comfortable. The advice merits careful reevaluation. Does it really make sense to create a deliberately unpleasant, countertherapeutic environment in a mental health unit? It is far better to allow a few unnecessary days in the unit by an inappropriate patient than to render the entire program less than optimally effective for all.

Failure to appreciate the chronicity of mental illness leads to a substitution of crisis intervention for regular follow-up care. Whenever patients are discharged from a mental health unit, their treatment plan should specify a program of regular therapeutic contact. Case-management strategies can help achieve continuity of care.

Treatment staff should be attentive to sources of stress in the patient's daily life. As already indicated, one significant source of stress in a jail is the process of trial and sentencing.

To discourage "malingering," some officials—even correctional mental health professionals—have recommended that mental health units not be made too comfortable. The advice merits careful reevaluation. Does it really make sense to create a deliberately unpleasant, countertherapeutic environment in a mental health unit? We know that the environment (*ambience*) itself is an essential part of treatment. Do we seriously want to reduce the effectiveness of a treatment program just to discourage some possible overuse? Rather, we should entrust skilled clinicians with the task of determining who needs to be admitted and who should be discharged.

It is far better to allow a few unnecessary days in the unit by an inappropriate patient than to render the entire program less than optimally effective for all. Also, patients who quickly develop severe symptoms on return to the general population should not be rashly labeled malingerers who just want to enjoy the comfortable mental health unit. Normal, mentally healthy people do not ordinarily seek the constant company of mental patients for "enjoyment and comfort."

All too often, standard correctional practices of discipline and punishment are inflicted on inmates known to be mentally ill. If the mentally ill patient is in a treatment program, improper behavior is best dealt with in a therapeutic manner by treatment staff. Punitive methods are not helpful in controlling the disruptive behavior of mental patients. The treatment team should always employ clinically appropriate responses to difficult and refractory behavior by patients.

For three reasons, placement of a mentally ill patient in segregation is a major area of concern: (1) the events that led to segregation may be indicative of a developing problem, (2) the stressful circumstances of the segregation environment may provoke further symptoms, and (3) the offending behavior may have resulted from the mental illness.

Given the high prevalence of mental illness in correctional populations, failure to fund appropriate levels of programming and staffing for mental health can be linked to a misperception of the nature of chronic mental illness. Consequently, without effective and humane treatment, management problems in the facility only increase.

CONCLUSION: AN ETHICAL IMPERATIVE

This chapter expands on the theme developed in the first three chapters—namely, that a clear foundation of ethical principles must serve to guide the practice of health care in correctional settings. Here we have explored the practical implications of ensuring a correct understanding of chronic mental illness and of basing our actions and policy advice on that understanding. As a consequence of what we have seen, it is incumbent on mental health professionals who work in the criminal justice system to advocate for a radical revision of the prevailing traditional paradigm in our society that consigns so many persons with serious mental illness to prison or jail in the first place. Better alternatives urgently need to be developed and implemented. Improving treatment strategies in correctional institutions is critically important for the immediate future, but long-term strategies need to transfer large numbers of these people into community treatment settings as well as prevent such persons from being arrested and incarcerated in the first place.

A failure to provide suitable housing and treatment for mentally ill prisoners inevitably leads correctional officials to cope as best they can, often by resorting to use of segregation units for housing of mentally ill persons who exhibit deviant, uncooperative, and sometimes violent behavior.[35] There is ample evidence that typical conditions of isolation, segregation, and sensory deprivation, especially when prolonged, are seriously harmful to the health and well-being of persons with mental illness. Moreover, living in these conditions is exceedingly painful and cruel. Such treatment cannot be called humane. It is decidedly within our knowledge and our power to alter this trend. The answer begins as simply as treating others as we ourselves would wish to be treated were our roles reversed.

Hence, there is an ethical imperative for health care professionals to work on both fronts: within the larger community to endeavor to encourage the formation of a set of ready alternative strategies in society to keep mentally ill persons out of the criminal justice system and within the correctional setting itself to create therapeutic environments (special residential treatment programs) as effective alternatives to segregation and isolation. This is consistent with our belief that mental illness should be treated rather than punished.

Chapter 7

A Patient or a Prisoner?*

Two mental health nurses at a large urban jail were fresh from attending their new employee orientation program. One was heard to remark, "I guess we just have to realize that we're not working in our own house. After all, like they told us, this is a jail, not a mental health unit. Custody makes the rules here. We don't." The other added, "But this is so very different from the way I was trained! It wasn't this way where I used to work." A more experienced jail nurse spoke up, "That's OK. I used to feel that way too. But you'll soon get used to it. We do have to remember that we're working with inmates here."

This scenario is not unusual. Although new employee orientations in too many system present the relationship between custody and health care in just this manner, something is decidedly wrong with this picture,

Should anyone care whether the person sitting in the holding tank and waiting for a medical appointment is called a "patient" or an "inmate"? What does it matter whether mental patients are being treated in a "jail mental health unit" or in a "mental health treatment unit located in a jail"? Does it really make a difference whether the nurse writes in the progress note "applied dressing to *inmate's* left wrist," or writes, "applied dressing to *patient's* left wrist"? In the abstract, they probably do

---

* The author, along with his friend Richard M. Campau, presented a paper on this topic at the 24th National Conference on Correctional Health Care in St. Louis, Missouri, on September 13, 2000. A subsequent article by Nancy Vitucci appeared in the Fall 2000 issue of *CorrectCare*, describing our presentation and quoting the response of long-time correctional psychiatrist Henry C. Weinstein: "'Inmate' and 'patient' are not just words. They are labels that carry perceptions and consequences. The label of 'patient' is important in that it 'medicalizes' the caring, treatment focus of our services versus the mission of the corrections side." Vitucci's article also quoted B. Jaye Anno, one of the founders of the National Commission on Correctional Health Care, who commented: "It will help set the professional tone for interaction between patient and provider."

not. Such distinctions might appear trivial, but in practice and in the real world they do make a difference and can have profound and far-reaching effects over the long term.

In any context, denigrating and insulting names tend to diminish respect for the person or category of persons who are being called these names. When classes of people are referenced by derogatory epithets along ethnic or racial or national lines, they are dehumanized. There is an old saying: "Give a dog a bad name and hang him." Habitual use of degrading terms and labels tends to reduce normal scruples about mistreating captured enemy soldiers or killing civilians. It is much easier to lob a bomb or grenade at a group of "%&@#!"s than to do so on real people who are much like we are. A common feature of wartime propaganda has been the promotion and use of debasing and dehumanizing nicknames for the enemy so as to override any instinctive hesitation on the part of military personnel to pull the trigger on a weapon aimed at another human being. Recall, for instance, what Americans called Germans, Japanese, and Viet Cong peoples when we were at war with their nations.

WHY CALL THEM "PATIENTS"?

The health care professional—whether a physician, dentist, nurse, pharmacist, psychologist, therapist, or social worker—has been taught the proper way to treat patients or clients. Medical students learn the principles embodied in the Hippocratic oath, commonly expressed as: "I will use treatment to help the sick according to my ability and judgment, but I will never use it to injure or wrong them."[1] A central tenet of this training is that "the patient is always my first and foremost concern and, above all else, I must not cause my patient any harm." Most persons who choose a healing and caring profession do so because they derive satisfaction and find intrinsic reward in relieving pain, saving lives, and restoring function and well-being to others. Health care professionals respond almost instinctively to assist and benefit their *patients*. Terms such as *prisoner, inmate, offender, delinquent,* or *detainee* simply do not elicit the same automatic response.

The word *patient* means "one who suffers or endures pain" and "one who receives care or treatment, especially from a doctor." In common parlance, the patient is the person whose illness or malfunction is to be treated and healed. The patient is seen as the beneficiary of health care services. Physicians, dentists, nurses, and other medical care staff customarily use the term *patient*. Psychologists, therapists, social workers, or substance-abuse counselors may prefer the term *client* or *recipient*. Some correctional systems prefer the term *residents*, and many juvenile facilities use the term *students*. Although this usage avoids the negative connotations of punishment and wrongdoing, words such as *resident* and *student* do not usually evoke the same healing responses from health care professionals as *patient* and *client*. The author does not quarrel with such usage if it is customary in community practice and will subsume these terms under the more general term *patient*.

The term *offender* has been adopted in some correctional systems. For some reason, it has even become the designation regularly used in the standards and policy pronouncements of the American Correctional Association—a fact that will likely further promote and consolidate its usage. Nevertheless, among these terms, the author regards *offender* as the one that is least desirable for use by health care staff because it focuses so explicitly on the person's history of wrongdoing, implying at least subliminally that he or she is bad and deserves punishment. This perception can undermine the clinician's disposition to respond as a healing professional. At least terms such as *inmate, prisoner,* and *detainee* directly focus on the individual's current status and only by implication suggest any history of wrongdoing.

Some readers may object that this discussion is splitting hairs and focusing too much on nuanced parsing of words and the minutiae of language, but it is indisputable that certain forms of expression carry pejorative overtones and their constant use negatively affects the overall environment. This leaves for thoughtful consideration whether such usage brings any countervailing benefit that outweighs its potentially harmful consequences. The author contends that it does not and advances the hypothesis that if rehabilitation is a valid goal of corrections, then all of us— whether correctional personnel or health care staff—should strive in every reasonable way to build and elevate the sense of personal worth and dignity of all human beings in custody while avoiding what needlessly tends to diminish and destroy their self-image.

There are, of course, times when it is not inappropriate for the doctor or nurse to speak of "inmates" or "prisoners," as when referring to the census of a facility or the capacity of a housing unit. But qua patient—that is, in the context of a person who is to receive medical treatment—they should be thought of and called "patients."

The point can be depicted graphically. What we call people affects how we think about them, and this helps shape the way we behave toward them. See Figure 7.1.

The overall approach and philosophy of the healing professions diverge widely from those of the correctional system.[2] Margaret Wishart and Nancy Dubler aptly termed the correctional environment "a non-health care space."[3] Dr. Michelle Staples-Horne phrased it this way: "The health care model can be perceived as foreign and often contradictory in a correctional setting."[4] Prisons are places of punishment. A punitive methodology tends to permeate their staff, buildings, and policies. Punishment, however, is antithetical to healing. Punishment is the deliberate and intentional infliction of harm. It often comprises confinement, deprivation of liberty, denial of privileges, and imposition of discomfort or pain—albeit

Figure 7.1
Language can influence behavior.

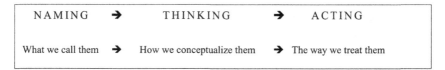

NAMING	→	THINKING	→	ACTING
What we call them	→	How we conceptualize them	→	The way we treat them

legally or for a purpose approved by society. Most correctional personnel rightly understand that although prisons are places *of* punishment, they are not places *for* punishment. Confinement to a prison—that is, the deprivation of a person's liberty—is precisely the punishment decreed by a court of law, and levying of additional punishment and suffering by staff is inappropriate. Still, by its nature, a jail or a prison is a punishing environment. In contrast, healing professionals must never harm their patients, or punish them, or act in any way except in their best interests. This attitude and orientation are part and parcel of a solemn promise and trust that must never be forgotten. If medical service providers were to do otherwise, none of us could ever place full confidence in their hands. People literally entrust their lives to their physicians.

Health care professionals respond almost instinctively to assist and benefit their patients. Terms such as *prisoner, inmate, offender, delinquent,* or *detainee* simply do not elicit the same automatic response.

Experience has shown that health care staff who customarily refer to their patients as *prisoners* or *inmates* or *offenders*, in speech and in writing, are at some risk of developing a diminished respect for the dignity and worth of their patients. Sometimes the consequences are obvious and unfortunate. Nurses and physicians can almost subconsciously become punishing in their demeanor, attitude, and behavior toward those whom they regularly degrade verbally. Chapter 2, "Areas of Significant Ethical Role Conflict," under "A Note of Caution," describes a tendency toward gradual erosion of the ethical principles central and sacred to health care professionals and suggests that there may be a dose-response relationship. The more closely and the longer they work with prisoners and correctional staff, the more rapidly and profoundly they are likely to be affected.

People may not even realize or find any cognitive dissonance with use of a word such as *inmate* because it is by now a long-established pattern and the feeling is, "No harm intended, no foul committed." But look again. They may have imperceptibly succumbed to some desensitization of their principles; even if not, their continued use of such terminology contributes to an environment that can negatively influence coworkers. It is prudent to choose the accepted terminology of the health profession and avoid terms with negative or toxic connotations.

This phenomenon deserves more research and is readily amenable to sociological measurement. Such a study could also attempt to discover the factors that offset this tendency in some persons and accelerate it in others. In any case, the phenomenon does appear to exist. This is not surprising, inasmuch as the health care component in any correctional system rarely comprises more than 15 percent of its staff, funding, policy, and program resources.

Correctional nurse Jamie S. Brodie, MSN, RN, FPN makes the following insightful and sobering observations:

Correctional facilities can be disorienting environments for nurses, who may feel like "fish out of water" when the setting lacks appropriate professional leadership, structure, and support of the values essential to professional nursing practice. There is danger of being coerced by the security system, especially when orientation and training focus too much on security issues and not enough on professional nursing practice. Professional isolation and the need to maintain boundaries and accommodate facility needs can erode the essential nurse-patient relationship that is the core of nursing practice. . . . Staff who view inmates as less worthy or as lesser human beings exhibit thinly disguised contempt which damages the quality and outcome of care.[5]

Brodie's comments remain true, even when health care staff do not engage in overt acts of punishment or cruelty toward prisoners. Should they occur, such events are symptomatic of an extremely serious problem and likely indicate major career dissonance. Practitioners who take delight in deliberately causing their patients to suffer were not suited in the first place to be health care professionals and have violated a very basic principle of professional ethics. A person with these tendencies is also not well suited for the position of correctional officer. Brodie, however, is referring to a more subtle and gradual erosion of ethical principles and boundaries, and he wisely cautions us that they can still impair the quality and integrity of the provision of health care services.

> In constantly calling attention to the penal condition that is implied by the term *inmate* or *prisoner* or *offender*, the health care provider signals that the individual is bad, has done wrong, deserves to be punished, and therefore is entitled to few rights or privileges. This not only serves to reinforce the person's already poor sense of self-worth but also is inconsistent with a therapeutic approach. It does not even have to be intended as such because the chosen words speak for themselves and carry a message that is detrimental to rehabilitation and treatment.

Terminology used by supervisors and staff can and does influence the way in which they carry out their function. Common signs of deterioration in the fabric of a healer's professional ethics are comments such as, "He missed his appointment, so I'll just put him on the bottom of the waiting list," "These convicts have nothing coming to them. They already get more benefits than they deserve," and "They're all just a bunch of addicts and whiners." It sometimes also shows up in the way kites and grievances are answered. An example of this attitude is failure to investigate or take the time to hear complaints and instead focusing only on how to show the grievant is wrong and that no remedy is required. Worse yet, find a technical defect in the complaint such as it being a day late and then dismiss the grievance out of hand without even considering its merits.

Failure of health care practitioners to be proactive and forthright in patient advocacy is another warning sign. Nurses, psychologists, and other health care staff who do not speak up when they see patients mistreated or when they find patients living in extreme distress and discomfort may have already succumbed to the belief that prisoners deserve whatever they get. On the other hand, concerned health professionals who learn that a patient's medication is unduly delayed or that a needed specialty appointment has been inadvertently or mistakenly canceled will intervene proactively on behalf of the patient and try to get the problem resolved promptly.

Judith Stanley of the NCCHC staff illustrated this point in a discussion about effective pain control:

It is distressing to be honest about this, but inadequate pain control is often a result of poor attitude and stereotyping. Correctional staff's negative experiences with drug-dependent persons, health staff memories of being "burned" by inmate-patients, the additional safeguards for use of strong pain medication—all contribute to a reluctance to prescribe for pain relief as would be done in community practice. Even with highly professional providers there may lurk unconscious motivation such as, "Well, this is an inmate who has done wrong and deserves to suffer."

Perhaps the best way to deal with personal biases is to forget for the moment that the patient is an inmate and ask, What is the appropriate professional response to the clinical distress? What ordinarily would be done in community practice? Offering over-the-counter meds for pain from end-stage-cancer, root canal, acute injury or surgery is not the current standard of care. Even if the patient is drug dependent, alternative pain medications are available and should be tried.[6]

Consider also the effect on patients' sense of personal worth and their image of the health care program itself when medical professionals fail to accord their patients the dignity of being called *patient* (which would imply a person with an illness or health condition requiring care, including appropriate evaluation and treatment). In constantly calling attention to the penal condition that is implied by the term *inmate* or *prisoner* or *offender*, the health care provider signals that the individual is bad, has done wrong, deserves to be punished, and therefore is entitled to few rights or privileges. This not only serves to reinforce the person's already poor sense of self-worth but also is inconsistent with a therapeutic approach. It does not even have to be intended as such because the chosen words speak for themselves and carry a message that is detrimental to rehabilitation and treatment. It also contradicts what the health care professional believes. An impaired sense of self-worth may have been a factor in the life of crime, but effective rehabilitation will not happen until this is effectively addressed.

Because of their history, context, and patterns of usage, words can come to convey or connote more meaning than their literal or etymological definition. Writing

"PT" or "patient" rather than "IM" or "inmate" in the medical chart, or asking "How many more patients are to be seen today?" instead of "How many more prisoners are out there?" is not a trivial difference. Persons who are consistently called *patient* are likely to be regarded and treated like patients—and therefore to behave like patients. Practitioners instinctively associate and apply the concepts of "care" and "do no harm" to their *patients* but not so easily or quickly to *inmates* or *offenders*. This recommended usage provides constant daily reminders of what treatment and caring are about.

When a newly hired nurse at a prison hospital walked past the room of a debilitated terminally ill patient, she saw that his pillow had fallen to the floor and he appeared extremely uncomfortable. She entered the room, picked up the pillow, fluffed it, placed it under his head, and proceeded to adjust the blanket while asking the patient if that felt any better. Her supervisor happened to be in the vicinity and took notice. She subsequently scolded the new nurse severely for "fluffing and buffing inmates!" Had the supervisor, also a nurse, forgotten what it means to care for a patient?

A social worker accepted a position to work on an outpatient mental health team at a maximum security facility. She walked out after the second day of new employee orientation, explaining that she felt she would be asked to compromise her professional principles because the training video she was required to watch admonished new staff "never to trust anything that an inmate tells you" and that "you need to forget everything they told you in school about caring for your patients. Here, you do your job, but you must never 'care for' the prisoners."

At one facility, the author was told, "The problem with too many health care staff is that they forget that their patients are inmates. That's why they should always refer to them as inmates—as a reminder." The supposition here is that if nurses and doctors treat their patients as though they were in the free world, they will not take the necessary precautions, keep the appropriate reserve, or limit their treatment to what is suited for inmates. However, whether in the free world or in corrections, medical staff should always exercise due precautions and reserve with any patient that they have reason to believe might be dangerous. Medical staff are unlikely to forget that they are in a correctional setting where security rules and policies must at all times be observed. If they do demonstrate a lax attitude with respect to security, they need to be counseled and, perhaps, scheduled for more training—or separated from the service. Similarly, physicians and other health providers must learn that it is acceptable to say "no" to their patients when, in their professional judgment, the requested treatment or procedure is not required or is not clinically appropriate. This is not dissimilar to a physician in the community advising a patient why a particular treatment or procedure is not recommended or that it is not a covered benefit by an insurer. "Inmate status" should never contraindicate proper care.

The reader is referred to Chapter 1, "Ethics in the Context of Correctional Health," and the discussion under "A Caring Approach."

IS IT A HEALTH CARE UNIT?

Is it a prison or a health care unit? Some glibly and simplistically answer, "We don't need to quarrel over terms. It is *both*. It is for *inmate-patients*" (using the hyphenated approach). "It is a *jail-infirmary*" or "It is a *prison-clinic*." They may also add that "security must come first" and that "everything depends on security." This rationalization, however, misses the point. "Security" does not diagnose or treat a dental abscess, a fractured ankle, or a bipolar disorder, yet each of these conditions must be treated in a safe and secure manner. In the correctional setting, this is ensured by adherence to the reasonable rules and regulations that were established for the sake of safety and security. The purpose of the medical clinic, mental health unit, or infirmary is to treat and heal. Although security is a necessary condition for good treatment to take place, it is not the purpose of treatment.

The author believes that hyphenated terms such as *inmate-patient* and *prison-clinic* are awkward and clumsy at best and reflect a degree of unresolved ambivalence. At worst, they are meant to inject the notion that the patients belong to an inferior class and are of diminished worth and dignity. Doctors do not usually refer to their "engineer-patients," "housewife-patients," or "carpenter-patients" because these compound designations are irrelevant to the art of healing, unlike terms that might be useful such as toddler-patients or nursing-home-patients or dialysis-patients. The positive and beneficial impact of the word *patient* is diluted when linked by a hyphen to a word that carries a negative or punitive connotation. However, an exception might be reasonable to distinguish, for example, an inmate-patient from other patients who are being cared for in a community hospital.

> The purpose of the medical clinic, mental health unit, or infirmary is to treat and heal. Although security is a necessary condition for good treatment to take place, it is not the purpose of treatment.

If the health services area is perceived to be first and foremost a part of the jail or prison and only secondarily as a health care unit, then the incongruence of certain undesirable practices may go unnoticed. As an example, officers in a mental health unit (viewed only as part of the prison) may routinely ticket and punish patients for failure to follow rules instead of referring unacceptable behaviors to the treatment team for a more appropriate therapeutic response. Rules applicable to a mental health unit should be different from those in effect throughout the rest of the institution. These rules need to be more consistent with the needs and limitations of mentally ill patients and more compatible with a therapeutic environment, while yet respecting important safety concerns. The daily schedule may also differ. There will be more attention to therapeutic activities, treatment planning, voluntary participation, informed consent, freedom of movement, and self-determination.

In an ideal health care unit, all of the furnishings and design are compatible with and tend to reinforce its therapeutic function. In correctional facilities, however, it too often happens that the health care program must "adapt" and "force-fit" itself into a setting that was designed and intended for other and quite different purposes.

> The author believes that hyphenated terms such as *inmate-patient* and *prison-clinic* are awkward and clumsy at best and reflect a degree of unresolved ambivalence. At worst, they are meant to inject the notion that the patients belong to an inferior class and are of diminished worth and dignity.

These remarks do not suggest that security precautions may be relaxed where health services are provided. Safety is every bit as important in an infirmary, a clinic, or a mental health unit as in the rest of the institution. It is never acceptable for health care staff to condone or enable the introduction of contraband or to facilitate an escape. The objectives of safety and security, however, should be achieved in a way that works to facilitate and support the effective and efficient delivery of quality health care services.

WHERE THE LINES GET CROSSED

In a few jails, nurses are actually sworn officers or deputy sheriffs. They wear the same uniforms and badges as the custody officers, sometimes even sporting the belt clip with handcuffs and the empty pistol holster while on duty in the jail's health care unit. The officer training these nurses receive is not a bad thing and does not compromise the quality of their nursing practice. The nurses with whom the author spoke appeared to be highly professional and competent. When asked, these nurses responded that their patients did not appear to have any problem relating because "They know I am a nurse." But two concerns remain. First, is there a role ambiguity conflict for the nurse who has no visible reminder of the nursing profession in the uniform worn? Second, some patients may be both confused and concerned about the role and the loyalties of the nurse who presents him- or herself outwardly as a custody officer. There are significant boundary issues here, and the lines are being unnecessarily blurred. The patient's legitimate and understandable question— not always explicitly formulated—is, "Will this nurse really act in my best interests? Can I fully trust this person to be a caring provider of health services?" To the extent that the already tenuous patient–provider trust is further compromised or called into question, the effectiveness of care invariably suffers.

In a few correctional systems, long-standing practices require all staff (including health care professionals, kitchen employees, teachers, mechanics, and clerical personnel) to demonstrate current proficiency in firearms and other security-related skills, even to the point of marching and drilling during their periodic training programs or practicing on a shooting range. Aside from being a costly diversion of time and effort for doctors, nurses, psychologists, and dentists that could be put to more productive use, it conveys the preeminence of security and the subservience of all other functions—as perhaps was long ago intended when the practice was first introduced. Surely, there is no reasonable expectation that a health care professional's marksmanship and weapons-handling ability will ever be used or relied on in a time of institutional crisis. Instead, these nurses and doctors will be carrying out important relevant priorities within their own field of specialty. Training and preparing to shoot (or otherwise harm) prisoners is so fundamentally opposed to the role and mission of health care professionals that it should never be part of their orientation, indoctrination, or job duties. (This is not meant to suggest any inherent ethical conflict or impropriety when correctional health care professionals elect to participate in hunting or marksmanship activities for recreation or sport.)

PATIENT ADVOCACY

Health care professionals are expected to act as advocates for their patients. This is particularly the case for patients whose conditions (age, mental capacity, or disability) impede them from adequately taking care of their own needs. The way in which one conceptualizes the person—whether as a *prisoner* or as a *patient*—can subconsciously influence the caregiver's inclination to act in the advocate role.

In a managed care setting,[7] nurses and physicians in a remote location (e.g., a central health care office of a state corrections department or the headquarters of a private contractual health care provider) typically review requests for costly medical procedures, consultations, or referrals. These requests are prepared and submitted by the patient's primary care provider. Because the person who will approve or disapprove the request has never seen the patient, the decision may depend on how well the primary care provider formulates the request. Haste, carelessness, omission of important details, and failure to describe previous unsuccessful treatment efforts will probably result in a denial. Not every request is meritorious, but the requester who believes a request has merit should be willing to include the necessary rationale and supporting documentation and be prepared to resubmit the request or to appeal the denial if the circumstances warrant. By the same token, a care provider should not submit a request for approval of treatment that he or she does not believe the patient really needs. The primary provider should say "no" to the patient when appropriate rather than pass the decision up to another level out of fear of disappointing the patient.

Every managed care system needs to have an appellate procedure because no formula considers all relevant variables. The primary care physician should initiate an appeal on behalf of the patient to obtain a treatment or diagnostic procedure that is deemed necessary. The process for selecting physicians to work in a prison or jail system should seek to find and retain those who instinctively assume an advocacy stance on behalf of their patients, not those who are pleased to find any rationale to deny care. (Even in the interest of cost containment, the prison is better served by doctors who are strong patient advocates because their approach will lead to fewer instances of negligent care or wrongful adverse outcomes in the long run.)

A LESSON FROM THE CAPTAIN

The captain with 25 years of experience at a large New England state correctional facility was addressing a group of auditors touring the medical inpatient unit at the facility—a group that included the author. Here is a close approximation of his words:

We must always remember that this is, first of all, a prison and, only secondly, a hospital. We keep reminding our medical staff of this. It's *not* a hospital first, and *then* a prison. If you get this mixed up, you start taking chances. You then forget that you have to watch your back all the time. You can never trust a prisoner. The prisoner has 24 hours a day to study the staff—to get to know their patterns, their every move, how they think. The inmate listens—eavesdrops—remembers everything he hears. Then someday, when you least expect it, he will use it against you.

To give the captain due credit, he did not suggest that health care staff should regard their clients as prisoners first and only secondarily as patients. And the captain had a valid point, one developed from long years of experience. He had seen fellow officers and other staff seriously injured by prisoners. He knew how quickly a problem can arise and situation get out of control. He understood the paramount importance of securing anything that could be made into or used as a weapon—and such instruments certainly abound in a medical area. What he said was true. The nurses, doctors, psychotherapists, and others who work in the medical unit must never, ever forget that they are working in a prison and that the security rules and policies exist for legitimate reasons—safety and good order. But his words could be misleading and convey an impression that was not intended. Certainly, not every inmate is always untrustworthy, and he did not say that one should never believe anything a prisoner says. The requirements of security and medical practice must always be appropriately balanced in the design and operation of a medical or mental health unit, and a proper awareness of the realities of the situation is critically important.

A storekeeper regards persons coming into the shop as customers and treats them accordingly. The actor or performer looks out over the lights and sees fans and an audience, not a crowd or a mob. It is not unethical for the jail or prison officer to refer to "prisoners" or "inmates," but the doctor and nurse must see them as "patients" first and foremost. To do otherwise is to adopt a style and approach that is ill-suited to their role.

To be crystal clear, nothing in this chapter is meant to suggest that health care staff should ignore or fail to take seriously the advice and legitimate concerns of security. Particularly in their first few months on the job, health care providers should be slow to criticize or question established patterns and routines. Their presumption should be that existing practices and rules have been developed for a good reasons that will eventually become clear as they learn more about the system. Of course, there can be exceptions. Some practices are so clearly out of place and so obviously wrong that they should not be followed, but these are rarely found in the formal orientation and training of new employees or in agency policies. They may, however, be passed on informally by "seasoned" correctional staff who have come to believe in a "tougher" approach. New health care employees are advised to bring their doubts and questions to a more experienced employee or supervisor whom they can trust as a mentor to help them gain a better perspective on these issues.

CONCLUSION

This chapter encourages strict adherence to the commonly accepted community terminology, calling patients "patients" and designating the space in which health care is provided with a clinically or therapeutically appropriate name. This practice should begin during the hiring process and the initial orientation of employees to the job, and it should be uniformly reflected in every policy and procedure as well as in the health record forms and similar documents. Supervisors must not only demonstrate good example in this respect but also insist on compliance. This does not mean that an occasional reference to an "inmate," "prisoner," or "offender" ought to be treated as a rule violation or misconduct, but regular usage of this nature by health care staff should be discouraged as incorrect or less than fully professional. Once the change in customary practice has taken place, its maintenance by example and timely reminders should not be difficult.

Implying that all health care professionals who use terms such as "inmate" and "offender" have abandoned the ethical principles of their profession and become punitive would be wrong. Nevertheless, the risk is real, and those working day after day in the environment of a correctional facility whose overt purpose includes punishment are counseled to avail themselves of every reasonable means to prevent being adversely and subtly influenced. Staff should endeavor to position themselves always in the mode of patient advocate. Health care professionals working in these environments need to be watchful and monitor their own responses carefully.

Self-deception is easily possible as one begins using uncritical or exaggerated thinking and adopts the old saws as justification: "Custody always comes first," "These people are getting better health care here than they did in free society," or "They have nothing to do all day but figure out how to manipulate the system." Long-standing habits in phraseology, wording, or oversimplistic statements should be carefully reviewed and revised as necessary. One place to look for inappropriate statements and terminology is in the videos, manuals, and lesson plans of employee orientation and training. Another is in the facility's health care policies and procedures. Each instance should be corrected as soon as feasible. Until that happens, the new employees or trainees should be provided a disclaimer that explains the preferred terminology and its rationale before viewing the training materials or reading the policy manuals.

Undoubtedly, there is a sense in which it is correct to say that this facility is first a prison and only secondarily a health care unit, or that this person is a prisoner who happens to be a patient or that not every prisoner is always trustworthy. Nevertheless, incorrect and possibly unintended overtones and implications can flow from statements such as these. They can be misleading and a source of confusion or erroneous perception, especially to the newcomer on staff. Over time, such usage may desensitize even the best health care providers with respect to their instinctive responsiveness to a patient's legitimate care needs.

Chapter 8

Organizing Correctional Health Care

COMMON MISSION WITH DIFFERENCES

After *public protection*, the most commonly cited mission of corrections is the *care and custody* of prisoners. This formulation clearly entrusts correctional officials with the *care* of inmates and not solely with their custody or confinement. Ensuring that their *health* needs are met is undeniably an essential aspect of their care.

It follows, then, that the policies and practices of a good correctional system must be consistent with the requirements of good health care. A properly managed correctional system, like a properly managed health care program, will assign a high priority to each of the following as a matter of principle:

- Safety and well-being of each person
- Safe and secure environment for staff and patients
- Orderly management of the institution
- Proper hygienic practices and sanitation
- Confidentiality of private and sensitive information
- Respect for dignity and basic human needs of inmates
- Emergency preparedness
- Prevention of harm
- Due attention to maintaining and improving program quality
- Adherence to ethical and professional standards
- Conservation of scarce resources by avoidance of waste and inefficiency

Each of these characteristics is critically important to the success of both correctional and health care programs. Neither system can properly achieve its mission in an unsafe or disorderly environment. Good hygienic practices and sanitation measures protect the health of staff, inmates, and visitors. To be successful, each discipline requires clear and consistent policies along with ongoing staff training and development that reflect due concern for human dignity and respect for fundamental human needs and rights. Each must have a quality-control program, a focus on preventing bad outcomes, a solid ethical and professional foundation, and an emphasis on efficient use of resources. Their priorities need to be balanced and optimized with mutual cooperation and respect by both the custody and health care sectors.

After public protection, the most commonly cited mission of corrections is the care and custody of prisoners. This formulation clearly entrusts correctional officials with the care of inmates and not solely with their custody or confinement.

Even though the two systems share elements of a common mission, they have some important and fundamental differences. Correctional and health care programs differ in their purpose, means employed to achieve that purpose, primary client served, use of coercive measures, type of employee training, and system of beliefs. The fact that they share similar priorities and goals does not mean that they will (or should) choose to implement them in exactly the same manner. They have decidedly different functions. This theme is elaborated further in Chapter 9, "Corrections and Health Care Working Together," where differences and similarities of health care and corrections are examined, and strategies for productive cooperation are explored in detail.

RESPONSIBLE HEALTH AUTHORITY

Who is the responsible health authority for a prison or county jail or youth correctional facility? In one sense, it is the governor of the state, the director of corrections, and the warden (or sheriff, county commissioner, and jail administrator) because the public responsibility and legal liability for what happens in their systems cannot be delegated. If a suit is brought alleging medical malpractice or violation of civil rights by a doctor or nurse, then the first-named defendant is often the governor or sheriff—the elected official who bears ultimate executive responsibility. This is true when the doctors and nurses as state or county employees ultimately are supervised by the governor, sheriff, or warden, but it is equally true when the agency has contracted the provision of health services to a private for-profit or not-for-profit vendor. A governmental agency cannot delegate or contract away its ultimate responsibility and liability, no matter how much language is inserted into the contract about holding the state harmless.

However, the term *responsible health authority*, as used throughout this book, refers specifically to the person who is duly charged, as the American Correctional Association (ACA) states, to make "decisions about the deployment of health resources and the day-to-day operation of the health services program" of a specific facility.[1] Essentially, the responsible health authority is analogous to the chief executive officer of a business or a corporation. The National Commission on Correctional Health Care (NCCHC) describes this individual's duties as broad and comprehensive, including arranging for every level of health care and ensuring "quality, accessible, and timely health services for inmates."[2] When the responsible health authority is not a physician, a licensed physician must be given the authority to supervise all medical judgments regarding the care of persons housed at a specific facility. This person is often designated as the responsible physician, medical director, or chief medical officer.

If mental health services are not under the direction of the designated responsible health authority, there must be a designated mental health clinician who is given this responsibility for clinical mental health issues at the facility.

Large correctional agencies generally have a designated system-wide health authority, whose responsibility it is to provide leadership and coordination over the responsible health authority at each facility, serve as liaison with top officials in the department, and be the ultimate advocate for patients at the highest levels within the agency. This same central health authority can also influence resource allocation, facilitate bulk-purchasing arrangements, and achieve a reasonable measure of consistency and uniformity of medical practice across facilities. In keeping with the standards, however, this individual does not substitute for the responsible health authority at each facility, and NCCHC insists this person must be on-site at the facility at least weekly. In a state that has contracted out its entire health services program, it may be the contracting entity that supplies the statewide central health authority. But here it is highly desirable for the state to designate its own statewide medical director to exercise final authority. The complex organization structure can vary, but it is key that there be accountability designated for responsible management.

Notwithstanding the language of the NCCHC and ACA standards that permit an *agency* to serve as the responsible health authority, it is always good policy to designate a named individual person to serve in this capacity. Even when the health services program is delegated to a health department or other agency, it is the author's position that a specific person in that agency needs to be assigned as the responsible health authority. If that person is not a physician, then a responsible physician also needs to be designated. Otherwise, the responsibility is diffused and weakened. Agencies do not think or decide.

Medical Autonomy

In its simplest terms, in *Estelle v. Gamble* the U.S. Supreme Court recognized the essence of medical autonomy. The Court said that deliberate indifference to the serious medical needs of prisoners can be manifested "by prison guards in intentionally denying or delaying access to medical care or intentionally interfering with the treatment once prescribed."[3] In other words, the medical autonomy of health care providers requires that nonmedical personnel refrain from any interference in strictly medical decisions. This concept is strongly endorsed in the standards. For the ACA: "Clinical decisions are the sole province of the responsible health care practitioner and are not countermanded by nonclinicians."[4] For the NCCHC, "Clinical decisions and actions regarding health care provided to inmates to meet their serious medical needs are solely the responsibility of qualified health care professionals."[5] And for the APHA, "Health care providers are the sole dispensers of medical decisions and should not be impeded by security staff or correctional administrators."[6]

Within reason, it is legitimate for correctional authorities to determine working conditions and schedules such as the place or time at which sick call will be held. As the experts and authorities responsible for custody and security, they may also impose reasonable restrictions. They may, for instance, prohibit any person from working at the facility who fails to meet the established security criteria or who violates the security regulations, and they may prevent health care staff from access to a given area until it is properly secured, delay medical transport of a high-risk inmate until adequate security provisions are made, or prevent the introduction of a potentially dangerous prosthetic device. They may also regulate the kinds and amounts of medications that inmates can keep on their persons or purchase in the commissary. The warden or jail administrator may determine, for example, that not enough security staff are on duty outside the regular day shift to permit a routine dental clinic operation during evening hours or on weekends.

In the community, a third-party payer may seek clarification or ask the rationale for a particular procedure that the doctor has ordered and may inquire whether a more conservative, less costly, or safer alternative is available. The correctional authority may also inquire as to the urgency or necessity for a medical decision or treatment order when it appears to inconvenience or conflict with correctional routine or when it is extremely costly. For example, on days that transportation officers are busy with court-scheduled movement, it is appropriate to ask the doctor to set priorities for the day's medical off-site appointments and to indicate whether there is urgent need to transport a particular patient on that day. It is not acceptable, however, for correctional officers to determine these priorities unilaterally or simply to leave medical transportation schedules unmet. Correctional authorities should not determine the time of day for distribution of medications, although they may express preferences within the time frames deemed clinically necessary by the responsible health authority.

Should a correctional official contravene or interfere with implementation of a medical order, the health care professional who becomes aware of this should evaluate the situation immediately. On determining that the health and well-being of the patient will be adversely affected, the health professional is obliged to pursue an advocacy role and promptly bring the matter to appropriate supervisory attention.

Generally, a direct confrontation with the officer is not advisable, but the issue should be promptly discussed by the proper parties at a higher level of authority in both ranks.

Rationale for Designating a Responsible Health Authority

Several reasons support designating a responsible health authority for each facility with duties that are clearly specified in a job description, policy, or contract:

- *Credibility.* The facility will fare better in court if health care decisions are made only by properly trained and licensed persons whose job descriptions assign them this responsibility.
- *Professionalism.* It is prudent to let the health professionals manage the health arena. They are the experts.
- *Recruitment.* It is easier to recruit good health care staff when their line of supervision and reporting is to an appropriate health care professional rather than to a correctional official.
- *Accreditation.* The accreditation standards of both the NCCHC and the ACA require it.
- *Legal liability.* Only licensed health professionals may legally exercise medical judgment on behalf of a patient, within the scope of practice authorized by their license. It would be illegal for anyone without an appropriate credential or license to interfere with or countermand the medical judgment of a licensed health care provider. Consequently, if the responsible health authority is not a physician, a responsible physician must be designated. If the mental health program is part of a different agency or program, a separate responsible health authority and responsible physician must be designated unless there is a clear agreement that the medical authority will accept and exercise overall comprehensive responsibility.

ACA's mandatory Expected Practice on Health Authority reads:

The facility has a designated health authority with responsibility for ongoing health care services pursuant to a written agreement, contract, or job description. Such responsibilities include: establish a mission statement that defines the scope of health care services; develop mechanisms, including written agreements, when necessary, to assure that the scope of services is provided and properly monitored; develop a facility's operational health policies and procedures, identify the type of health care staff needed to provide the determined scope of services; establish systems for the coordination of care among multidisciplinary health care providers; and develop a quality management program.

The health authority may be a physician, health services administrator, or health agency. When the health authority is other than a physician, final clinical judgments rest with a single, designated, responsible physician. The health authority is authorized and responsible for making decisions about the deployment of health resources and the day-to-day operations of the health services program.[7]

The essential NCCHC standard explicitly requires the responsible health authority to be on-site at least weekly. However, except for the smallest facilities, this would appear to be a minimalist solution. Although it may be difficult to set a universal threshold, consideration of the responsibilities of this individual suggests that a substantial presence is appropriate and necessary. In its commentary to this standard, the NCCHC defines a responsible physician as "a designated MD or DO who has the final authority at a given facility regarding clinical issues."[8]

Role of Responsible Health Authority

The health authority has *facility-specific* responsibility as previously indicated. Global responsibility for an entire correctional system does not suffice. The responsible health authority (and responsible physician) should be on-site regularly and frequently. In a very small facility, this may require only a few hours a week. A large correctional system may have a central statewide health authority who supervises and directs the health care staff at all of the facilities, but there is still a need for a local responsible health authority and responsible physician for each individual facility (or small cluster of facilities) who is on-site frequently and for long enough to be genuinely familiar with the details of its operation. This is the local person who interfaces directly with the facility administrator whenever the occasion requires; who knows the health care staff and their assignments, capabilities, limitations, and circumstances; who is familiar with the setting and circumstances of the inmates; who likely knows at least the patients who suffer from significant chronic illness; and who is prepared to intervene with timely guidance, direction, or mediation as needed.

The responsible health authority should have immediate access to any health record, log, report, or other relevant documentation. This is the person who directs all arrangements for care, interprets to the warden or jail administrator the concerns of health care staff, and relates the concerns of the warden to health care staff. This is also the person who ensures that medical equipment is working and is properly maintained; that supplies are ordered and delivered; that health care staff are hired, adequately trained, present, and ready for duty; and that doctors' orders are properly carried out.

It is important for the responsible health authority (and, indeed, all key health care staff) to become well acquainted with the layout of the facility, the characteristics of its inmates, and the circumstances or conditions in which they are confined. For this reason, regular visitation by the health authority and responsible physician to the various housing units; the recreation, work, program, and dining areas; and especially the segregation units is critically important. In large facilities, these tours may be conducted also by other physicians who rotate specific areas among themselves so that the visits are more frequent, but the responsible physician covers the entire facility on a regular basis. These tours can identify potential barriers to access, problems with environmental sanitation and safety, and other factors relevant to the inmates' health and well-being. They also afford opportunities for improving the efficiency and quality of health care service delivery.

Systems that fail to designate facility-specific responsible health authorities or responsible physicians place themselves in a precarious situation. The chief medical officer or statewide medical director then bears the de facto responsibility but lacks intimate knowledge of the day-to-day operational pattern and practice at each site. This creates an unacceptable situation for many of the problems that can arise.

What about clusters of facilities that are situated in close proximity? What about satellite facilities? What about correctional camps? Certainly a responsible health authority or responsible physician may cover more than a single facility such as adjacent or nearby institutions, camps, or satellite units. The guiding principle should be that the health authority or responsible physician routinely visits each unit at least weekly, actually reviews medical charts there, and periodically spends sufficient serious time with the health care staff and correctional authorities to have a current, firsthand impression of the status of the program. In other words, the responsible health authority and the responsible physician need to exercise genuine responsibility over the health services program at that specific location. The function of responsible health authority or responsible physician cannot be properly discharged by remote control or be delegated except for brief periods such as during vacations and leaves of absence.

Role of the Medical Director

Because many duties of the responsible health authority are administrative in nature, it is often desirable to elect the option of having a separate responsible physician. This arrangement allows assignment of most administrative functions to a person who has special training and qualifications in budgeting, supervising, and managing. In many systems, this person is also the director of nursing.

> The responsible physician must serve as advocate for the health and well-being of patients.

The responsible physician or facility medical director must be viewed as more than a doctor who writes prescriptions for medication. In their quest for cost savings, some systems have limited the role of physicians to seeing and prescribing care for patients who are referred by nurses. In much the same way, psychiatrists sometimes see only those patients whom psychologists, social workers, or nurses refer to be evaluated for treatment with psychotropic medication. Thereafter, they might see these patients briefly every 30 to 90 days solely for medication renewal. Denying correctional physicians a broader role and responsibility is a false economy.

Above all else, the responsible physician must serve as advocate for the health and well-being of patients. For example, the responsible physician should serve as the public health officer for the facility and exercise due concern for sanitation, safety, infection control, nutrition, environmental hazards, medication distribution, hazardous waste, and the sources of stress for those housed there. Physicians who do not feel qualified or current in some of these technical areas should devote the time to research and learn what is essential for carrying out these public health responsibilities. The responsible physician should meet regularly with the health care staff and with the institution head and also should be involved in quality-improvement and peer-review activities. By so doing, the medical director also promotes and ensures a safe work environment for correctional staff. Similarly, the psychiatrist must be involved in treatment planning decisions and have an active concern for the conditions of confinement of mentally ill patients rather than just be content to review and renew their medications.

ORGANIZATIONAL MODELS

Diverse organizational models exist in jails, prisons, and youth facilities across the nation. Whatever the historical, philosophical, or legal rationale for these arrangements, they may work well or they may work poorly. They may achieve some purposes and fail quite miserably by other standards. What is abundantly clear is that there is no single best or correct way to do things. Almost any arrangement could work satisfactorily given the right players, good leadership, and the will or incentive to succeed. However, experience shows that, all else being equal, some forms of organization tend to succeed better than others. Here we shall examine a few general types or models of organization and offer reflections on each.

Interdisciplinary coordination is also relevant to this discussion and is applicable to any organizational model that is adopted. Most correctional programs embrace both medical and dental services under the same health authority. A great many combine their medical, dental, and mental health programs under a single health authority. Not many, however, now incorporate their substance-abuse rehabilitation program into the health services division, even though there are persuasive reasons to consider this approach. All health disciplines share a great deal in common, and despite their specific differences they have much to be gained by sharing key resources and leadership, at least at the highest levels. This approach can also foster an interdisciplinary team approach that encourages and better enables clinicians to coordinate their treatment planning and delivery efforts efficiently for the greatest benefit of the patients.

No Central Health Authority

Although relatively rare today, before 1980 many state correctional systems had no central health authority at all. Typically, health professionals were hired by and responsible to the wardens of individual prisons. The health care service was viewed as just one more program offered by a prison like education, religious services, a barber shop, the commissary, the law library, recreation, hobby craft, and work assignments.

In a study undertaken by the National Commission on Correctional Health Care in 1989, B. Jaye Anno found that, of 35 states responding, only 10 were still operating without a central health authority.[9] In a follow-up study in 1999 with 28 states responding, Anno found that six states reported that the head of correctional health services was a correctional administrator. However, six other states that had reported no central director of health care in 1989 were not among the responders in 1999.[10]

It was under this type of system that some of the most serious deficiencies in correctional medical and mental health services were allowed to develop. See Chapter 1, "Ethics in the Context of Correctional Health," under "A Brief Historical Perspective" for further details. They involved widespread use of inmates in the delivery of health services, employment of impaired or unlicensed physicians, seriously inadequate equipment and supplies for diagnosis and treatment, and blatant denial of access to care for serious medical needs. When these appalling conditions finally reached the attention of the courts and the public, the revolution in correctional health care practices of the 1970s and 1980s began to take place. See Chapter 4, "Legal Issues in Correctional Health Care," under "A Break in the Hands-off Era," for further documentation of these developments.

Unless the medical services program in a large prison system has a strong central health authority, it generally lacks the stature and leverage required to insist on conditions essential to good medical practice. There will be little consistency across institutions if each facility is essentially autonomous. Interpersonal relationships will tend to have greater influence over outcomes than will policy. Efficient management practices and cost-effective bulk-purchasing strategies are difficult to implement without a centralized structure. Faced with other pressing monetary needs, health care issues may not rate highly among the warden's priorities.

Edward Brecher and Richard Della Penna, physicians who were charged by the Law Enforcement Assistance Administration of the U.S. Department of Justice to look at the New York prison system and other correctional systems around the country, described the problem in 1975 as one in which health care personnel, on the one hand, have no involvement in planning or budgeting and have no real authority to implement improvements; on the other hand, they are simultaneously "free to let things slide with little or no fear of supervisory intervention" from the warden or any other source. They described how the monies appropriated for health care services, where not independently identified, were "buried without trace in the overall budget requests of each correctional institution," making it impossible for legislatures to intervene in favor of better health care even when they wished to do so. "Health care personnel in such an organizational structure are at the same time impotent to foster improvement and free to tolerate deterioration. This is a recipe for chaos. A change in this organizational structure is the most important initial step which any state can take toward improving correctional health care— more important even than increasing appropriations."[11] They then recommended a structure in which there is a statewide health care administrator who is is responsible directly to the commissioner of corrections and has direct administrative authority to give orders and demand compliance and in which the budget and funding for health services is identified and fully visible. Moreover, "[e]ach correctional institution should similarly have an administrator responsible for health care activities in that institution. He should have direct access to the warden or director. In all professional matters, however, he should report directly to the statewide health care administrator."

In documenting the extensive systemwide deficiencies and substandard conditions in medical and health service delivery that prevailed in the Michigan Department of Corrections in 1974, Faiver concluded: "It is quite apparent in the wide ranging view and insight we have been afforded that the lack of such overall program direction and coordination is largely responsible for the significant variations found in facilities, levels and quality of services provided."[12] In fact, a key recommendation from this Michigan study was the establishment of a central health care office to direct and administer the statewide correctional health care program:

It is recommended that a special office be established with responsibility for administration of state correctional health services. Care should be taken to assure that the office will be independent from routine departmental operations and will have full authority to implement the new health care system.

A central authority shall be designated as responsible for developing and maintaining a comprehensive and effective health care system for persons served by the Michigan Department of Corrections. . . . Health care in the correctional system must be adequately financed with a clearly identifiable budget. . . . [T]here is great need for a Director of the overall health care needs of the Department. His responsibility would be to direct, supervise and coordinate the entire state-wide program of correctional health care. He would plan and carry out needed improvements in budget planning, operation, methodology, new equipment and services, repair and maintenance procedures, etc., to achieve and maintain an acceptable level of quality. . . . There is needed preferably an experienced medical (physician) health care administrator to direct the program. If a qualified and experienced physician cannot be found, then a qualified and experienced hospital and/or public health administrator should be provided.

With the whole-hearted support of Governor William Milliken, implementation of this recommendation was accomplished by Director Perry M. Johnson, who later served as president of the American Correctional Association. Simultaneously, a substantial appropriation of new line-item funding for prison health services, facility by facility, was enacted.

The recommendation made by the Medical Advisory Committee on State Prisons in Massachusetts in 1971 had a similar purpose: "The establishment of an agency separate from the Department of Corrections to be responsible for the administration and delivery of health services to state correctional institutions."[13]

Similarly, the recommendation made by the Kentucky Public Health Association in 1974 stated:

The health care and environmental aspects of all penal institutions should be coordinated through a central office at the state level, an Office for Forensic Health (OFH) within the Department for Human Resources. The OFH should be provided with sufficient staff, have authority to set standards and to inspect the penal institutions and to initiate corrective action when individuals responsible for operating the institutions fail to do so in an approved manner.[14]

Based on her research and national survey of the organizational structure in state prisons, Anno commented on the traditional model (with no central health authority) as follows:

The traditional organizational model of correctional health services does not serve anyone well—not the correctional administrator who wants to provide good health care, not the health professional who wants to serve patients' needs, not the director of the DOC who wants to avoid lawsuits, not the taxpayer who wants the most efficient utilization of public funds, and not the inmate who is less likely to have his or her health needs adequately served under this model.[15]

As indicated, few if any state correctional systems lack a central health authority today. However, in view of more recent trends, another note of caution must be sounded. In their haste to shed the burdens of managing a health care system through privatization, some states have imprudently delegated all responsibility to contractual health services providers. A state should never to relinquish its role as overseer and monitor—tasks that require diligent and ongoing watching and planning and considerable technical expertise. Left to themselves, private health care corporations may tend to diminish services or forgo quality to increase profits.

Outside Public Health Authority

In some county and local jails and juvenile facilities, responsibility for medical services has been given to the county health department and responsibility for mental health services has been assigned to the community mental health services agency. An example of this is the New York City system of jails, for whose inmates the New York City Department of Health and Mental Hygiene has been responsible for medical, mental health, substance, dental, discharge planning, and transitional health care services. According to Anita Cardwell and Maeghan Gilmore of the National Association of Counties, "This helps facilitate a comprehensive public health approach to health services for the incarcerated population."[16]

A variant of this is an arrangement with a university medical school to manage a state correctional health care program. Notable examples are the states of Georgia and Texas. Similarly, some state prison systems have arranged for their state mental health departments to provide some or all of the mental health services. The rationale offered for these approaches is that the selected health agency has specific expertise as well as a public responsibility, may be able to achieve certain efficiencies, and may have a recruiting advantage. A close working relationship with correctional authorities is required. Usually, the county commission or state legislature appropriates funding separately to each agency. Less often, the correctional agency has the money in its budget and purchases the services from the health agency.

Success of this arrangement requires genuine commitment by the involved health agency so that the correctional activities are not viewed as lowest among its priorities and also to ensure that the correctional program is not looked on as a source of revenue to subsidize other agency functions. The locus of responsibility within the agency needs to be clearly defined so that it does not become a vague and amorphous arrangement but resides in a competent and designated person who remains engaged in the process, is aware of all salient issues, and actively exercises a leadership and advocacy role.

Need for Patient Advocacy

The issue of patient advocacy is a concern that must be addressed forthrightly at the outset when an arrangement with another agency is being considered. The outside agency (public health department, mental health department, university medical school) can easily find itself "trapped" if its staff are required to work under professionally unacceptable or ethically compromising conditions, such as with inadequate or substandard equipment and materials, without due access to their patients, or with unreasonable restrictions placed on their exercise of clinical judgment. Health providers must be assured that they will be permitted and even encouraged to serve in a patient advocacy role, fully knowing that this could extend to raising concerns about impediments to the practice of good health care or about excessively harsh conditions of restraint and confinement of patients, especially the mentally ill. If the outside health agency goes along with and tacitly condones what it finds to be unacceptable without making a continued and sincere effort to improve the conditions and the quality of the health program, then it is failing to fulfill its own mission and principles.

One possible solution is to appoint at the outset a high-level executive from the correctional department and from the outside health agency with the understanding that they will meet regularly and have free access to each other at any time to raise and mediate issues encountered by their respective staffs. It should be mutually acknowledged that this advocacy role is of paramount importance and will be in the best interests of the correctional agency if it is carried out well. In addition, the topics of patient advocacy and conditions of confinement affecting health of inmates should be routinely and explicitly addressed in quality-improvement efforts conducted by the outside health agency. This approach will avoid sources of friction and impediments to efficient provision of services in the workplace and provide a constructive and workable mechanism for advocacy.

If the outside health agency goes along with and tacitly condones what it finds to be unacceptable without making a continued and sincere effort to improve the conditions and the quality of the health program, then it is failing to fulfill its own mission and principles.

Risk of Excessive Fragmentation

Correctional health services programs are often divided into distinct and virtually autonomous organizational units such as medical, mental health, and dental services. Despite a superficial attractiveness of this arrangement, such fragmentation does not promote a holistic approach because no single provider is looking at the entire individual from the perspective of health. Communication is rendered more difficult because each program typically wants to maintain its own separate medical record for the patient. It is also less efficient because bulk purchasing and coordination of similar functions such as data and record keeping, purchasing, supervision, and budgeting are less readily accomplished.

Although these practice disciplines are typically separate in the free world, the critical difference is that free citizens choose their own doctors, dentists, psychologists, and hospitals. If they do not like them, they are free to choose someone else. Coordination thus becomes the patient's own primary responsibility. In the correctional setting, the patient does not have these choices. If the physician prescribes a medication that conflicts with medication ordered by the dentist or psychiatrist, then a court may determine that the correctional system selected these providers and therefore ought to have known that this particular combination of medications was contraindicated. Unless providers are sharing a single medical chart, this can be difficult to accomplish.

To minimize these deficiencies, we concur with Anno's recommendation that a single responsible health authority for the department of corrections should be responsible for coordinating mental health, dental, and medical services and also work closely with representatives of any outside agency to ensure that services are not duplicated and that pertinent information regarding patients is properly shared. Similarly, where one or more services are contracted out to vendors while the department of corrections operates the remaining services, a health services director needs to be designated to oversee the contract services as well as supervise services provided by the department of corrections.[17]

One state with a large correctional population encountered serious problems largely because of excessive fragmentation. The correctional department provided the medical and dental services, except that the physicians and midlevel practitioners were all hired and supervised by a for-profit managed care company that also handled all off-site and specialty care services and the statewide pharmacy program. The state mental health department provided mental health services. This fragmentation was further compounded by the decision to regionalize the correctional health program geographically into quasi-autonomous segments. The central medical leadership in the department of corrections was not strong enough to hold this large and complex system together. The staff complement of the central office of health care had been drastically reduced from previous levels in view of the regionalization and outsourcing. Little effective monitoring of the private contractor's performance took place. Moreover, the mental health department did not bring a frequent central office presence to the institutions and did not exercise a strong patient advocacy role regarding the conditions of confinement of mentally ill patients. The quite predictable problematic results led to highly publicized instances of poor patient care, some tragic deaths, protracted federal court involvement, and excessive costs.

Coordination by a Central Health Care Authority

Perhaps the most common arrangement today for large correctional systems is the appointment of a central coordinating health authority (a position filled by a health care professional who reports to the director or deputy director of the department of corrections). This person exercises oversight, planning, and monitoring of health care operations at the institutions. In this model, health care personnel may be hired by and under the supervision of the warden of each institution, although the central health authority usually plays a significant role in recruiting and selecting staff, determining and negotiating the budget, defining specific job descriptions, and ordering supplies.

Although this approach can and sometimes does work well, success is variable from institution to institution and from system to system and depends in large part on the chemistry and style of the individual institution head and the medical staff at each location. Sometimes, an outwardly "compatible" match may be less than satisfactory, as with an overly authoritarian warden and an overly compliant health services administrator. Similarly, a mediocre physician and a mediocre warden may get along quite well socially but provide inadequate services. When an important unresolved issue exists, the warden and the central health coordinator may need to bring their dispute to the agency director for resolution.

LINE AUTHORITY FROM A CENTRAL OFFICE OF HEALTH CARE

In some state systems, the central health authority's role is stronger and includes line authority to hire, fire, supervise, and direct the institutional health care staff. These systems tend to achieve more uniformity across institutions and greater consistency in the criteria for treatment or for the medical transfer of inmates. They can also more readily take advantage of efficiencies in bulk purchasing, contracting for services, and regionalization of costly services. In a county jail, the sheriff or jail administrator employs a medical director or health administrator to hire and supervise the health care staff. In prison systems, it is ideal for this central health authority to be a deputy director or a bureau chief who reports directly to the head of the department of corrections.

This view is also supported by Anno: "The importance of health services in the DOC's total mission—as well as the technical expertise required to make appropriate administrative decisions regarding personnel, service levels, equipment, and supplies—argues for a separate division with direct access to the head of the DOC."[18]

Except for its financing arrangements, many of the administrative aspects of a large correctional health care program more closely resemble a hospital operation than a prison or jail system. This is true of the types of personnel employed, methods of recruitment, credential verification, types and sources of supplies and equipment (and their maintenance requirements), and formats employed for utilization data, expenditure reporting, and quality improvement. Consequently, it is possible to achieve even greater efficiencies when the central health authority is given a dedicated personnel officer and business officer to ensure that transactions such as recruiting, hiring, purchasing, and cost reporting are performed appropriately for the highly specialized requirements of a health care system. Given their other priorities, it can be very difficult for the personnel office or business office of individual institutions to meet the legitimate specialized needs of a large health program in a consistent and timely manner.

With a strong central health authority, continuing efforts must be made to include the institutional wardens as important players who have a significant investment in the successful outcome of the program. After all, the warden is the institution's chief executive officer and his or her cooperation is essential to the successful implementation of health services. Conversely, the way in which health services are managed can affect the institution's operation and the efficient accomplishment of its mission. It would be overly simplistic to conclude that the only way to enlist the warden's commitment and cooperation and ensure that the health care program will fit smoothly into the institutional operation is to give the warden ownership—in other words, direct supervision and control over the health care program—perhaps even over the health care budget. It is equally counterproductive to ignore or bypass the warden and attempt to control a program of the magnitude and significance of health care within each facility from a central office. At worst, this can invite active noncooperation. At best, it fails to enlist an important ally and partner. Either way, the efforts will be more costly and less effective. Partnership and teamwork, based on mutual respect and a common mission, are crucially important.

In practice, the institution head should ratify and cosign every health care policy and procedure that involves or affects administrative, security, or safety issues in any way. This ensures consistency and avoids any plausible claim by a correctional employee that the policy was not binding. It is not necessary that the warden cosign strictly clinical policies and procedures such as nursing protocols, practice guidelines, chronic disease treatment protocols, and pharmacy formularies.

Similarly, the responsible health authority should cosign institutional policies and procedures that are directly related to or affect health care, including the health care aspects of the disaster plan, the training curriculum, the food service, and the environmental safety and sanitation policies. This approach ensures that both points of view have been considered and encourages a high quality and efficiently managed correctional health care system.

One organizational model that can work well begins with an overall central health services administrator with line authority over all health care staff in the system. Alongside this person and perhaps administratively accountable to the health services administrator would be the system's medical director or chief medical officer. Reporting to the medical director are the chief mental health authority, the chief dentist, and possibly the chief of substance-abuse rehabilitation—all at the central office level. The health unit administrator at each institution reports to the central health services administrator.

It is good to keep a line of clinical responsibility through physician, dentist, and mental health staff within their respective disciplines up to the central office position. Thus, clinical direction, setting of clinical guidelines, and final selection of professional staff for mental health services would ultimately rise to the level of the central chief psychiatrist. The overall system medical director would rarely if ever countermand the clinical directives of this person but would play a major role in selection of the chief of mental health services or the chief of dental services and would have authority with respect to coordinating decisions that affect multiple disciplines.

CONCLUSION

Like the warden who sets the overall tone for the operation of any correctional facility, it is the responsible health authority and responsible physician who, more than anyone else, are called to inspire and cultivate through word and example a strong ethical orientation among the other health care professionals working in the facility. Clinical staff should have a clear understanding that their highest duty is to the health and well-being of their patients, with all that this implies. In addition, due care and diligence must be taken to ensure that, in hiring health care professionals, only those are selected who, in addition to being competent and well skilled in their profession, espouse and exhibit strong ethical principles and values consistent with the healing disciplines, in particular, patient advocacy, caring, dedication, and respect for the dignity and worth of their patients.

This book began with an emphasis on the commonality of mission shared by corrections and health care, despite their significant and recognized differences. As was pointed out in Chapter 2, "Areas of Significant Ethical Role Conflict," under "A Note of Caution," unresolved tension between the methods and culture of correctional and clinical staff can promote a gradual erosion of the clinicians' ethical principles, but this can also result from a phenomenon some have described as correctional fatigue, akin to what is more widely known as employee burnout. In

Chapter 9, where the similarities and differences between corrections and health care will be more fully explored, a detailed set of strategies for cooperation will be presented. This chapter subscribes to the view that clear role definition and careful delineation of lines of responsibility can go far toward easing tensions and enabling achievement of the proper mission of both sets of actors in this complex arrangement on whose success so many lives literally depend. It can also enhance employee morale and job satisfaction, thereby reducing the tendency to burnout. The author sees proper organizational alignment as key to enabling and enhancing the achievement of an ambience in the correctional workplace where the practice of ethical principles is more consistently and effectively encouraged and facilitated.

Besides the ethical perspective, there is also a public health role that medical staff must exercise in bringing its expertise and perspective to issues of safety, hygiene, sanitation, prevention of contagious disease, and reduction of stress and tension, as these may affect inmates, staff, visitors, or the public. For this public health role to be carried out effectively, it is important to assign a primary locus of responsibility—and that is seen to be the responsible physician.

Chapter 9

Corrections and Health Care Working Together

CORRECTIONS AND HEALTH CARE

How do we facilitate and inform an ongoing dialogue and communication between health care professionals and correctional authorities about health-related ethical principles and their practical application in the work setting? This is the central focus of the final chapter.

The priorities of wardens and correctional officers have much in common with those of doctors and nurses. The list below shows twelve concerns that should rank very high among the priorities of every well-managed correctional system as well as of every properly managed health care system.

Shared Priorities of Well-Managed Correctional and Health Care Systems

- Safe and secure environment
- Well-being of prisoner population
- Good hygiene and sanitation
- Respect for human dignity and worth
- Quality improvement
- Cost effectiveness
- Public safety
- Good order
- Emergency preparedness
- Due confidentiality
- Prevention of harm
- Adherence to ethical standards

The respective parties should have little disagreement about any of the items listed here and this fact establishes solid common ground on which to frame the discussion. The mission of corrections is the *care and safe custody* of incarcerated persons. The mission of the correctional health care team, in common with corrections, is the *safe delivery of care* to incarcerated persons.

RECOGNIZING DIFFERENCES

Having established that corrections and health care share a common mission, it follows that they need to work together. There are, however, significant and abiding differences. To be able to collaborate effectively, we should first identify and understand these differences. Various elements are listed, and the two systems are compared in Table 9.1. Both differences and similarities are displayed.

Purpose

In addition to *societal protection* and the *care and custody of inmates*, the correctional agency is also expected to carry out society's desire for *punishment of wrongdoers*. Other than monetary fines, the principal form of punishment ordered by courts in the United States is deprivation of personal liberty through incarceration under correctional authority. Some less restrictive punitive modalities such as probation, parole, electronic tether, and community service are also commonly placed under correctional supervision. In slightly more than half of all states, the death penalty can be imposed, and its implementation is carried out under correctional supervision.

> The clear and avowed primary purpose of the health care profession is to promote the health and well-being of the incarcerated population, never to inflict harm or punishment.

It is no surprise, then, that discipline of correctional inmates is generally enforced through the threat and use of punitive sanctions. When a rule is broken, a ticket or citation is issued. Due process is followed. A sentence is given and carried out—typically a restriction of privileges or confinement in segregation. In some instances, the period of incarceration can be extended by forfeiture of good time. Additional duties or physical exercises are sometimes assigned as punishment, especially in boot camps.

The health care profession, on the other hand, is a healing profession. Its clear and avowed primary purpose is to promote the health and well-being of the incarcerated population, never to inflict harm or punishment. This fact alone constitutes a

Table 9.1
Selected Comparisons between Cultures of Corrections and Health Care

	Corrections (Custody)	Correctional Health Care
Public Mission	Protection of society by the confinement of lawbreakers	Protection of public health by control of infection and harmful behavior
Individual Mission	Care and custody of inmates	Care and well-being of individual patients
Principal Purpose	Confinement (punishment) Public safety Rehabilitation from crime	Healing and health maintenance Rehabilitation of health and function
Principal Means	Restrictive measures Regimentation Rehabilitative programs Counseling and education	Diagnosis and treatment Therapeutic milieu Rehabilitative programs Counseling and education
Coercive Measures	Coercion, regimentation Limited choice, restraint Direct orders	Informed consent Least restrictive environment Persuasion and encouragement
Punitive Sanctions	Loss of privileges Segregation or lockdown Security level increase Extra duty or exercise Forfeiture of good time	None. Instead, the following are used: Counseling and education Time-out Focused therapeutic activities Medical restraint or seclusion
Primary Client	Society	Individual patient
Principal Style of Training	Paramilitary Follow orders Policies and procedures	Scientific and clinical basis Professional judgment Practice guidelines and protocols
System of Beliefs	Inmates are untrustworthy Security always comes first Direct orders must be obeyed	Doctors must listen to their patients Patient–provider trust is paramount Patient well-being comes first Practice health care in safe setting Best to elicit voluntary compliance

profound and fundamental difference between the two systems. In terms of rehabilitation, the focus includes physical health and well-being, adoption of a healthy life style, mental hygiene, behavioral health and healthy patterns of thinking, and substance-abuse rehabilitation. Often, remedial health and life-style education is imperative because so many inmates arrive with significant deficiencies in hygiene, sanitation, nutrition, infection, and high-risk behaviors. Improving sense of self-worth is also an essential component.

In addition, correctional agencies are usually recognized as having the important responsibility of rehabilitating those in their custody, helping them to lay aside a life of criminal behavior and become productive and contributing members of society. In many cases, this involves providing or supplementing the fundamental tools they will need. Basic and advanced academic education or vocational skill education is frequently needed. Other tools include social skill development, language skills (including literacy), workplace behavior and attitudes, principles of fairness and respect for others, family skills, appreciation of one's own dignity and self-worth, and rehabilitation for substance dependence.

Means Employed

To fulfill their mission, correctional agencies essentially use three strategies: restriction, regimentation, and rehabilitation. First, *restrictive measures* include practices such as confinement, restraint, and deprivation of privileges. Although the prison itself constitutes confinement, even more severe forms occur in segregation, lockdown, and isolation, which are frequently employed as punitive sanctions. Second, *regimentation* is commonly employed through the firm and consistent imposition of rules and established routines. Correctional managers may view "individualization" as an invitation to disorder and therefore instinctively resist variances and exceptions. Third, many correctional systems wisely devote resources to a *rehabilitation* component, which may include programs related to substance abuse, academic or vocational education, life-skills training, social and family skills, guidance counseling, and reentry preparation, although resources dedicated to these services are often limited. Unfortunately, rehabilitation programs tend to be trimmed back or abandoned whenever funding is scarce or when political dialogue and debate turn more punitive, as in "My opponent obviously doesn't stand for 'law and order' and for 'getting tough on criminals,' but I do. So, vote for me!"

Health care, in contrast, uses *preventive* and *therapeutic* measures to attain its objectives: medication, surgical intervention, therapeutic milieu, counseling, education, persuasion, prostheses, rehabilitation, immunization, therapy, and other forms of individual and group treatment. It never punishes or condones the use of punishment to achieve its purpose. Even when therapeutic seclusion or restraint is ordered by medical or psychiatric staff, as may be the case for a severely agitated psychotic patient, it is because this has been explicitly determined to be the least-restrictive means available to prevent serious harm to self or others, and it may be employed only for as long as needed to accomplish its purpose. It is never to be employed punitively.

Outside of the classification and disciplinary processes, health care staff in many jails and prisons constitute the primary source of approval for individual accommodations (special diet, lower bunk, prosthetic and orthotic devices, lay-in, and work restrictions). Often these accommodations are central to the provision of necessary health care. But the act of recommending individual accommodations at times unfairly places health care staff in conflict with the culture and expectations of the correctional system, especially when some perceive it as "coddling" or catering to the prisoners. For instance, prisoners ought to be issued properly fitted shoes by institutional staff whenever needed and only receive a prescription for an orthopedic shoe when a physical abnormality requires this accommodation. The mattresses and bed springs of prisoners should not cause back problems; if they do, repair or replacement is in order, and the doctor should not be called on to prescribe a bed board. Similarly, prescribing blankets for warmth should rarely be a medical concern unless prison issue is deficient.

Coercive Measures

Many correctional practices intentionally or unintentionally tend to negate or diminish individual responsibility. The lives, activities, and behavior of inmates are closely regimented. Prisoners are generally afforded few opportunities to exercise free choice and then only within tight limits. Rules are promulgated and enforced to promote conformity and consistency, ostensibly for reasons of efficiency and good order, but also perhaps, at least implicitly, as punishment. Officers are taught to enforce rules equally to all inmates and not to accord "special treatment" to any individuals.

The concept of *least-restrictive environment* or *least-restrictive* measures must always guide health professionals' treatment decisions.

In contrast, good health care practice must respect and encourage the free and informed choice of each patient with regard to the treatment given. Only in the most exceptional circumstances—as when a patient is not mentally competent—can treatment be administered without voluntary consent. The patient is or should be actively involved in making the treatment decisions reflected in his or her care plan. And the patient, even though a prisoner, retains the right to accept or refuse the prescribed treatment. Health care professionals are taught to develop and use an individualized treatment plan[1] for each patient rather than try to accommodate all within the same general treatment method.

The concept of *least-restrictive environment* or *least-restrictive measures* must always guide health professionals' treatment decisions. Restraint and involuntary treatment are allowed only when this is determined necessary, as for a mentally ill patient who is imminently dangerous to self or others, and less restrictive measures are known to be ineffective. This contrasts with the correctional environment, which itself is constraining. Even so, the "least restrictive" rule applies also in corrections. It is a cardinal rule that use of excessive force is always wrong. Moreover, there is a guiding principle, expressed in the public correctional policy of the American Correctional Association (ACA): "the sanctions and controls imposed by courts and administered by corrections should be the least restrictive, consistent with public and individual safety and the maintenance of social order."[2]

Punitive Sanctions

In corrections, rule violations may be punished by loss of privileges (such as commissary, television, recreation, or visitation), confinement in segregation, lockdown in one's own cell, forfeiture of good time, or assignment of extra duty or physical exercises. Due process is required, and policies outline the applicable disciplinary hearing and redress procedure.

Punitive sanctions, on the other hand, are not employed by health care staff. In a health care unit such as an infirmary, mental health ward, or intermediate mental health unit, a therapeutic response should be employed to manage inappropriate behavior. This may consist of counseling by treatment staff, instruction in proper behavior, teaching techniques for controlling behavior (as in anger-management training), involvement in structured and supervised therapeutic activities, time-out, or even medical seclusion or medical restraint when deemed necessary for brief periods to prevent injury to self or others. These measures are never punitive. A medical seclusion or restraint, for example, may be employed only when it is determined to be the least-restrictive effective alternative, and it is never imposed for a predetermined period of time, as might be the case with time assigned to segregation, but is ended as soon as the patient no longer constitutes a threat.

Primary Client Served

The principal client of corrections is *society itself*, which it serves by humanely and securely confining accused and convicted wrongdoers away from the community and, to the extent possible, by facilitating and promoting their rehabilitation before the term of incarceration is completed and they are released back to the community. At the extreme, this duty to its primary client may even be construed to justify the use of lethal force by correctional officers when deemed necessary to prevent the escape of a dangerous criminal.

The primary client of a health care service, in contrast, is the *individual patient*, whose health and well-being always hold a preeminent place for the care provider. As a consequence, medications may not be used to control the dangerous behavior of a healthy inmate. Nor may health care staff reveal confidential information or cooperate in procedures that could bring harm or punishment to the patient, except in extraordinary circumstances. An example of such a circumstance would be the duty of a psychologist to reveal information received in confidence from a client if the client has disclosed a credible threat to the life of another party. Health care providers also have a duty to protect the public health, and sometimes this requires a balancing of individual and public goods.

Style of Staff Training

Paramilitary style training is commonly used for correctional employees. They are drilled and taught and expected to obey all orders without hesitation and to adhere strictly to laws and agency policies. Quick, dependable, and uniform response by officers is necessary for their own safety, the safety of coworkers, and the safety of the public at large. The agency bears liability for the consequences of employees' actions when they are on duty. Ongoing training is mostly carried out in brief segments of a few hours at a time. It closely adheres to a prepared lesson plan and may be presented in a classroom setting, by video, or in a computerized interactive module. Sometimes initial or recurring training for officers is conducted at a correctional training academy in courses lasting five days or even longer. The training is narrowly focused for specific learning objectives and the mastery of established practices. Correctional policies, procedures, and post orders are minutely detailed and leave little room for judgment and discretion. Correctional systems tend to follow a command-control approach, where those in charge know best. They operate in a world that leans toward certainty, so any deviation from the routines presented in policy and training is frowned on because it can lead to breaches in security or loss of control.

Not only correctional officers but also doctors and other health care professionals must follow laws and rules. Both groups must exercise good judgment at all times, but there is a significant difference of emphasis. Most training for health care professionals is both academically and clinically based. Independent study, guided self-study, direct observation, hands-on clinical experience, and research-oriented approaches are common. Doctors are expected to use their knowledge and skills to diagnose and treat a patient's condition based on their best scientific understanding and professional judgment. They may exercise clinical judgment within a broad range of discretion. Nurses, psychologists, pharmacists, and other health professionals, in varying degrees, also exercise professional judgment predicated on proper application of the general principles and scientific knowledge base of their profession or discipline to an individual patient's needs and condition, within the scope of practice permitted by law and regulation in that state. Rather than command control, health care professionals are taught and expected to exercise judgment within a set of practice guidelines. They are trained to be comfortable with uncertainty and must remain able to make real-time course corrections and adjust their diagnostic impression and treatment protocol whenever indicated by a change in the patient's clinical condition. They instruct and persuade rather than command their patients.

This does not imply that correctional officers are not allowed to exercise discretion. To the contrary, there are numerous situations in which they are expected to use good judgment. One example is illustrated by the ACA's public correctional policy on use of force, which encourages policies and procedures that "provide ongoing specialized staff training designed to teach staff to anticipate, stabilize and diffuse situations that might give rise to conflict, confrontation and violence and that ensures staff's competency in the use of all methods and equipment in the use of force."[3] It is when this advice is not followed that tense situations can all too quickly escalate into open conflict and violent outbursts that result in injury. Correctional institutions should avail themselves of a valuable internal resource in the person of their own skilled mental health professionals, who often can provide beneficial assistance both in staff training and in offering real-time collaboration in actual conflict-resolution situations without resorting to use of force or risking the escalation of aggression and violence.

System of Beliefs

Certain "beliefs" pervade every discipline. For example, some security training classes have taught that staff should never believe anything an inmate says. Some have insisted that an officer must never back down once a direct order is given to an inmate.

Health care professionals, in contrast, are trained to listen attentively to each of their patients, both to elicit clues about the nature and origin of the illness and to discover the effect of prior remedies. Physicians, dentists, nurses, and mental health workers would not be able to treat their patients effectively if they accepted the premise that the symptoms and history described by their patients are routinely untrue or untrustworthy. Particularly in mental health settings, treatment staff prefer to offer encouragement and direction and then wait for the patient to comply rather than attempt to achieve compliance by force. The health practitioner seeks to give the patient an opportunity to make an informed choice rather than issue a direct order. Overly simplistic application of the aphorism "Security always comes first" can result in unintended and unfortunate outcomes if the legitimate requirements of the medical and mental health disciplines are ignored, are not respected, or are inappropriately overridden.

> Particularly in mental health settings, treatment staff prefer to offer encouragement and direction and then wait for the patient to comply rather than attempt to achieve compliance by force.

Warden Art F. Beeler and Gary N. Junker described this phenomenon as a "Clash of Cultures."

The "Clash of cultures" arises because of divergent beliefs and experiences, especially between correctional and medical staff. . . . The culture of the correctional staff is rules-oriented and paramilitary. The staff learn through experiences on the job and are taught through tradition. . . . On the other hand, medical staff are academic in nature and often have specializations in certain areas. They are used to peer support and feedback as well as autonomy from management. The cultures create barriers and points of divergence between the staffs, which differ in dress, years of schooling, language and vocabulary, and salary.[4]

Psychologist Erik Schlosser sums up the differences between correctional staff and mental health care staff especially well and offers the following insights:

Correctional staff see their mission as maintaining order through the use of reward and punishment. Inmates are viewed as people not to be trusted, who have done wrong and are likely to repeat past behaviors. Correctional staff are exposed routinely to the dirtier parts of correctional work, such as violence and abuse and the games inmates engage in, which can jaundice their view of inmates.

Mental health staff see inmates as potential clients. Clients receive mental health services to become more stable and change problematic behaviors. While mental health staff are aware of the games and behaviors of inmates, the focus is on their potential for change."[5]

Overly simplistic application of the aphorism "Security always comes first" can result in unintended and unfortunate outcomes if the legitimate requirements of the medical and mental health disciplines are ignored, are not respected, or are inappropriately overridden.

According to Schlosser, "custody issues that mental health staff can address include whether an inmate is a risk to self or others, will be a management problem, and whether this is the best place for this inmate given the resources of this particular unit." Addressing these questions enables mental health staff to assist correctional staff in their mission and helps correctional staff see mental health staff as partners. Schlosser further states:

[C]orrectional staff see inmates more than mental health staff do. Correctional staff are in a unique position to observe inmate behaviors in various settings, while mental health staff tend to be limited to observations in clinic settings. Information on an inmate's sleep pattern, appetite, energy level, social interaction and significant changes in behavior can help mental health staff to assess an inmate more accurately. Tell correctional staff that they are your eyes and ears out there; this can help them to view their work in a new light.[6]

INTERDEPENDENCE

What follows is only a partial listing of the many ways in which custody and health care are mutually interdependent. It serves to illustrate the vital importance of cooperation and joint problem resolution. Each is obvious and requires little or no comment here, and some readers may be able to suggest other dependencies that they have encountered.

To summarize, it should come as no surprise that the disparity in background, training, orientation, beliefs, and methodology can frequently cause a degree of mutual stress and discomfort. Nevertheless, as each side observes the generally successful activities of the other within their own primary sphere of activity, the unease and discomfort level should decrease. Officers working on a mental health unit can observe how talk therapy and patience can successfully resolve a tense and potentially dangerous situation with a patient who is acting out, even though the officer in other circumstances might have traditionally handled the matter far differently. Health care staff can learn to appreciate the minute attention to security details by correctional staff, an area in which they might have been too casual on their own. Both parties can learn from each other but also need to respect the valid differences in style, approach, and expertise.

How Health Care Depends on Custody and Institutional Services

- To ensure a safe work and living environment
- To locate, summon, and allow (or escort) prisoners to go to health clinic
- To provide transportation for patients to off-site care appointments
- To remain at the bedside of patients who are hospitalized
- To serve nutritious meals
- To prepare and properly serve special medical diets
- To organize and conduct point-of-arrival health screening
- To transmit promptly all sick-call requests and urgent complaints
- To detect and report promptly any signs and symptoms of suicidal ideation
- To conduct suicide risk surveillance
- To monitor intoxicated prisoners
- To monitor mentally ill patients
- To monitor and protect other vulnerable inmates
- To report signs and symptoms of physical and mental distress
- To avoid discouraging patients from seeking care
- To act as competent first responders, as in first aid, CPR, and suicide precautions
- To provide key control
- To provide a clean and sanitary living and working environment
- To maximize fire safety

- To provide, in the typical nonprivatized operation, business office services (financial accounting, budget, invoice payment, contract management)
- To provide, in the typical nonprivatized operation, personnel office services (human resource functions of recruitment, preemployment testing, payroll, benefits, training, grievances)
- To provide security screening of prospective health care staff
- To respond to any emergency or crisis situation
- To maintain a reliable communications infrastructure—telephone, radio, fax, Internet, intranet
- To provide a structure for orientation and training of employees

How Custody Depends on Health Care

- To keep the inmate population healthy
- To advise on health and hygiene and nutrition issues
- To intervene and advise in a medical crisis
- To advocate on behalf of patients' health needs
- To provide emergency medical treatment to an injured or sick officer, visitor, or inmate
- To establish a reliable program for management of chronic illness
- To conduct receiving health screening and intake health appraisals so as to discover and document the health status of each new arriving inmate
- To advise on infection control and containment of outbreaks of contagious disease
- To monitor and treat mentally ill patients
- To monitor health status of segregated inmates
- To monitor health status of restrained inmates
- To manage reasonably the costs of health care services
- To advise on conditions that may be hazardous to health
- To establish and maintain linkage with off-site providers of care and off-site sources of medical equipment and supplies
- To maintain a dependable medical on-call system for off-hours response
- To determine the nature of special diets and who requires them
- To determine who requires suicide watch, the precautions to be observed, and when the patient can be taken off the watch

Dr. Kenneth P. Moritsugu, former medical director of the Federal Bureau of Prisons, eloquently summarized the theme of this chapter:

It has always been my belief that there is no health care decision that doesn't have some type of impact on custody. There are very few custody decisions that don't have an impact on health care, or access to health care. For us to pretend that we are in two Balkanized areas, and that we can make our decisions on health care independent of what goes on in corrections or that corrections can go on and make independent decisions in terms of custody that do not have an impact on health care and health care provision is a big fallacy.[7]

WORKING TOGETHER

With basic differences such as those described previously, one well might ask if it is even possible for these two systems to work together. Some fundamental differences in purpose, methods, training, approach, policy, and procedure will necessarily exist even in well-run systems. Under less than ideal circumstances, these differences can proliferate and engender resentment, resulting in half-hearted cooperation or passive aggressive behaviors on the part of staff of both disciplines. The following strategies have proved effective in promoting a sound and productive working relationship between security staff and health care staff.

An attempt should be made to bridge the gap between the professional "cultures" of health care staff and of correctional staff. The combination of differences in mission, purpose, primary client, measures employed, style of training, and belief systems can be lumped together and cumulatively termed the *cultures* of the two disciplines. They are, indeed, distinct as has been pointed out. A fundamental premise of this book is that, properly understood, there is no intrinsic or essential contradiction between the principles and requirements of corrections and of health care and that neither discipline should find it necessary to violate its professional ethics.

This premise finds support in the ACA public policy, which wisely encourages including "correctional officers who work in health care units as active participants in the multidisciplinary treatment team."[8]

Strategies

First, both parties need to recognize and appreciate the important *similarities* in their mission and purpose. Both disciplines are responsible for the care and safety of inmates, and both professions emphasize personal dignity, humane treatment, and safety. Each also has a concern for the well-being of society. This common ground provides both a basis and an incentive for reaching decisions together.

Second, both corrections and health care should appreciate their extensive network of interdependence.

Third, it is equally important to recognize and respect the real *differences*. Parties that begin with fundamental differences in philosophy, purpose, and policy are not always going to agree.

Fourth, total and lockstep agreement is neither necessary nor even desirable. Not all differences are negative. Each system has its skills and strengths. These should be recognized as well, because they are mutually complementary.

Fifth, all staff should respect and acknowledge the *professionalism* and good intentions of those with different points of view. This should be the first presumption. Only in a context of mutual respect does an effective working relationship become possible. The American Correctional Association's *Standards Manual* recognizes the important principle of medical autonomy for clinical decisions, saying "Clinical decisions are the sole province of the responsible health care practitioner and are not countermanded by nonclinicians."[9] The commentary to the standard quite appropriately also states:

> The provision of health care is a joint effort of administrators and health care providers and can be achieved only through mutual trust and cooperation. The health authority arranges for the availability of health care services; the responsible clinician determines what services are needed; the official responsible for the facility provides the administrative support for making the services accessible to offenders.

The National Commission on Correctional Health Care (NCCHC) uses nearly the same words: "Clinical decisions and actions regarding health care provided to inmates to meet their serious medical needs are solely the responsibility of qualified health care professionals."[10]

Sixth, so that the parties can work harmoniously and effectively together, it is neither required nor helpful that one group *dominate* or subordinate the other. To dominate—in other words, to impose one's point of view on another—is to act according to the belief that "might makes right." When a domineering structure acts to crush the weaker party, even when the stronger party is right, inevitably everyone loses. Each issue has at least two sides. Rarely is there a simplistic black–white dichotomy. An appreciation of the various perspectives and nuances of a difficult and complex situation enables the best solutions to be identified and implemented.

It is a fundamental premise of this book is that, properly understood, there is no intrinsic or essential contradiction between the principles and requirements of corrections and of health care.

There is, of course, real danger that, in practice, the perspective of corrections will tend to dominate because (1) it regards and describes itself as the "landlord" (to the "tenant" health care program), (2) it typically controls 85 percent or more of the resources and staff of the agency, and (3) it is a paramilitary style organization. It is, however, worth noting that correctional institutions were not built or established for the purpose of affording medical treatment. Nor were the army and navy created to provide health care to military personnel; they were established to fight wars, just as jails and prisons are built to confine offenders. Yet each of these institutions must also make suitable accommodations for the correct and proper delivery of health care services if they are to survive and function effectively.

Both disciplines bring to the table their own expertise, professional ethics, and goals. These approaches, on a practical level, are neither irreconcilable nor incompatible. When reasonable persons come together in shared and mutual respect, it is possible to reach decisions that meet the highest and best purposes of each and simultaneously satisfy the fundamental requirements of each. Neither side uniquely possesses the complete truth. A deliberated solution, cooperatively reached, is nearly always better than any choice that either side alone could have made and imposed. This belief is an undergirding principle of all that is said here. Were it not so, this book would have little purpose other than to advise on how one or another side should strive to dominate.

Dialogue and Respectful Deliberation

As indicated, some of the best solutions arise from dialogue. In Michigan in the early 1980s, a topic of concern was the excessive time spent by physicians in prescribing bed boards. Even the carpentry shop complained. Officers argued that they did not know who had legitimate back complaints and insisted that physicians make that determination. Finally, Perry M. Johnson, then director of corrections, having listened to the heated debate among wardens and representatives of health care, calmly said: "It sounds like the real reason the doctors are having to prescribe bed boards is because the bed spring supports are defective. So, let's fix or replace the defective beds." This project kept the maintenance staff occupied for a few months, but bed boards were no longer required, and complaints of back pain greatly decreased.

Reasoned and respectful deliberations lead to the wisest and best solutions. Each party should view itself as providing a service to the other (who can be regarded as a client or customer whose needs they attempt to satisfy). How can services such as health care, transportation, escort, security and safety, classification, training, infection control, environmental health, sick call, maintenance, food service, personnel, or accounting performed by one party best meet the needs of the other? This is a central and explicit approach of total quality management (TQM) or continuous quality improvement (CQI) programs. It is also an essential strategy for working together as a team.

Examples abound. When health care staff are not consulted in the planning and design of the clinic for a new or remodeled facility, the space is usually found to be inadequate or ill-proportioned with resulting inefficiencies for staff for many years ahead. When a new computerized management information system or scheduling program is being designed for the facility, health care staff should be involved early in the planning process so that the product will be suited also to the needs of health care without costly retrofitting. A change in the schedule of health care events such as sick call, medication pass, and segregation rounding can have unsatisfactory or disruptive consequences if appropriate dialogue with custody has not taken place beforehand. Disaster-planning efforts and drills cannot meet their full objectives unless the health care system has been actively involved at all levels in the planning, implementation, and evaluation of the exercise.

Each party needs to be considerate and attentive to reducing the burden of the other party, especially since neither side starts with an excess of resources. It would alleviate the burden on officers if clinicians could see patients at the correctional facility instead of at an off-site location whenever this is feasible. Downtime for the dentist is reduced if two or three patients can arrive at the clinic waiting room prior to count time and remain secured in the clinic until count has been cleared. The optometrist or orthopedic surgeon should be scheduled to hold on-site clinics at a time of day that does not conflict with the regular count or an institution-wide mobilization drill. All appropriate diagnostic and treatment procedures should be performed on-site before referring a patient to an off-site specialist, outside of an emergency.

When a correctional facility practices an emergency scenario or mobilization, health care activities come to a standstill—perhaps for several hours. It does not need to be this way. A reasoned discussion among the proper parties might recognize that the mobilization itself could be practiced under even more realistic conditions if certain essential health care functions were allowed to proceed—as they undoubtedly would during a prolonged lockdown situation. Thus, medication pass and selected call-out functions might take place, possibly at a slower pace or at a different location and with additional officer escort beyond that ordinarily required. Patients could be seen by the physician or dentist for routine care or follow-up of chronic conditions, even during the mobilization drill. This approach affords an excellent opportunity for all staff to cooperate in evaluating and refining the procedures so that essential medical care will be provided safely and efficiently in the event of a real emergency.

These and other solutions have proved satisfactory in some settings and are likely to prove so again. Whether they are equally appropriate for a particular location or circumstance is best determined through study and discussion by an interdisciplinary team of persons from that facility who have responsibility for these areas. Although the principles and reasoning presented in this reference manual should apply to most situations, collaborative discussion of specific needs and applications will usually suggest the most appropriate variations and creative solutions.

Medical staff occasionally prescribe treatments or interventions for patients that some security staff may find objectionable. Staff must then bring their conflicting interests and concerns to the attention of their supervisors. When necessary, legitimate medical requirements will need to be accommodated by extraordinary or enhanced security measures. At other times, acceptable alternative treatment interventions are available that do not place an extra burden on security. These occasions provide opportunities for cooperative attainment of mutual goals and should not be allowed to become interdisciplinary power struggles in which one party wins and the other loses.

> If good and principled professionals quit their jobs and abandon a program because of discomfort with its shortcomings, they are likely to be replaced by staff who do not have the same high professional and ethical principles. Then things will only get worse. Sometimes it requires a critical mass of good people to effect needed improvements.

To summarize, in an atmosphere of mutual trust and respect, a correctional system and its health care program can readily work in cooperation, despite their basic differences. Both parties will need to plan and reason together collaboratively to work out ways to meet the highest purposes and the mission of both agencies.

This being said, no health care professional should ever continue to work in a system in which she or he is forced to compromise the principles of professional and medical ethics. However, a careful distinction should be made. This is different from a situation in which one is unable to do all that a health care professional feels should be done for the patients but is still able to accomplish some good. The reality is that, if good and principled professionals quit their jobs and abandon a program because of discomfort with its shortcomings, they are likely to be replaced by staff who do not have the same high professional and ethical principles. Then things will only get worse. Sometimes it requires a critical mass of good people to effect needed improvements. The insightful comments of correctional psychologist Joel Dvoskin[11] on this important subject are discussed in Chapter 2, "Areas of Significant Ethical Role Conflict," under "Should I Quit My Job?"

COOPERATING IN TRAINING

This chapter does not address security training requirements for correctional officers nor does it address clinical training requirements for the various health professions. It comments only on the crossover areas: *health-related training for correctional officers* and *security-related training for health care staff*. The policy manual used by each correctional system or facility specifies the minimum required training for initial orientation, specific job assignments, and annual in-service training of all staff.

Health Aspects of Officer Training

In addition to their required initial and annual training requirements relating to security, all officers, deputies, youth counselors, and caseworkers are ordinarily trained in inmate management, report writing, supervision, and communication. They should also be trained in specific health-related topics. Some of this training is best provided by qualified health care staff because of their expertise and familiarity with the circumstances of the facility. All of the training materials for officers related to these topics should be periodically reviewed and approved for adequacy, completeness, clarity, accuracy, and currency by the responsible health authority and not merely by the warden or other correctional authority.

The ACA explicitly requires all new correctional officers to receive 120 hours of training during their first year of employment on several specific topics that include *suicide intervention and prevention*. The ACA standard also requires that before commencing employment, all new full-time employees complete 40 hours of training that includes the following health-related topics: *universal precautions, occupational exposure, personal protective equipment,* and *biohazardous waste disposal.*[12] In addition, the ACA requires "designated correctional staff" to be trained to respond to health-related situations within four minutes and to receive training each year on:

recognition of signs and symptoms, and knowledge of action required in potential emergency situations; administration of basic first aid, certification in cardiopulmonary resuscitation (CPR) in accordance with the recommendations of the certifying health organization; methods of obtaining assistance; signs and symptoms of mental illness, violent behavior, and acute chemical intoxication and withdrawal; procedures for patient transfers to appropriate medical facilities or health care providers; [and] suicide intervention.[13]

The NCCHC requires that "a training program, established or approved by the responsible health authority in cooperation with the facility administrator, guides the health-related training of all correctional officers who work with inmates," and explicitly includes the following mandatory topics for training:

a.) Administration of first aid; b.) Recognizing the need for emergency care and intervention in life-threatening situations (e.g., heart attack); c.) Recognizing acute manifestations of certain chronic illnesses (e.g., asthma, seizures), intoxication and withdrawal, and adverse reactions to medications; d.) Recognizing signs and symptoms of mental illness; e.) Procedures for suicide prevention; f.) Procedures for appropriate referral of inmates with health complaints to health staff; g.) Precautions and procedures with respect to infectious and communicable diseases; h.) Cardiopulmonary resuscitation.[14]

Another NCCHC standard further specifies that officers who will be administering or delivering prescription medication must be trained in *matters of security, accountability, common side effects,* and *documentation of administration of medicines.* This training must be approved by the responsible physician and the facility administrator or designee.[15]

The training of security staff should include at least the following health-related topics. Although the list is lengthy, it is hardly an exhaustive list of relevant topics, but it is considerably more comprehensive and detailed than what the published national standards explicitly require. However, few recognized experts in the field of correctional health would challenge the importance or relevance of the topics presented here:

- Knowing appropriate precautions for blood-borne pathogens and airborne diseases.
- Preventing transmission of infectious diseases.
- Maintaining good hand hygiene for themselves and promoting good hand hygiene among the inmate population.
- Recognizing signs and symptoms of mental illness and developmental disability.
- Recognizing signs and symptoms of suicidal ideation and knowing the appropriate intervention strategies.
- Recognizing signs and symptoms of acute and chronic physical illness.
- Recognizing obvious symptoms of active tuberculosis.
- Knowing and practicing nonviolent and nonconfrontational approaches to management of the mentally ill or intellectually disabled.
- Using the automated external defibrillator (AED).
- Administering CPR as a first responder.
- Being prepared for disaster.
- Recognizing the need for emergency care in life-threatening situations.
- Knowing the proper first-aid treatment for persons who have been exposed to chemical agents or electrical stun disablers.
- Recognizing signs and symptoms of alcohol or barbiturate withdrawal, particularly in jails and receiving facilities.
- Recognizing risky behavior related to physical exercise.
- Knowing how to manage mentally ill patients properly.
- Being familiar with and sensitive to the special issues faced by persons who have been victims of physical or sexual violence in the past.
- Understanding ectoparasite control.
- Understanding relevant health care policies.
- Knowing and understanding procedures for urgent and routine access to health care.
- Knowing the appropriate medical call out and escort procedures.
- Knowing that officers are obliged to maintain in confidence all patient medical information that they may learn or discover in the course of their duties.
- Knowing the limits of medical confidentiality.
- Knowing how to behave in the medical area (for example, having due respect for patient privacy and confidentiality and being careful not to distract the nurses from performing their duties).
- Using strategies for conflict avoidance and conflict resolution vis-à-vis health care staff.

The amount of time required for this component of the training will vary, but generally 24 to 48 hours (in addition to the hours spent in obtaining or updating CPR certification) will be appropriate for the initial training and 16 to 24 hours can satisfy an annual or biennial update.

Additional hours of training specific to the officers' area of assignment may also be required. These should be mandated, not only for officers regularly assigned to these special units but also for any officer who is likely to be called on as a replacement on one of these units. When applicable, these additional types of training may include the following:

- Knowing how to perform medical arrival or point-of-entry screening, including procedures for appropriate disposition and referral.
- Knowing how to distribute medications.
- Knowing how to transport patients with physical or mental health problems.
- Being familiar with and sensitive to the special gender-related issues of incarcerated women.
- Being familiar with and sensitive to the special emotional and developmental issues of incarcerated juveniles and adolescents of either gender.
- Being familiar and sensitive to the special physical and psychological problems of elderly persons.
- Being familiar with and sensitive to the special physical and emotional needs of the disabled or infirm. This should include training by competent personnel in the proper and safe way to assist persons suffering impairment affecting ambulation and transfer and with activities of daily living. (Competence to provide this training will require some specialized expertise in the fundamental principles of body mechanics and kinetics so as to minimize risk of injury to themselves and to the patients.)
- For those assigned to work in prison hospice units, being familiar and sensitive to the needs of the terminally ill and the bereaved.
- Knowing basic principles of working on a mental health unit.
- Using principles of safe exercise and proper use of exercise equipment.
- For those officers who will be supervising prison industry areas and potentially hazardous work details, using machinery and hazardous equipment safely.
- Understanding basic principles of a substance-abuse rehabilitation program, particularly for those officers who will work in residential substance-abuse treatment programs.
- Observing basic operational principles of cleanliness, hygiene, and sanitation for those assigned to inspect food service, housing, bathrooms, and water and air handling systems.

The officer-training program should explicitly incorporate efforts to encourage officers to be respectful and supportive of the medical and mental health programs and the substance-abuse rehabilitation programs in their facility.

Security and Institutional Aspects of Health Care Staff Training

Health care staff, including part-time and contractual employees, require adequate training in institutional policies and in security-related matters. Some of this training is more authoritatively, more credibly, more accurately, and more efficiently provided by experts in security than it can be by health care staff.

Appropriate topics include the following:

- Being familiar with the institution; knowing how to get from place to place safely.
- Understanding relevant institutional and departmental policies.
- Knowing the do's and don'ts of safe and proper behavior in dealing with inmates.
- Understanding games inmates play.
- Understanding what contraband is and how to properly search for it.
- Knowing rules of behavior for inmates.
- Knowing rules for misconduct reporting. (Although it is not advisable for health care professionals to be routinely involved in writing tickets or reporting disciplinary infractions, this practice may occasionally become necessary when a health care staff member is the only person to observe a breach of security or a behavior that exposes others to danger.)[16]
- Understanding the importance of and observing key control practices.
- How to store and handle toxic, caustic, and inflammable supplies and how to document their use (inventory control).
- Knowing how to deflect, disengage from, or deescalate rather than aggravate or escalate potentially tense situations.
- Using nonviolent and nonconfrontational intervention techniques.
- Recognizing and responding to signs and symptoms of suicidal tendencies.
- Responding to disaster situations and to institutional emergencies and mobilizations.
- Understanding specific job duties.
- Knowing how to respond to kites and grievances if applicable.
- Recognizing and reporting abusive staff behavior.
- Practicing strategies for avoiding and resolving conflict with correctional officials.
- Specific training relevant to interacting with and meeting the needs of special populations housed at the facility such as juveniles, women, elderly, disabled, or mentally ill.

Cross training on some of these topics can contribute to a better understanding of each other's areas and responsibilities and also improve cooperation and communication. It even may be feasible to offer some sessions to a blend of participants representing both health care staff and security staff.

It is not recommended that health care staff be trained to perform shakedowns of persons or housing units. This is clearly not an appropriate function for medical and mental health staff and can involve a conflict of interest and a confusion of roles. Nor is it the highest and best use of their time and skills. This is discussed in greater detail in Chapter 2, "Areas of Significant Ethical Role Conflict," under "Shakedowns Performed by Health Professional Staff." For similar reasons, health care staff should not participate in weapons training afforded to correctional officers.

As previously mentioned, there are notable differences in the typical methodology of training used for correctional officers and health care professionals. Few correctional systems have taken this into account and instead subject their health care professionals to the same classroom didactic methods that are used for officers. Worse still, some of those directing the training programs seem not to have made use of the vast body of knowledge currently available in the field of adult education. Many techniques traditionally employed with schoolchildren are not especially useful or effective with adult learners.

At best, this is inefficient. Instead of requiring health care professionals to attend a one- to two-week (or longer) new employee orientation, alternative approaches such as a few days of classroom exposure, plus guided self-instruction with selected readings, followed by a written or oral test may be more effective. Given the salary paid to physicians and dentists while attending these courses, there can be potential monetary savings.

Not only the training curriculum and materials used by correctional trainers of health care personnel but also the actual teaching presentation should be periodically reviewed and approved by the responsible health authority. Some trainers are fond of using "scare tactics" and consider it their mission to "put the fear of the Lord" into these new noncustody employees. They have been known to overstate things in extreme terms for the shock value. They may say things such as "You need to stop being 'do-gooders.' That 'caregiver' approach just doesn't work in a prison." It is awkward when health care supervisors need to tone down some of this rhetoric later with the new staff because they risk giving the impression that what the trainers said is to be taken with a grain of salt. Medical authorities should sit in occasionally for portions of the lectures and videos to know exactly what is being taught, especially when they discover evidence of these practices while debriefing new staff after their orientation.

SOME TOUGH QUESTIONS

We provide here some additional suggestions for successful collaboration between corrections and health care.

Sample Questions Wardens Might Ask of Their Health Care Staff

- Is all of this off-site transportation really necessary?
- I want good health care, but how can we make it easier for my officers?
- How private do health care encounters need to be?
- Do we really need to send so many persons to the hospital? How can we cut this number down?
- Why does your nursing staff take so long to pass medications?
- What are your recommendations on how we can better prevent suicide?
- How can we improve our infection-control program and reduce risks for correctional staff?

Sample Questions Medical Directors Might Ask of the Warden

- Is all of this isolation or restraint really necessary? Are we not further exacerbating their rage and hostility by excessive confinement, isolation, or restraint?
- Are we punishing illness? Should we try instead to give therapeutic approaches a chance, especially with the mentally ill, and not hobble them with the additional stress of an overly restrictive environment?
- How can we improve cell-side health encounters in the high security units?
- Do health care staff really need to call them *inmates*? We prefer the word *patients*.
- How can we work together to improve living conditions for our large number of elderly prisoners?

TWO EXAMPLES OF PRODUCTIVE COOPERATION

The following true stories clearly illustrate how a spirit of trust and cooperation contributes to good outcomes, especially when something out of the ordinary occurs.

Rhabdomyolysis

Rhabdomyolysis[18] is defined as the rapid breakdown (-*lysis*) of skeletal muscle tissue (*rhabdomyo-*) because of injury to muscle tissue. The injury may have any of several precipitating causes, including a crushing injury, electrical shock (as with a stun gun or taser), or severe burns. (Other factors include a genetic predisposition, some psychotropic medications, snake bites, infections, drug overdose, and prolonged seizures.) It can also be caused by excessive repetitive exercise such as when untrained people undertake vigorous or competitive exercise in hot, humid weather.

Damaged muscle fiber releases breakdown products of muscle cells into the bloodstream. Some of these, especially myoglobin, are toxic to the kidneys and can lead to acute kidney failure. Treatment is with intravenous fluids and dialysis. If untreated, it can be fatal.

Anyone, regardless of age, gender, race, or ethnicity, can develop rhabdomyolysis—even otherwise healthy persons who are in excellent physical condition. However, persons with the sickle-cell trait or disease are at greater risk than others for experiencing rhabdomyolysis. This fact is relevant because a large proportion of inmates are black, and it is this ethnic group that accounts for the majority of persons in the United States who have the sickle-cell trait.[19] About one in 12 African Americans carries the sickle-cell trait.[20]

Sickle cell disorder is a condition that causes the production of crescent-shaped blood cells. Largely as a result of their shape, the blood cells cannot flow as easily through veins and arteries and are unable to carry as much oxygen and nutrients to muscles as do normal blood cells. Therefore, when the muscles are demanding more oxygen and nutrients than the blood can supply during heavy or extreme exercise, the muscle tissue begins to break down, leading to rhabdomyolysis.

Picture a group of prisoners in the day room or exercise area. It is a hot day. One prisoner dares another to match his performance at push-ups, chin-ups, squats, or laps around the gym. The competition is fierce, and the cheers and jeers of enthusiastic onlookers urge the participants to continue well beyond the normal number of exercise repetitions—perhaps 300 or 400 times. This form of extreme exercise can bring on rhabdomyolysis, especially if the participants are ill-conditioned and not trained in exercise techniques, if temperature and humidity are high, and if the participants are poorly hydrated, The risk is many times greater for a person who has the sickle-cell blood disorder.

The symptoms of rhabdomyolysis include dark brown, tea-colored urine, muscle soreness, tense and swollen muscles, pain with movement, confusion, difficulty walking, decreased urinary output, and arrhythmia. It is a medical emergency, and the patient must go to the hospital for immediate intervention.

This is an area in which the alertness and cooperation of correctional officers is critically important. In one Florida jail, an observant officer alerted a nurse to unusual complaints of an inmate following his involvement in an excessive exercise competition involving hundreds of push-ups. The nurse evaluated the patient, was concerned, and contacted the physician who ordered immediate hospitalization. Because of the quick actions and the mutual trust of the officer and nurse, the patient survived. A postincident critique took place, and medical staff assisted the jail administrator in modifying the facility policy and training modules so that officers (1) would appropriately discourage excessively strenuous or prolonged exercise activity and (2) would not dismiss signs of postexercise exhaustion too quickly. One way to help promote these cooperative relationships is for medical staff to educate officers and recreation supervisors to recognize the risk factors and early signs and symptoms of rhabdomyolysis and to discourage and prevent this type of exercise competition because it can too quickly turn fatal. It may take as long as 12 to 24 hours for a person to develop symptoms, so officers should report any such incidents or suspicious symptoms to medical staff immediately for follow-up.

Correctional staff should also be aware that an electrical shock, such as that imparted by a taser, has been known to bring on rhabdomyolysis.[21]

Emergency Vodka

The author well recalls an instance that eloquently illustrates how the mutual respect and wholehearted cooperation between the medical director and the warden contributed to the successful management of a highly unusual crisis and minimized the damage. Briefly, some of the inmates obtained access to a bottle of the fluid used in those days to operate a spirit duplicator or ditto machine. It was largely methanol (wood alcohol), a form of alcohol that is highly toxic if taken internally.

One Sunday morning, an unusually large number of inmates began to show severe symptoms, and the nurses became alarmed. They phoned the medical director, who arrived at the facility a short time later. He quickly determined that the problem was methanol toxicity, and he knew that the treatment of choice was inges-tion of quantities of ethanol (drinking alcohol). Ethanol is an effective antidote to methanol, and it essentially delays the process of methanol metabolizing into form-aldehyde and formic acid, both toxic substances that can quickly cause coma, blindness, and death.

Because alcoholic beverages were not stocked in the prison pharmacy or in the commissary, the physician phoned the warden, explained the situation, and imme-diately obtained permission to have drinking alcohol brought into the prison. Then he called his wife and asked her to bring whatever liquor they had at home. She brought two or three bottles of vodka. This was not enough, but Michigan had a law prohibiting the sale of alcohol on Sunday. So he then phoned the author, who contacted an acquaintance who served on the Michigan Liquor Control Com-mission, secured permission for a liquor store to supply whatever quantity was needed, and jumped in the car to drive the 40 miles to Jackson and deliver a case of vodka to the prison.

Ultimately, 13 prisoners were sent to various hospitals and placed on dialysis. Two eventually became blind, but there were no fatalities. Scores of prisoners lined up to drink the vodka that was being offered in the infirmary. The mutual trust of the warden and physician and their willingness to move without hesitation or unnecessary delay into uncharted territory in managing this crisis undoubtedly saved many lives and avoided an even greater tragedy.[22]

SELECTED PROBLEMS FOR COOPERATIVE RESOLUTION

Integrated strategic planning is essential to good health care service delivery and management. Examples of areas that overlap the responsibilities of both cor-rections and health care include sanitation, food and diet, safety, reduction of injury and illness risk, access to care, efficient use of time, housing and care of mental health patients, receiving screening, infection control, and minimization of need for using segregation and restraint. Neither sector can achieve satisfactory results alone in any of these areas.

Ensuring Safety and Security within Clinic Areas

No nurse or other health professional wants to feel unsafe or uneasy on the job. Neither do they want officers shadowing their every move and intruding themselves unnecessarily into the midst of patient encounters. There needs to be a proper bal-ance. The nurses are busy and should not be unnecessarily distracted from their duties. By the same token, nurses must remain sufficiently attentive and not hesi-tate to request officer presence should any concern arise. Patients should not be wandering through or aimlessly lingering in the clinic area once their clinical encounter has been completed. Officers need to be concerned with the details of prisoner movement to and from the clinic. Successful achievement of a safe and secure clinic environment requires a constant and mutual cooperation.

What Should We Call "Them"?

A few wardens still insist that even nurses and doctors refer to their patients as "prisoners," "inmates," or "offenders," and some may even require staff to address inmates in this fashion. To these wardens, I would respectfully invite a reading of Chapter 7 of this book ("A Patient or a Prisoner?") followed by a face-to-face meeting with their medical director and health administrator. Those who still remain determined to insist on the "prisoner" nomenclature perhaps have good reasons and should not be judged as doing anything wrong. The health professionals will then need to employ other ways to remind each other of their primary function as caring, healing professionals who, above all, advocate for their patients' best interests and well-being.

The flip side may also be relevant: what should they call "us"? Probably "Ms. Jones," "Mr. Smith," "Doctor," "Nurse," "Sir," or "Ma'am" are best. Calling health professionals by their first name or nicknames suggests overfamiliarity and disrespect. Some staff prefer not to carry their surnames on name tags to preserve anonymity, but this is precisely why it may be a good idea. How can the patient identify the provider to others? As "the redhead nurse" or "the bald man" or "the tall lady"? A person is entitled to know who is treating him or her, and anonymity breeds distrust. Therefore, use of last names on ID tags is suggested, perhaps also with the first initial and the professional designation (MD, DO, RN, MSW, and so forth) or the title (physician, nurse, nurse practitioner, social worker, psychologist). Posted professional licenses ought to have the licensee's home address blacked out, and staff should be counseled against sharing their telephone numbers or e-mail addresses with inmates. Proper boundaries must be respected, and it is usually better if all staff adopt the same protocol. Hence, there is need for interdisciplinary discussion and reflection to determine the most prudent course.

Security Housing Units and Other Forms of Severe Isolation

Security housing units (SHUs) and supermax programs may be necessary, although not everyone agrees. The resolution of this question is beyond the scope of this book. But could some changes be considered, for example, to the typical restrictions on exercise and social interaction? Could there be two periods of 45 minutes to one hour out of cell daily, seven days a week? Could some social interaction, albeit restricted and monitored in some cases, be arranged for even the most securely housed? Could the mentally ill be removed from these isolation units and be placed in a secure therapeutic environment, at least on a trial basis?

If mentally ill patients are being housed for long periods in these types of units, perhaps we are punishing them for their illness—a rather discomforting conclusion but one that may be true. Is there not a better way? This topic is discussed in some detail in Chapter 3, "Other Challenging Topics in Ethics," under "Housing the Mentally Ill in Isolation or Supermax Settings." This is a major concern, and the issues are involved and complex. Outside consultation and technical assistance are available if needed.

What about the problem encountered so often in these types of units in which a nurse or psychologist must crouch down by the food slot to pass medications or converse with the patient? Again, there has to be a better way. If the best minds in corrections and health care at a facility get together and reason about it creatively, they will certainly find a solution—possibly one that is unique to their setting—that will simultaneously satisfy the concerns for safety and good order while meeting the essential requirements for patient health and well-being. They might even be more successful if they were to include a member of the engineering or building maintenance staff or perhaps even a professional architect in one of their meetings to discuss this topic. Requiring a nurse and patient to yell at each other through the food slot or the crack by the hinged end of the door, or to wave frantically through the window of the cell door, is an unreasonable solution, results in inadequate health care, and is inexcusably disrespectful to health care staff and patients alike. Policy changes and procedural solutions may be enough, but often an engineering solution will, in the long run, prove to be not only more effective in resolving the problem but also more efficient in use of day-to-day staff time.

Physician On-Call Arrangement

Why are there so many trips to the emergency room? Perhaps not at all of them are necessary. Do they tend to occur principally on weekends and evenings when no health professional staff are on duty? Would it be cost-effective to pay a doctor or a physician assistant to come in when called on weekends or at night to evaluate whether a patient can be treated there or really needs to go off-site? Or would it be helpful to add another shift of on-site nurse coverage?

On-Site Specialty Care

Are there frequently used specialty services that could be provided on-site so as to reduce the need to transport patients to off-site locations? Depending on the needs of the facility population, optometry, orthopedics, physical therapy, psychiatry, infectious disease, podiatry, or OB-GYN specialty consultations may be efficient solutions and might be scheduled weekly, monthly, or at other intervals, depending on expected needs.

Privacy of Clinic Encounters

Ordinarily, it is not necessary for an officer to be in the same room during a health care encounter. On rare occasions this may be necessary. Then the officer becomes bound by the identical rules of confidentiality that bind health care staff in the event private patient information is unavoidably overheard or observed. This admonition should be taken seriously, explicitly stated in correctional policy, and included in officer training.

It is perfectly reasonable for a particular inmate on a given day to be designated as requiring an officer (or two) in close proximity during a clinical encounter, as long as this decision is based on a justifiable expectation of dangerous or assaultive behavior. Less acceptable (harder to defend) is a policy requiring all prisoners belonging to a particular class to have this precaution—for example, all maximum security prisoners or all segregation prisoners. This is a matter of judgment for the security experts, but the patients' privacy should be respected insofar as is reasonably possible and consistent with safety concerns.

Sometimes only visual privacy or auditory privacy is required. Sometimes both should be provided. That depends on the type of procedure and the perceived dangerousness of the patient. Privacy can be of sight, sound, or both.

Officers in the booking area or receiving health screening area or in the clinic should routinely remain a respectful distance away so that the patient may feel free to talk with the health care provider and answer the screening questions without the officer being close enough to hear. Often it is reasonable for the officer to stand at least 10 to 12 feet away or just outside the partly open door and where a loud voice would immediately be heard but normal conversation does not carry.

Health Classification

Many systems and institutions find it useful to classify inmates according to health status or need. In its simplest form, a health classification indicates whether an inmate is suited (1) for any housing or job, (2) for some housing and jobs according to specified limitations, or (3) not suited for any job or only suited for special housing.

The above nomenclature is nonrevealing yet highly useful. It is not necessary to state the precise nature or diagnosis of the injury or illness of an inmate when specifying that she or he should not be given an assignment that requires lifting more than 10 pounds or climbing more than five stairs or that requires something other than a lower bunk. If the classification is "No restrictions on job or housing assignment," no further inquiry is needed before making an assignment to kitchen duty or to the upper bunk.

Of course, use of a classification system such as this places a burden on health care staff to keep the designated status of each inmate up-to-date. One way of doing this would require the physician, midlevel practitioner, or nurse at each clinic encounter to note whether any new finding or treatment requires a revision of the current classification. Although this may seem to be an onerous task, in reality it is probably less of a burden than would be the case if every change of housing assignment or job required review by health care staff to ascertain that this individual has no particular problem. Once a status is determined, it is likely to remain stable for long periods.

If desired, this classification method can be much more sophisticated. It should be tailored to the specific situation and intended use of the facility (or of the larger correctional system), keeping in mind that a good system should (1) help ensure that persons with special health needs will be accorded proper accommodations, (2) protect the confidentiality of health-related information, and (3) reduce, if possible, the amount of time and paperwork that would otherwise be required to ensure appropriate assignments. When the classification code is entered as a variable on the computerized inmate-tracking system, it can help avoid wrong placements and assignments.

Transporting Prisoners

Handcuffs, especially when applied for extended periods such as during transport from one facility to another, can become extremely uncomfortable. Their usage should be reviewed with medical staff. Given certain health conditions, their use may be ill advised, and some suitable compromise may need to be reached through dialogue between security and medical personnel.

On longer trips, some patients may require access to their medications *en route*. Nurses should provide detailed instructions for the transport officer in these cases. Similarly, patients who are diabetic or hypoglycemic may require an appropriate snack or meal at certain times that would not ordinarily be the meal time for the other passengers.

Pregnant women should not be unnecessarily or tightly shackled during transport and not at all during labor. Both ACA and NCCHC standards address this important consideration. The ACA prohibits

the use of restraints on female offenders during active labor and the delivery of a child. Any deviation from the prohibition requires approval by and guidance on methodology from the medical authority and is based on documented serious security risks. The medical authority provides guidance on the use of restraints on pregnant offenders prior to active labor and delivery.[23]

In addition, the ACA's public policy states, "Waist restraints should not be used during pregnancy at any time. Leg restraints should be used only in extreme circumstances during transport and never during labor and delivery. Electronic restraint devices should not be used during pregnancy, labor and delivery."[24]

NCCHC states:

The use of restraints is potentially harmful to the expectant mother and fetus, especially in the third trimester and during labor and delivery. Restraint during transport to the hospital or during labor and delivery should not be used except when necessary due to serious threat of harm to the patient, staff, or others. The diagnosis of active labor can be difficult to make, and should be made by a qualified health professional. If restraints are deemed necessary, abdominal restraints, leg and ankle restraints, and wrist restraints behind the back should not be used.[25]

Especially when transporting mentally ill or special needs inmates, both security staff and health care staff should ensure that these patients are appropriately prepared for the move, and they should cooperatively endeavor to prevent such transfers from arriving at the destination facility in the evening or on weekends or holidays when professional mental health staff may not be available to assess their condition promptly on arrival.

The best resolution in each of these instances is one that gives due attention to all relevant factors and the concerns of both custody and health care.

Security Constraints That Impair Cost-Effective Health Care

Maximum security facilities often place a limit of one, two, or three inmates who can be in the health care area at a time, or they may require two escort officers and belly chains to move an inmate across the yard to the clinic. These requirements can work havoc on an appointment schedule, increasing provider downtime and reducing the number of patients a provider can see in a day.

What can be done? Sometimes nothing. If this is the reality, it must be accepted. But health care staff need to find ways to remain productive during these "wait" periods instead of simply accepting it as unavoidable lost time. For example, a dentist might work on prosthetic cases, do paperwork, or reorder supplies while waiting for the next patient. A nurse or dental aide could autoclave instruments, prepare medications, clean equipment, reorder supplies, review kites or grievances, set up patient schedules, check inventory, or do a tool control inventory of sharps and instruments. The medical director could do chart reviews. But this type of task rearrangement and efficiency planning can go only so far. At some point it is certainly legitimate for health care providers to ask security staff to reconsider some of the barriers. A "critical path analysis" in TQM mode may identify bottlenecks that were not previously recognized as such by the staff who are directly involved but that are remediable.

Another example: keep-on-person (KOP) medications can reduce staff time for medication distribution but at some added risk (or concern) for security staff regarding presence of contraband. Some institutions have created "pill boards" that display each type of pill, tablet, and capsule identified in the formulary and commonly used as KOP medications. This facilitates officer recognition of a legitimate medication should a question arise. The use of blister packs is another possible solution.

In some housing units, patients can line up to get their medications when the nurse arrives. In segregation units, a small window in the door at face height that can be opened from the corridor might greatly expedite face-to-face contact and medication pass.

Requiring a corrections officer to escort mentally ill inmates from a mental health unit to the medical clinic, visiting area, barber shop, or other destination sometimes also causes delays that could be avoided if a mental health worker could be authorized and properly trained to perform this function. The mental health workers are better acquainted with their patients and may be more trusted by them. They have had extensive training and experience on how to handle mentally ill persons.

Would the creation of medical exam rooms in the high-security housing units be able to reduce the number of patients needing to be escorted to the clinic? Can call-out appointments be scheduled better? Each situation is somewhat different, but it is still appropriate to question and rethink long-standing practices.

Rehabilitation—Start with Respect for Dignity and Self-Worth

As stated in the beginning of this chapter, prison systems, although battered by rapid growth and diminishing budgets, still have prisoner rehabilitation as one of their purposes. How could they not given that the vast majority of prisoners will sooner or later be released back to society? Even with severe budget constraints, it behooves them to see what can be done, with input from the health care and corrections professionals alike, to help victimized and traumatized persons and educationally deficient individuals come to grips with their situation and begin to build worthwhile lives? We know that they need to begin to believe in themselves—to know that they are worth it. How can we help them improve their sense of self-respect and personal dignity? What are we doing that detracts from this? Are there strong reasons for continuing in this direction? What can we do to change it? Would it not be appropriate for the wardens and their training staff to say forthrightly to the nurses and doctors and psychologists that "we want you to demonstrate proper professional care and concern, understanding, and respect to each of your patients? We would also like you to show us how to do this better."

Even when formal rehabilitation programs—such as education, counseling, substance-abuse treatment—are often the first to go in a budget shortage, it is good to know that some basic and effective rehabilitation can be accomplished with so little extra cost.

CONCLUSION—SPEAKING OUT LOYALLY

Now that we have seen in some detail many of the specific issues around which tension can arise between corrections and health care, we can perhaps better appreciate the sheer necessity of good strategies to help the parties work together. Collaborating does not mean lockstep, arm-in-arm camaraderie. This author believes there should be a healthy tension, not one that is toxic, malicious, or pernicious. Staff or care providers must never be afraid to speak truth to power. One should not back down or compromise on principle. In this relationship, some tension, stress, and challenge will be evident. This is as it ought to be. Doctors must be advocates for their patients. This is their first and highest responsibility. The medical director and the health care staff are responsible for the health and well-being of the incarcerated population, but in a very real sense so also are the warden (superintendent, institution head) and collectively the entire correctional team. Everyone, doctor and warden, nurse and officer alike, will have failed in their mission to the extent that the health needs of the inmate population are not properly addressed. Therefore, we have urged ongoing respectful dialogue and principled challenges of any conditions and practices that should be reevaluated or changed. Such disagreement is not disloyal. Its intent is for the betterment of the entire program, and constructive critique should not be regarded as an attack or as negative criticism.

Doing good things on the job is not enough. It is also important to have the courage and fortitude to speak up on behalf of those who have no power to speak for themselves. Recall the famous words attributed to Edmund Burke: "All that is necessary for the triumph of evil is that good men do nothing." Or as stated more recently by Mohandas Gandhi, "Noncooperation with evil is as much a duty as cooperation with good."[17] When health care professionals become aware of abuse or of conditions that are detrimental to the health of the inmate population—or to individual members of that population—they become complicit in the problem if they fail to speak up.

Speaking up effectively implies more than just blurting out one's opinions to whomsoever will lend an ear. It means saying the right things to the right people at the right time in the right way. It means choosing one's words carefully— removing from them any sting of anger, accusation, or superiority. One should not begin a discussion with the attitude that "I'm right, and you're wrong." Always assume the other party has both goodwill and good intentions. Try to understand and appreciate the difficult decisions and consequences that had to be faced in reaching a position. Seek to identify the highest and most central principles and needs of each professional point of view. Then see how to bring them together. What emerges as the solution may be a surprise to both sides, but it will likely be better than a unilateral decision by either side.

"All that is necessary for the triumph of evil is that good men do nothing."
—Edmund Burke

Often those with decision authority have not been made aware of the conditions at ground level. Or they may have naïvely believed that such unfortunate conditions were unavoidable. They may have seen but not appreciated the full extent, severity, or significance of the problem. Here is where the patient advocate can be helpful by bringing these conditions factually and persuasively to the authorities. Always have your facts straight. Do not be accusatory. Do not overstate your case or exaggerate. If it is important enough to bring up, the facts should speak for themselves and need no embroidery.

Epilogue

This book was long in preparation, but the effort was inspired and sustained by a felt hope that some correctional administrators and officials and some correctional health care professionals might find these reflections helpful. The author would always welcome feedback and suggestions. They can be sent to me directly or via Jessica Gribble, acquisitions editor at ABC-CLIO/Praeger: jgribble@abc-clio.com.

This book has examined many difficult and often controversial topics, sometimes entertaining or advancing points of view with which good and reasonable people may choose to disagree. The author has tried to lay out his reasoning at all times and cite a standard or two or sometimes an authority or a piece of research in support of that position when they are available. At times, he went outside of or beyond the standards and said what he thought best, given his experience, information, and belief.

In going out on a limb, he knowingly accepts the risk of being wrong or being out of synch with the time and realizes that not all of his positions will be universally accepted. But standards of decency have a way of evolving, and where we are is not necessarily where we were or where we will be. We may hope that things will be a certain way because it appears right and good, even though we know that in a practical sense the world is not fully ready for this. But it could become ready if we bring up the issues for constructive discussion.

If the reader feels a visceral disagreement with a stand that is advocated in this book, the author only asks that you take a moment to see if there is perhaps at least a shred of truth in what is proposed. Perhaps you can improve on it without rejecting its basic principle. But please do not just reject it out of hand because "that's not the way we have been doing it." Take another look at the way you use restraints, how you supervise suicidal persons, how you confine the mentally disturbed, what treatment access your segregated prisoners have to the health care staff, and whether the safety of your institution requires strip searches and body cavity searches to be conducted without probable cause. Look again at whether more can be done to enhance due respect for the dignity of each man, woman, and child in custody. If you still disagree with some of the opinions or recommendations, perhaps the book will at least promote productive dialogue and reflection on these difficult topics.

It is good that professional standards, including those used in the accreditation process are not static or permanent. They are alive and dynamic. The U.S. Supreme Court has recognized that its decisions must reflect society's evolving conscience and awareness of decency and humanity. Similarly, each round of accreditation should become, as the pole vaulter or high jumper experiences each time the bar is raised another notch, a challenge and a beckoning to attain an ever-higher level of quality and achievement. *Ad astra per aspera*, said Seneca, the ancient Roman philosopher, humanist, and statesman; loosely translated, he meant "Let us keep striving to reach the stars through whatever difficulties we may face."

Those who have attempted to write a book will perhaps understand how one can feel, at various times, so engaged in the work that little else matters while at other times experience a nagging desire that it be quickly finished because there are so many other things you want to do in life. And when you do manage to take a break, an overwhelming feeling of guilt sends a reminder: "I really should be working on the book." So this sometimes conflicted feeling has continued, although I doubt it is really abnormal or unusual. Truly, I am happy to be arriving at the finish line. And I look forward to spending more time with other passionate interests: flying my little Cessna Cardinal, to "slip the surly bonds of earth and dance the skies on laughter-silvered wings . . . ,"[1] or communicating over shortwave ham radio via Morse code—both hobbies of well over a half century, or for my wife and me to travel, or to probe deeper into the challenges of family genealogy. Most of all, however, I welcome the opportunity to spend more time with my dear wife, engaging children, loving grandchildren, and with my siblings, other family, and friends.

Notes

PREFACE

1. Russian novelist 1821–1881, who spent four years in a Russian prison.

INTRODUCTION

1. Danielle Kaeble et al., "Correctional Populations in the United States, 2014," *Bureau of Justice Statistics* (December 29, 2015) NCJ 249513.

2. "Mass Incarceration: The Whole Pie 2016," *Prison Policy Initiative*.

3. B. Jaye Anno et al., *Correctional Health Care: Addressing the Needs of Elderly, Chronically Ill, and Terminally Ill Inmates* (Washington, DC: National Institute of Corrections, February 2004).

CHAPTER 1

1. Edward M. Brecher and Richard D. Della Penna, *Health Care in Correctional Institutions* (Washington, DC: U.S. Government Printing Office, 1975), 7, 8, 56.

2. Kenneth L. Faiver [research director and principal author], *Key to Health for a Padlocked Society: Design for Health Care in Michigan Prisons* (Lansing, MI: Office of Health and Medical Affairs, March 1975), 314, 315, 322. Due credit must be given to members of the Governor's Advisory Committee for State Correctional Health Care and to three talented staff members who contributed to the research and the writing of the report: T. Richard Currier, Joseph A. Droste, and Peter L. Grenier.

3. B. Jaye Anno, *Correctional Health Care: Guidelines for the Management of an Adequate Delivery System* (Chicago: National Commission on Correctional Health Care, 2001), 12.

4. *Protecting Inmate Rights: Prison Reform or Prison Replacement?* Report of the Ohio Advisory Committee to the United States Commission on Civil Rights (February 1976), 116, 117.

5. "Report of the Survey Team of the Washington State Medical Association," (December 15, 1971). In *Medical and Health Care in Jails, Prisons, and Other Correctional Facilities: A Compilation of Standards and Materials* (Washington, DC: American Bar Association and American Medical Association, August 1974): 142qq, 142uu.

6. *Newman v. Alabama,* 349 F. Supp. 284 (October 4, 1972).

7. *Battle v. Anderson*, 376 F. Supp. 402 (E. Dist. OK, 1974).

8. Plato's *Republic* (circa 390 BC) Book 1, 352d. (Translated by the author from original Greek).

9. Daniel N. Lerman, "Second Opinion: Inconsistent Deference to Medical Ethics in Death Penalty Jurisdictions." *Georgetown Law Journal* (August 2007), 1941–1978.

10. Felicia G. Cohn, "The Ethics of End-of-Life Care for Prison Inmates," *Journal of Law, Medicine and Ethics* 27(3) (Fall 1999), 252–259. The author trusts that he has not distorted or altered Dr. Cohn's meaning by attempting to abbreviate her excellent presentation. The reader is encouraged to peruse her original published article.

11. Here Cohn follows the social contract theory of John Rawls, referenced as J. Rawls, *A Theory of Justice* (Cambridge: Harvard University Press, 1971).

12. Cohn, "Ethics of End-of-Life Care," 254.

13. Cohn, "Ethics of End-of-Life Care," 255–256.

14. Cohn, "Ethics of End-of-Life Care," 257.

15. Fyodor Dostoevsky, *The House of the Dead: Prison Life in Siberia*, a novel written in 1861–1862. Available through Project Gutenberg.

16. Cohn, "Ethics of End-of-Life Care," 259.

17. Stanley L. Brodsky, "Ethical Issues for Psychologists in Corrections." In *Who Is the Client? The Ethics of Psychological Intervention in the Criminal Justice System,* edited by John Monahan (Washington, DC: American Psychological Association, 1980), 63–92.

18. Tom L. Beauchamp and James F. Childress, *Principles of Biomedical Ethics*, 4th ed. (New York: Oxford University Press, 1994), 189.

19. World Medical Association, "International Code of Medical Ethics." Adopted October 1949, last amended at 57th WMA General Assembly at Pilanesberg, South Africa, October 2006. *World Medical Association Bulletin* 1(3), 109, 111.

20. E. Haavi Morreim, *Balancing Act: The New Medical Ethics of Medicine's New Economics* (Boston: Kluwer Academic Publishers, 1991), 1.

21. Readers interested in pursuing this topic further may read with profit case examples in which both sides of the ethical deliberations are presented articulately; for example, in Chris Hansen and Gordon C. Kanska, "Ethical Problems: Cases and Commentaries," *Journal of Prison Health* 1(2) (Fall–Winter 1981), 97–104.

22. Rev. John P. Foglio, DMin, was professor of medical ethics and spirituality at the College of Human Medicine, Michigan State University.

23. David L. Thomas and Nicholas Thomas, "Bioethics in Corrections," *Correctional Health Today* 1(1) (2009), 52.

24. Patricia N. Reams et al., "Making a Case for Bioethics in Corrections," *Corrections Compendium* 24(12) (November 1997), 1ff.

25. John Stuart Mill, *On Liberty* (London: Longman, Roberts, & Green, 1859).

26. NCCHC (2014) P-H-02 (essential) on "Confidentiality of Health Records," *Standards for Health Services in Prisons 2014* (Chicago: National Commission on Correctional Health Care, 2014).

27. Nancy N. Dubler, ed., *Standards for Health Services in Correctional Institutions*, 2nd ed. (Washington, DC: American Public Health Association, 1986), 111.

28. ACA, ACI (2003) 4-4396 (mandatory) on "Confidentiality," *Standards for Adult Correctional Institutions*, 4th ed. (Lanham, MD: American Correctional Association, 2003) as updated in the *2014 Standards Supplement: Adult Correctional Institutions ACI*, 4th ed. (Alexandria, VA: American Correctional Association, 2014); and ACA, *ACI* 4-4414 on "Transfers" as updated in the *2014 Standards Supplement*.

29. Jill Doner Kagle and Sandra Kopels, "Confidentiality after Tarasoff," *Health and Social Work* 19(3) (August, 1994), 217. *See also Tarasoff v. Board of Regents of the University of California*, 551 P. 2d 334 (1976).

30. Dubler, ed., *Standards for Health Services*, 111; *see also* APHA, *Standards for Health Services in Correctional Institutions*, 3rd ed. (Washington, DC: American Public Health Association, 2003), 57.

31. *See* John Monahan, "The Prediction of Violent Behavior," *American Journal of Psychiatry* 141 (1984), 5–8.

32. Arthur F. Southwick, *The Law of Hospital and Health Care Administration* (Ann Arbor, MI: Health Administration Press, 1978), 203–204.

33. APHA, *Standards for Health Services*, 3rd ed., 6.

34. *Schloendorff v. Society of New York Hospital*, 211 N.Y. 125, 105 N.E. 92 (1914).

35. William P. Isele, "Right to Treatment/Right to Refuse Treatment," *Corrections Today* (June 1983): 90.

36. Robert P. Vogt, "When an Inmate Refuses Care," *CorrectCare* (Summer 2005), 8.

37. *Vitek v. Jones,* 445 U.S. 480, 494–96, 100 S. Ct. 1254 (1980).

38. *Baugh v. Woodard*, 808 F. 2d 333, 335 n. 2, 4th Cir. (1987); and *Witzke v. Johnson*, 656 F. Supp. 294, 297–98, W.D. Mich. (1987).

39. Mark R. Munetz, Patricia A. Galon, and Frederick J. Frese III, "The Ethics of Mandatory Community Treatment," *Journal of the American Academy of Psychiatry and Law* 31 (2003), 175.

40. "Forced Psychotropic Medications Reviewed by Courts," *CorrectCare* 8(2) (May 1994), 4, 6.

41. *Sell v. United States,* 539 U.S. 166 (2003), 123 S. Ct. 2174 (2003).

42. Liz Rantz, MD, "Ask ACHSA: A Regular Column Responding to YOUR Questions," *CorHealth Newsletter* (Spring 2008), 3.

43. Institute of Medicine, *Crossing the Quality Chasm* (Washington, DC: The National Academies Press, 2001), 3.

44. Mary Muse, "Caring: an Integral Aspect of Nursing." Paper delivered at the National Conference on Correctional Health Care, Orlando, FL (October 19, 2009).

45. Mary Muse credits this "Caring can occur with curing" principle to Jean Watson, RN, PhD.

46. Mary Muse, "Caring: an Integral Aspect of Nursing" and "Examining Correctional Nursing Practice and Moral Distress." Papers presented at the National Conference on Correctional Health Care, Orlando, FL (October 19 and 20, 2009).

47. S. J. Weiskopf, "Nurses' Experience of Caring for Inmate Patients," *Journal of Advanced Nursing* 49(4) (2005), 336–343 (cited by Schoenly).

48. Lorry Schoenly, "Chapter 2. Ethical Principles for Correctional Nursing," in *Essentials of Correctional Nursing,* edited by Lorry Schoenly and Catherine M. Knox (New York: Springer, 2013), 29–30.

49. Jamie Scott Brodie, "Caring, the Essence of Correctional Nursing," *Tennessee Nurse* 64(2) (2001), 10–12 (cited by Schoenly).

50. Schoenly, "Ethical Principles," 30.

51. Jean Watson, *Human Caring Science: A Theory of Nursing*, 2nd ed. (Boston: Jones & Bartlett, 2012). Cited and adapted by Schoenly, "Ethical Principles," 31.

52. Sue Smith, "Stepping through the Looking Glass: Professional Autonomy in Correctional Nursing," *Corrections Today* 67(1) (February 2005), 54–70.

53. Rebecca Bay, "Medical Management of Transgender, Transsexual, and Gender Dysphoria: Time for Policy Revisions." Paper presented at National Conference on Correctional Health Care, Orlando, FL (October 20, 2009) [from notes taken by the author].

54. Rodney L. Fry, "Transsexualism: A Correctional, Medical or Behavioral Health Issue?" *CorrectCare* (Winter 2003).

55. Bay, "Medical Management."

56. NCCHC, "Transgender, Transsexual, and Gender Nonconforming Health Care in Correctional Settings." Position Statement adopted by the National Commission on Correctional Health Care Board of Directors October 19, 2009, and reaffirmed with revision April 2015.

57. George R. Brown and Everett McDuffie, "Health Care Policies Addressing Transgender Inmates in Prison Systems in the United States," *Journal of Correctional Health Care* 15(4) (October 2009), 280–281, 288.

58. Wisconsin, Act 13 (302.386[5m]).

59. *Fields v. Smith* (previously *Sundstrom v. Frank*), 2010 Westlaw 1929819 (E.D. Wis.).

60. ACLU, "Federal Court Upholds Transgender Peoples' Right to Access Medical Treatment in Prison," August 5, 2011.

61. *Phillips v. Michigan Department of Corrections*, 731 F. Supp. 792, Dist. Court, W.D. Mich. (1990).

62. *Obergefell v. Hodges,* 135 S. Ct. 2584 (2015).

63. Rodney L. Fry, "Transsexualism."

64. NCCHC (2014) P-I-03 on "Forensic Information" states that "Health services staff are prohibited from participating in the collection of forensic information."

65. NCCHC (2014) P-I-03 on "Forensic Information."

66. ACA *JCF* (2009) 4-JCF-4C-63 on "Contraband Control," *Performance-Based Standards for Juvenile Correctional Facilities,* 4th ed. (Alexandria, VA: American Correctional Association, 2009).

67. ACA *ACI* (2003) 4-4193 on "Control of Contraband."

68. NCCHC (2014) P-I-03 on "Forensic Information."

69. Dubler, ed., *Standards for Health Services*, 112.

70. APHA, *Standards for Health Services*, 3rd ed., 5.

71. Including, at one time, the National Commission on Correctional Health Care and the American Public Health Association (Nancy N. Dubler, ed., *Standards for Health Services in Correctional Institutions,* 2nd ed., 1986). The (now outdated and superseded) NCCHC *Standards for Health Services in Prisons* (1992) at Standard P-10; *Standards for Health Services in Jails* (1996) at Standard J-66; and *Standards for Health Services in Juvenile Detention and Confinement Facilities* (1995) at Standard Y-66 stated: "Body cavity searches conducted for reasons of security should be done in privacy by outside health care providers (as noted above) or by correctional personnel of the same sex as the inmate [juvenile] who have been trained by a physician or other health care provider to probe body cavities (without the use of instruments) so as to cause neither injury to tissue nor infection."

72. ACA *ACI* (2003) 4-4193 on "Control of Contraband."

73. An interesting discussion of ethical issues related to strip searches, body cavity searches, and religious beliefs is found in Peter C. Williams and Joan Hirsch Holtzman,

"Ethical Problems: Cases and Commentaries," *Journal of Prison Health* 1(1) (Spring–Summer, 1981), 44–54.

74. World Medical Association, "WMA Statement on Body Searches of Prisoners." Adopted by 45th World Medical Assembly at Budapest, Hungary, October 1993, and editorially revised by 170th WMA Council Session at Divonne-les-Bains, France, May 2005.

75. *Mary Beth G. v. City of Chicago*, 7th Cir. 1983, 723 F. 2d at 1272.

76. *John Does 1-100 v. Boyd*, 613 F. Supp. 1514, 1522, D.C. Minn. (1985).

77. *Justice v. City of Peachtree City*, 961 F. 2d 188, 192, 11 Cir. (1992).

78. *Trop v. Dulles,* 356 U.S. 86, 101 (1958): ". . . the evolving standards of decency that mark the progress of a maturing society."

79. Peter C. Williams and Joan Hirsch Holtzman, "Ethical Problems: Cases and Commentaries," 54.

80. Pamela Dole, "Spotlight," *Hepp News* 2(6) (June 1999), 5 (Providence, RI: Brown University School of Medicine).

81. John Monahan, *The Clinical Prediction of Violent Behavior* (Northvale, NJ: Jason Aronson, 1995); Henry J. Steadman, "The Right Not to Be a False Positive: Problems in the Application of the Dangerousness Standard," *Psychiatric Quarterly* 52(2) (Summer 1980), 84–99.

82. An excellent treatment of this subject is found in Robert B. Greifinger, "Commentary: Is It Politic to Limit Our Compassion?" *Journal of Law, Medicine and Ethics* 27(3) (Fall 1999), 235–236.

83. Joel A. Dvoskin, "What are the Odds on Predicting Violent Behavior?" *The Journal of the California AMI.*

84. Robert Hilton, "Crushing Medications" *CorrectCare* 7(4) (November 1993), 12.

85. Cohn, "Ethics of End-of-Life Care," 253.

86. ACA *ACI* (2003) 4-4258 on "Supervision."

87. ACA *ACI* (2003) 4-4256 on "Admission and Review of Status."

88. NCCHC (2014) P-E-09, *Segregated Inmates* (essential).

89. Robert B. Greifinger, "Five Steps toward an Ethical Practice," *CorrectCare* (Fall 2009), 3.

90. ACA *ACI* (2003) 4-4320 on "Therapeutic Diets."

91. ACA *ACI* (2003) 4-4264 on "General Conditions of Confinement" as updated in the *2014 Standards Supplement.*

92. *McNabb v. Department of Corrections*, 180 P. 3d 1257 (Washington, 2008).

93. Marc F. Stern, "Force-Feeding for Hunger Strikers," *CorrectCare* (Spring 2009), 18; *see also* News Briefs, "Force-Feeding of Inmate Deemed Legal," *Corrections Today* (June 2008), 20.

94. *Singletary v. Costello,* 665 So. 2d. 1099, Fla. App. 4th Dist. (1996).

95. *Thor v. Superior Court of Solano County (Howard Andrews, Real Party in Interest)*, 855 P. 2d 375—1993—Cal. Supreme Court.

96. World Medical Association, *Declaration of Tokyo*, "Guidelines for Physicians Concerning Torture and Other Cruel, Inhuman or Degrading Treatment or Punishment in Relation to Detention and Imprisonment." Adopted by the 29th World Medical Assembly, Tokyo, Japan, October 1975, and revised at the 173rd WMA Council Session, Divonne-les-Bains, France, May 2006.

97. World Medical Association, "Declaration of Malta on Hunger Strikers." Adopted by 43rd World Medical Assembly at Malta, November 1991, and last revised by the WMA General Assembly at Pilanesberg, South Africa, October 2006.

CHAPTER 2

1. ACA, *ACI* (2003) 4-4365 (mandatory) on "Health Appraisal," *Standards for Adult Correctional Institutions,* 4th ed. (Lanham, MD: American Correctional Association, 2003) as updated in the *2014 Standards Supplement: Adult Correctional Institutions ACI,* 4th ed. (Alexandria, VA: American Correctional Association, 2014).

2. ACA, *ACI* (2003) 4-4400 (mandatory) on "Segregation" as updated in the *2014 Standards Supplement.*

3. NCCHC (2014) P-A-08 (essential) on "Communication on Patients' Health Needs," *Standards for Health Services in Prisons 2014* (Chicago: National Commission on Correctional Health Care, 2014).

4. Eugene V. Boisaubin et al., " 'Well Enough to Execute': The Health Professional's Responsibility to the Death Row Inmate," *CorrectCare* 8 (Fall 2004), 8.

5. C. Gregory Smith and Woodhall Stopford, "Health Hazards of Pepper Spray," *North Carolina Medical Journal* 60(5) (September–October 1999), 268.

6. M. A. McDirmid, U.S. Department of Labor, Occupational Safety and Health Administration, Letter to Jay Bagley, Administrator, Utah Occupational Safety and Health Division, November 1993. (Cited in Smith and Stopford, "Health Hazards of Pepper Spray," 271.)

7. Silas Norman, Medical Director of the State Prison of Southern Michigan in Jackson, Michigan, Memorandum to Kenneth L. Faiver on March 4, 1988.

8. Lt. Col. John Medici, U.S. Army Chemical Corps (ret.), "Emergency Response to Incidents Involving Chemical and Biological Warfare Agents" (Quincy, MA: National Fire Protection Association, 1997).

9. Smith and Stopford, "Health Hazards of Pepper Spray," 271–272.

10. Craig Haney, "Second Report to the Court," in *Osterback v. Moore,* Case No. 97-2806-CIV-HUCK.

11. B. Jaye Anno, *Correctional Health Care: Guidelines for the Management of an Adequate Delivery System,* 2001 ed. (Chicago: NCCHC, 2001), 84.

12. ACCP, Code of Ethics, American College of Correctional Physicians (2016); ACHSA, Code of Ethics, American Correctional Health Services Association (2016).

13. Scott A. Allen, Robert L. Cohen, and William J. Rold, "Dual Loyalties: Our Role in Preventing Inmate Abuse," *CorrectCare* 20(3) (Summer 2006), 1, 16–17.

14. Nancy N. Dubler, ed., *Standards for Health Services in Correctional Institutions,* 2nd ed. (Washington, DC: American Public Health Association, 1986), 3.

15. ACA, *ACI* (2003) 4-4190 on "Use of Restraints."

16. ACA, *ACI* (2003) 4-4191 (mandatory) on "Use of Restraints" as updated in the *2014 Standards Supplement.*

17. ACA, "Public Correctional Policy on Use of Force," as amended in 2010, *ACA Public Correctional Policies* (Alexandria, VA: American Correctional Association, 2012).

18. Brian McCormick, "Ethics Panel Spells Out Physician Role in Executions," *American Medical News* (December 28, 1992): 6.

19. Dubler, ed., *Standards for Health Services,* 114.

20. APHA, *Standards for Health Services in Correctional Institutions,* 3rd ed. (Washington, DC: American Public Health Association, 2003), 5.

21. "Health Groups Oppose A.G. on Executions," *CorrectCare* 7(1) (January–February 1993), 3, 7; "Health Care Associations Join to Oppose Participation in Executions," *CorrectCare* 8(2) (May 1994), 5.

22. ANA, Position Statement: "Nurses' Role in Capital Punishment"(Silver Spring, MD: American Nurses Association, January 28, 2010).

23. ACCP and ACHSA, Code of Ethics.

24. NCCHC (2014) P-I-07 on "Executions."

25. World Medical Association, *Declaration of Tokyo,* "Guidelines for Physicians Concerning Torture and other Cruel, Inhumane or Degrading Treatment or Punishment in Relation to Detention and Imprisonment." Adopted by the 29th World Medical Assembly, Tokyo, Japan, October 1975, and revised at the 173rd WMA Council Session, Divonne-les-Bains, France, May 2006.

26. Atul Gawande, "When Law and Ethics Collide—Why Physicians Participate in Executions," *New England Journal of Medicine* 354(12) (March 23, 2006), 1221–1229.

27. Janet Weiner et al., *Breach of Trust: Physician Participation in Executions in the United States.* American College of Physicians, Human Rights Watch, National Coalition to Abolish the Death Penalty, and Physicians for Human Rights (1994).

28. General Assembly of North Carolina, House Bill 442 of 2007.

29. American Civil Liberties Union, *2015 Legislative Report Card.*

30. Florida Statute 922.105(6).

31. An enlightening commentary on this topic is found in Gawande, "When Law and Ethics Collide."

32. Gregory D. Curfman, Stephen Morrissey, and Jeffrey M. Drazen, "Physicians and Execution," *New England Journal of Medicine* 358 (January 24, 2008), 403–404.

33. AMA, "Chapter 9: Opinions on Professional Self-Regulation," *AMA Principles of Medical Ethics,* Title 9.7.3 "Capital Punishment" (Chicago: American Medical Association, 2016), 124.

34. *AMA Principles of Medical Ethics,* Title 9.7.3 Capital Punishment, 124–125.

35. Atul Gawande, "When Law and Ethics Collide."

36. Atul Gawande, "When Law and Ethics Collide."

37. Death Penalty Information Center, "One Year After Botched Execution, Many States Still Haven't Resumed Executions."

38. Lee Black and Robert M. Sade, "Lethal Injection and Physicians: State Law vs. Medical Ethics," *Journal of the American Medical Association* 298(23) (December 19, 2007), 2779.

39. "Brief for the Petitioner," *Baze v. Rees,* 553 U.S. 35, 128 S. Ct. 1520 (2008) at 12, 17.

40. "Brief for the Petitioner," *Baze v. Rees.*

41. APhA, *Code of Ethics for Pharmacists* (Washington, DC: American Pharmacists Association, 2016).

42. APhA, *Code of Ethics for Pharmacists.*

43. Curfman et al., "Physicians and Execution."

44. American Pharmacists Association, House of Delegates, motion introduced by William Fassett (February 11, 2015).

45. APhA House of Delegates Adopts Policy Discouraging Pharmacist Participation in Execution."

46. National Coalition to Abolish the Death Penalty (NCADP). "APHA votes to oppose participation in execution."

47. Richard Wolf and Jayne O'Donnell, "Pfizer Rules on Lethal Injection Drugs May Limit Death Penalty Executions," *USA Today* (May 13, 2016).

48. National Coalition to Abolish the Death Penalty (NCADP). "Drug-maker Akorn bans use of midazolam for executions."

49. *Washington v. Harper,* 494 U.S. 210 (1990).

50. *Sell v. United States*, 539 U.S. 166 (2003).

51. Douglas Mossman, "Is Prosecution 'Medically Appropriate'?" *Mossman Macro,* New England School of Law, p. 74.

52. Mossman, "Is Prosecution 'Medically Appropriate'?" 75.

53. Mossman, "Is Prosecution 'Medically Appropriate'?" 73.

54. *Ford v. Wainwright*, 477 U.S. 399, 409–10 (1986).

55. Paul S. Appelbaum, "The Parable of the Forensic Psychiatrist: Ethics and the Problem of Doing Harm," *International Journal of Law and Psychiatry* 13 (1990), 258.

56. American Academy of Psychiatry and the Law, *Ethical Guidelines for the Practice of Forensic Psychiatry*, Section II.

57. D. A. Sargent, "Treating the Condemned to Death," *Hastings Center Report* 16(6) (December 1986), 5–6.

58. Neil J. Farber, et al., "Physician's Willingness to Participate in the Process of Lethal Injection for Capital Punishment," *Annals of Internal Medicine* (November 2001), 887.

59. AMA, *Principles of Medical Ethics,* Title 9.7.4 "Physician Participation in Interrogation," 125.

60. AMA, *Principles of Medical Ethics,* Title 9.7.3 "Capital Punishment," 123.

61. AMA, *Principles of Medical Ethics,* Title 9.7.3 "Capital Punishment," 124.

62. NCCHC, "Competency for Execution," *Position Statement.* Adopted by National Commission on Correctional Health Care Board of Directors on October 30, 1998, and reaffirmed in October 2012.

63. NCCHC, "Competency for Execution," *Position Statement.*

64. United Nations, "Principles of Medical Ethics Relevant to the Role of Health Personnel, Particularly Physicians, in the Protection of Prisoners and Detainees against Torture and Other Cruel, Inhuman or Degrading Treatment or Punishment." Adopted by United Nations General Assembly Resolution 37/194 of 18 December 1982, Principles 3 and 4. Copyright © 1982 United Nations. Reprinted with the permission of the United Nations.

65. World Psychiatric Association, *Declaration of Madrid.* Approved by the General Assembly of the World Psychiatric Association on August 25, 1996.

66. Frederic Grunberg, "Patients and Society: The Double Allegiance of Psychiatrists," *Bulletin*, Canadian Psychiatric Association (October 2002).

67. Alfred M. Friedman and Abraham L. Halpern, "The Psychiatrist's Dilemma: A Conflict of Roles in Legal Executions," *Australian and New Zealand Journal of Psychiatry* 33 (1999), 620–635; cited in Grunberg, "Patients and Society."

68. Rubens Laiño, "Ethics in Prison Health Care," Second World Congress on Prison Health Care, Ottawa, Canada (August 31, 1983). (From a 16-page copy of Dr. Laiño's presentation issued by the Canadian Secretary of State to Conference attendees.)

69. *Cf.* Frederick R. Parker, Jr. and Charles J. Paine, "Informed Consent and the Refusal of Medical Treatment in the Correctional Setting," *Journal of Law, Medicine and Ethics* 27(3) (Fall 1999), 245.

70. U. S. Central Intelligence Agency, "Death Investigation—Gul Rahman."

71. U. S. Central Intelligence Agency, *OMS Guidelines on Medical and Psychological Support to Detainee Rendition, Interrogation, and Detention.* (December 2004) Approved for release 6-10-2016.

72. For further comment, cf. *Doing Harm: Health Professionals' Central Role in the CIA Torture Program: Medical and Psychological Analysis of the 2014 U.S. Senate Select Committee on Intelligence Report's Executive Summary,* Physicians for Human Rights

(December 2014); cf. also Sarah Dougherty and Vincent Iacopino, "CIA Documents Show How Deeply Doctors and Health Professionals Were Involved in Torture," Physicians for Human Rights (July 25, 2016).

73. AMA, "Chapter 9: Opinions on Professional Self-Regulation," *AMA Principles of Medical Ethics,* Title 9.7.5 Torture, 126.

74. *AMA Principles of Medical Ethics,* Title 9.7.4 "Physician Participation in Interrogation," 125.

75. *AMA Principles of Medical Ethics*, Title 9.7.5 "Torture," 126.

76. World Medical Association, *Declaration of Tokyo.*

77. World Medical Association, "World Medical Association Supports Doctors Refusing to Participate in Torture," 49th WMA General Assembly at Hamburg, Germany (November 17, 1997), Universidad de Navarra.

78. NCCHC, "Correctional Health Care Professionals' Response to Inmate Abuse," Position Statement, adopted by National Commission on Correctional Health Care Board of Directors, October 2012.

79. APHA, *Standards for Health Services,* 3rd ed., 5.

80. NCCHC, "Correctional Health Care Professionals' Response to Inmate Abuse," Position Statement.

81. ACA Code of Ethics, adopted by the Board of Governors and Delegates Assembly in August 1994 (Alexandria, VA: American Correctional Association).

82. Lawrence McCullough and Richard Stubbs, *Ethical Challenges of Physician Executives* (Tampa, FL: The American College of Physician Executives, July 1995), 22.

83. Robert L. Cohen, "Statement before the Commission on Safety and Abuse in America's Prisons" (Newark, NJ: July 20, 2005).

84. Review of Burnout: Stages of disillusionment in the helping professions; Burnout and health professionals: Manifestations and management; and Stress, health and psychological problems in the major professions. No authorship indicated. *Family Systems Medicine*, 2(4) (1984), 444–448.

85. José Manuel García-Arroyo and María Luisa Domínguez-López (2014). "Subjective Aspects of Burnout Syndrome in the Medical Profession," *Psychology* 5, 2064–2072.

86. Lorry Schoenly, "Moral Distress and Correctional Nursing," CorrectionalNurse.net.

87. Bonnie Sultan, "Working Behind the Wall: Mental Health of Correctional-Based Staff," PsychAlive.

88. Caterina Spinaris, Michael Denhof, and Gregory Morton, *Impact of Traumatic Exposure on Corrections Professionals,* White paper, NIC Cooperative Agreement 12CS14GKM7. December 21, 2013, 17-18.

89. Spinaris, Denhof, and Morton, *Impact of Traumatic Exposure,* 22, 23, 28.

90. Joel A. Dvoskin, "Confessions of an Incrementalist," *Public Service Psychology* (American Psychological Association: Spring 1999).

CHAPTER 3

1. Ian Urbina, "Panel Suggests Using Inmates in Drug Trials," *The New York Times* (August 13, 2006).

2. This research is described in Alf S. Alving et al., "Procedures Used at Stateville Penitentiary for the Testing of Potential Antimalarial Agents," *Journal of Clinical Investigation* 27(3) Pt. 2 (May 1948), 2–5.

3. Andrew Goliszek, *In the Name of Science: A History of Secret Programs, Medical Research, and Human Experimentation* (New York: St. Martin's Press, 2003), Chapter 4.

4. Wayne D. LeBaron, *America's Nuclear Legacy* (Commack, NY: Nova Publishers, 1998), 105.

5. Allen M. Hornblum, *Acres of Skin: Human Experiments at Holmesburg Prison* (New York: Routledge, 1998).

6. Ian Urbina, "Panel Suggests Using Inmates."

7. Robert E. Hodges et al., "Clinical Manifestations of Ascorbic Acid Deficiency in Man," *American Journal of Clinical Nutrition* 24 (April 1971), 432–443.

8. Ethan Blue, "The Strange Career of Leo Stanley: Remaking Manhood at San Quentin State Penitentiary, 1913–1951," *Pacific Historical Review* 78(2) (May 2009), 210–241. For additional examples, see also Jessica Mitford, "Experiments behind Bars: Doctors, Drug Companies, and Prisoners," *Atlantic Monthly* 23 (January 1973), 64–73; and Jessica Mitford, *Kind and Usual Punishment: The Prison Business* (New York: Alfred A. Knopf, 1973), 138–168.

9. Frederick R. Parker Jr. and Charles J. Paine, "Informed Consent and the Refusal of Medical Treatment in the Correctional Setting," *Journal of Law, Medicine and Ethics* 27(3) (Fall 1999), 247.

10. ACHRE, "Chapter 9. Prisoners: A Captive Research Population: Introduction," *Final Report of the Advisory Committee on Human Radiation Experiments.* Washington, DC: National Archives and Records Administration (1995), 1.

11. NCPHS, *The Belmont Report: Ethical Principles and Guidelines for the Protection of Human Subjects of Research.* National Commission for the Protection of Human Subjects of Biomedical and Behavioral Research, National Institutes of Health, Office of Human Subjects Research (April 18, 1979), 5–9.

12. NCPHS, *Report and Recommendations: Research Involving Prisoners.* National Commission for the Protection of Human Subjects of Biomedical and Behavioral Research (1976), 13.

13. NCPHS, *Report and Recommendations*, 5.

14. *Trials of War Criminals before the Nuremberg Military Tribunals under Control Council Law* (Washington, DC: U.S. Government Printing Office, 1949), 10(2), 181–182.

15. NCPHS, *Report and Recommendations*, 16–17.

16. 45 *Code of Federal Regulations* (CFR) §46.306(a)(2)(i)–(iv) (10-1-09 ed.).

17. Office of Human Subjects Research Protection (OHSRP), *Institutional Review Board Guidebook: Chapter VIII—Special Classes of Subjects*, Section E—Prisoners: Regulations (last updated 1993). Washington, DC: U.S. Department of Health and Human Services, OHSRP.

18. OHSRP, "Standard Operating Procedure/Policy Approval & Implementation." February 25, 2016.

19. *Henry Fante et al. v. Department of Health and Human Services et al.*, U.S. District Court, Eastern District of Michigan, Southern Division, Civil Action No. 80-72778 (1981).

20. David Vulcano, "Research Involving Prisoners in Non-Prison Settings: FDA and OHRP Regulations," *Journal of Clinical Research Best Practices*, 6(1) (January 2010). This article contains helpful algorithms to determine the applicability of the complex federal requirements for research involving prisoners.

21. ACHRE, "Chapter 9: Prisoners: A Captive Research Population: History of Prison Research Regulation," *Final Report*, 5.

Also see Lawrence O. Gostin, Cori Vanchieri, and Andrew Pope, eds., *Ethical Considerations for Research Involving Prisoners*, Institute of Medicine (Washington, DC: National Academy Press, 2006), 67.

22. ACHRE, "Chapter 9: Prisoners: A Captive Research Population: History of Prison Research Regulation," *Final Report,* 4–5.

23. ACHRE, "Chapter 9: Prisoners: A Captive Research Population: History of Prison Research Regulation," *Final Report*, 5.

24. Gostin, Vanchieri, and Pope, *Ethical Considerations*, xi.

25. OHSRP, *Institutional Review Board Guidebook.*

26. ACA, *ACI* (2003) 4-4402 (mandatory) on "Research," *Standards for Adult Correctional Institutions,* 4th ed. (Lanham, MD: American Correctional Association, 2003) as updated in the *2014 Standards Supplement: Adult Correctional Institutions ACI*, 4th ed. (Alexndria, VA: American Correctional Association, 2014).

27. ACA, "Public Correctional Policy on Research and Evaluation," reaffirmed in 2012, *ACA Public Correctional Policies* (Alexandria, VA: American Correctional Association, 2012).

28. NCCHC (2014) P-I-06 on "Medical and Other Research," *Standards for Health Services in Prisons 2014* (Chicago: National Commission on Correctional Health Care, 2014).

29. NCCHC (2014) P-I-06 on "Medical and Other Research."

30. World Medical Association, *Declaration of Helsinki*, "Ethical Principles for Medical Research Involving Human Subjects," originally adopted in June 1964, it has since undergone nine revisions, the most recent by the 64th WMA General Assembly at Fortaleza, Brazil, October 2013.

31. Council for International Organizations of Medical Sciences (CIOMS), *International Ethical Guidelines for Biomedical Research Involving Human Subjects*, prepared in collaboration with the World Health Organization (WHO), Geneva, 2002, 49.

32. United Nations, "International Covenant on Civil and Political Rights," Article 7, Office of the United Nations High Commissioner for Human Rights, adopted December 16, 1966.

33. Gostin, Vanchieri, and Pope, *Ethical Considerations*, xi.

34. OHSRP, "Guidance: Special Subject Populations: Prisoners," Office of the Human Research Protection Program, UCLA (last updated October 24, 2011).

35. *Cf.* Gostin, Vanchieri, and Pope, *Ethical Considerations*, 8–9.

36. Gostin, Vanchieri, and Pope, *Ethical Considerations*, 10, 12, 14.

37. Osagie K. Obasogie, "Prisoners and Clinical Trials: Cruel and Unusual Ethics?" *Genetics and Society* (June 29, 2007).

38. Keramet Reiter, "Experimentation on Prisoners: Persistent Dilemmas in Rights and Regulations," *California Law Review* 97(2) (April 9, 2009), 506.

39. Reiter, "Experimentation on Prisoners."

40. Gostin, Vanchieri, and Pope, *Ethical Considerations*, 117.

41. Gostin, Vanchieri, and Pope, *Ethical Considerations*, 21.

42. Lawrence O. Gostin, "Biomedical Research Involving Prisoners: Ethical Values and Legal Regulation," *Journal of the American Medical Association* 297 (February 21, 2007), 737–740.

43. Newton E. Kendig, "Introduction," *Journal of Correctional Health Care* 14(4) (October 2008), 260–262. Nearly this entire issue of the journal is devoted to exploring a suitable research agenda to improve inmate health. Dr. Kendig is the assistant director of the Health Services Division of the Federal Bureau of Prisons.

44. These topics were mentioned in the several papers published by David Paar, Carol Bova, Jacques Baillargeon, William Mazar, and Larry Boly; by Kenneth L. Appelbaum;

and by Janet Fraser Hale, Arthur M. Brewer, and Warren Ferguson in this same issue of the *Journal of Correctional Health Care, 263–268.*

45. ACA, *ACI* (2003) 4-4402 (mandatory) on "Research."

46. Reiter, "Experimentation on Prisoners."

47. OHRPP, "Standard Operating Procedure/Policy—14C," Office of Human Subjects Research Protections, Department of Health and Human Services, National Institutes of Health.

48. World Medical Association, *Declaration of Helsinki.*

49. Kendig, "Introduction."

50. David Paar et al., "Infectious Disease in Correctional Health Care: Pursuing a Research Agenda, *Journal of Correctional Health Care,* 14(4) (October 2008).

51. Kenneth L. Appelbaum, "Correctional Mental Health Research: Opportunities and Barriers," *Journal of Correctional Health Care,* 14(4) (October 2008), 269–277.

52. Janet Fraser Hale, Arthur M. Brewer, and Warren Ferguson, "Correctional Health Primary Care: Research and Educational Opportunities," *Journal of Correctional Health Care,* 14(4) (October 2008), 278–289.

53. "Pinel, Philippe" *Complete Dictionary of Scientific Biography* (New York: Charles Scribner's Sons, 2008).

54. Jeffrey L. Metzner, "Mental Health Considerations for Segregated Inmates," *CorrectCare* (Fall 2015), 14.

55. APA, "Position Statement on Segregation of Prisoners with Mental Illness," American Psychiatric Association. Approved by Board of Trustees, December 2012; approved by the Assembly, November 2012.

56. Fred Cohen, excerpt from written statement titled "Isolation in Penal Settings," submitted by Fred Cohen to the Commission on Safety and Abuse in America's Prisons. July 19, 2005, Newark, NJ.

57. Kenneth L. Appelbaum, "American Psychiatry Should Join the Call to Abolish Solitary Confinement," *Journal of the American Academy of Psychiatry and Law,* 43:406-15, 2015, 407.

58. Hope Metcalf et al., *Administrative Segregation, Degrees of Isolation, and Incarceration: A National Overview of State and Federal Correctional Policies* (Liman Public Interest Program, Yale Law School, June 25, 2013) 4.

59. ACA, "Public Correctional Policy on Correctional Mental Health Care," as amended in 2009.

60. Dean Aufderheide, "Mental Illness in Administrative Segregation: How to Bulletproof Your Program Against Litigation," *CorrectCare* (Spring 2013), 14–16.

61. Craig Haney, "Second Report of Professor Craig Haney" (December 2003), 10, 13. In *Osterback v. Moore,* Case No. 97-2806-CIV-HUCK (S.D. Florida, 2001).

62. Keith R. Curry, "Letter to Donna Brorby, Esq." (March 19, 2002), 6, 7.

63. Maureen L. O'Keefe et al., *One Year Longitudinal Study of the Psychological Effects of Administrative Segregation* (Colorado Springs: Colorado Department of Corrections and University of Colorado, 2010).

64. This improvement was noted among all of the study groups and consequently cannot be counted as an effect of being in administrative segregation.

65. Philip Bulman, "The Psychological Effects of Solitary Confinement," *Corrections Today* (June–July 2012), 58–59.

66. Daniel Rose also supervised the construction of the prison. This prison, closed in 2002, was the inspiration for the novel and movie *The Shawshank Redemption.*

67. Jeffrey D. Merrill Sr., *Maine State Prison: 1824–2002* (Charleston, SC: Arcadia, 2009).

68. Keramet Reiter, Statement of Keramet A. Reiter before the U.S. Senate Committee on the Judiciary, Subcommittee on the Constitution, Civil Rights and Human Rights, February 21, 2014.

69. *Jones 'El et al. v. Berge et al.*, 164 F. Supp 2d 1096 (2001) at 1.

70. Stuart Grassian, "Testimony on Impact of Isolation," written testimony for the Commission on Safety and Abuse in America's Prisons (July 19, 2005), 1–2.

71. Stuart Grassian, "Psychiatric Effects of Solitary Confinement," redacted from a declaration submitted in September 1993 in *Madrid v. Gomez*, 889 F. Supp. 1146 and presented as an attachment to testimony before the Commission on Safety and Abuse in America's Prisons (July 19, 2005): 1–2, 13.

72. Cited in Sasha Abramsky, "Return of the Madhouse," *The American Prospect Magazine* (February 11, 2002).

73. Daniel P. Mears, *Evaluating the Effectiveness of Supermax Prisons,* U.S. Department of Justice (January 2006).

74. F. E. Somnier and I. K. Genefke, "Psychotherapy for Victims of Torture," *British Journal of Psychiatry* 149 (1986), 323–324 (cited in brief of professors and practitioners).

75. Hans Toch, "Men in Crisis: Human Breakdowns in Prisons" (Chicago: Aldine, 1975) (cited in brief of professors and practitioners).

76. Toch, "Men in Crisis," 54.

77. "Brief of Professors and Practitioners of Psychology and Psychiatry as Amicus Curiae in Support of Respondent," *Reginald A. Wilkinson v. Charles E. Austin* (March 3, 2005). The authors of this report included Stanley L. Brodsky, PhD; Carl Clements, PhD; Keith R. Curry, PhD; Karen Froming, PhD; Carl Fulwiler, MD, PhD; Craig Haney, PhD, JD; Pablo Stewart, MD; and Hans Toch, PhD. Other relevant information is available from Gretchen Borchelt, "Break Them Down: Systematic Use of Psychological Torture by U.S. Forces," Physicians for Human Rights (May 2005).

78. *Wilkinson v. Austin*, 544 U.S. 74 (2005) 372 F. 3d 346, affirmed in part, reversed in part, and remanded.

79. David C. Fathi, "The Common Law of Supermax Litigation," *Pace Law Review*, 24 (2004), 676.

80. Rice, Marnie E. and Grant T. Harris, "Treatment for Prisoners with Mental Disorders." In *Successful Community Sanctions and Services for Special Offenders: Proceedings of the 1994 Conference of the International Community Corrections Association*, edited by Barbara J. Auerbach and Thomas C. Castellano (Lanham, MD: American Correctional Association and International Community Corrections Association, April 1998).

81. Curry, "Letter to Donna Brorby, Esq.,"9.

82. ACCP, "Restricted Housing of Mentally Ill Inmates: Position Statement," adopted by the Society of Correctional Physicians Board of Directors, July 9, 2013.

83. 18 U.S. Code §114.

84. John F. Stinneford, "Incapacitation through Maiming: Chemical Castration, the Eighth Amendment, and the Denial of Human Dignity," *University of St. Thomas Law Journal* (2006), 566–567.

85. *Buck v. Bell*, 274 U.S. 200 (1927).

86. Stinneford, "Incapacitation through Maiming," 575–576.

87. Stinneford, "Incapacitation through Maiming," 578, 597–598.

88. AMA Code of Medical Ethics, American Medical Association (revised June 2001).

89. AMA, "Court-Initiated Medical Treatments in Criminal Cases," *CEJA Report 4-A-98* (American Medical Association Council on Ethical and Judicial Affairs, 1998), 1.

90. AMA, "Chapter 9: Opinions on Professional Self-Regulation," *AMA Principles of Medical Ethics,* Title 9.7.2. Court-Initiated Medical Treatment in Criminal Cases (Chicago: American Medical Association, 2016), 123.

91. AMA, "Court-Initiated Medical Treatments" (1998), 3.

92. AMA, "Court-Initiated Medical Treatments" (1998): 4. Here AMA has included a brief quote from John M. W. Bradford and Anne Pawlak, "Double-Blind Placebo Cross-over Study of Cyproterone Acetate in the Treatment of Paraphilias," *Archives of Sexual Behavior* (October 1993).

93. Carl C. Bell, "An Ethical Conundrum in Correctional Health Care," *CorrectCare* (Spring 2012), 4–5.

94. Margaret E. Clarke and W. Benton Gibbard, "Overview of Fetal Alcohol Spectrum Disorders for Mental Health Professionals," *Canadian Child and Adolescent Psychiatry Review* 3 (August 12, 2003), 57–63.

95. National Institute on Alcohol Abuse and Alcoholism.

CHAPTER 4

1. *Ruffin v. Commonwealth of Virginia,* 62 Va. (21 Gratt.) 790, 796 (1871).

2. *Spicer v. Williamson,* 191 N.C. 487, 490, 132 S.E. 291, 293 (1926).

3. "Justice, Texas Style," *Newsweek* (October 6, 1986), 50. The U.S. Supreme Court decision in *Ex parte Hull* [312 UA 546 (1941)] describes another instance.

4. See also William C. Collins, *Correctional Law for the Correctional Officer,* 5th ed. (Alexandria, VA: American Correctional Association, 2010).

5. *Ex parte Hull,* 312 U.S. 546 (1941).

6. *Monroe v. Pape,* 365 U.S. 167 (1961).

7. Margaret D. Wishart and Nancy N. Dubler, *Health Care in Prisons, Jails, and Detention Centers: Some Legal and Ethical Dilemmas* (New York: Montefiore Medical Center, 1983), 9.

8. Robert D. McKay (The McKay Commission), *Attica: the Official Report of the New York State Special Commission on Attica* (New York: Bantam Books, 1972), 63.

9. *Newman v. Alabama,* 522 F. 2d 71 (1974).

10. Ian D. Forsythe, "A Guide to Civil Rights Liability under 42 U.S.C. §1983: An Overview of Supreme Court and Eleventh Circuit Precedent," Orlando, FL (undated). San Antonio, TX: The Constitution Society.

11. Ellen J. Winner, "An Introduction to the Constitutional Law of Prison Medical Care," *Journal of Prison Health* 1(1) (Spring–Summer 1981), 70, 71.

12. *Estelle v. Gamble,* 429 U.S. 97 at 116 (1976).

13. Ian D. Forsythe, "Guide to Civil Rights Liability."

14. 42 U.S.C. §1997 (May 23, 1980).

15. Erwin Chemerinsky, *Federal Jurisdiction* (New York: Aspen, 2003), 464.

16. *Bivens v. Six Unknown Agents of the Federal Bureau of Narcotics,* 403 U.S. 388 (1971).

17. Erwin Chemerinsky, *Federal Jurisdiction,* 587–609.

18. Douglas C. McDonald, *Managing Prison Health Care and Costs* (Washington, DC: National Institute of Justice, 1995), 42.

19. *Wilson v. Seiter,* 501 U.S. 294, 111 S. Ct. 232 (1991), in "U.S. Supreme Court Redefines 'Deliberate Indifference,'" *CorrectCare* 5(3) (July, 1991), 1, 14.

20. John Boston, "Court Rules on Smoking Case," *CorrectCare* 8(2) (May, 1994), 7, 14.

21. The author is indebted to the following persons who reviewed and provided helpful comments for the section on the PLRA contained in his earlier book, *Health Care Management Issues in Corrections* (ACA, 1997): Hon. Richard Alan Enslen, Chief Judge, U.S. District Court, Western District of Michigan; Paul R. Belazis, Esq., Court Monitor for *Inmates of Wayne County Jail v. County Commissioner*; and William J. Rold, Esq, a civil rights and prisoner's rights attorney.

22. 42 U.S.C. § 1997e *et seq.*

23. Josh Kurtzman, "Overcoming the Exhaustion Requirement of the Prison Litigation Reform Act," *Young Advocates E-Newsletter*, American Bar Association (January 7, 2016).

24. Human Rights Watch telephone interview with Terry Kupers on November 14, 2008, "No Equal Justice: The Prison Litigation Reform Act in the United States," *Human Rights Watch* (June 16, 2009), 26–27.

25. *Minix v. Pazera*, 2005 WL 1799538, N.D. Ind. (2005).

26. Michael J. Dale, "Lawsuits and Public Policy: The Role of Litigation in Correcting Conditions in Juvenile Detention Centers," *University of San Francisco Law Review* (32) (Summer 1998), 675, 681.

27. Jessica Feierman, "Testimony of Juvenile Law Center, Youth Law Center, National Center for Youth Law, and Center for Children's Law and Policy for the House Judiciary Subcommittees on Crime, Terrorism and Homeland Security and Constitution, Civil Rights and Civil Liberties" (November 8, 2007).

28. Catherine Megan Bradley, "Old Remedies Are New Again: Deliberate Indifference and the Receivership in *Plata v. Schwarzenegger*" (June 29, 2007).

29. Margo Schlanger and Giovanna Shay, "Preserving the Rule of Law in America's Prisons: The Case for Amending the Prison Litigation Reform Act," *American Constitution Society for Law and Policy* (March 2007), 1.

30. The following cases are cited by Schlanger and Shay: *Martin v. Hadix,* 527 U.S. 343 (1999); *Miller v. French*, 530 U.S. 327 (2000); *Booth v. Churner*, 532 U.S. 731 (2001); *Porter v. Nussle*, 534 U.S. 516 (2002); *Woodford v. Ngo*, 126 S. Ct. 2378 (2006); *Jones v. Bock*, 127 S. Ct. 910 (2007). See also *Inmates of Suffolk County Jail v. Rouse et al.,* 129 F. 3d 649, 654, 1st Cir. (1997) and *Cody v. Hillard,* 304 F.3d 767, 776 (8th Cir. 2002).

31. John J. Gibbons and Nicholas de B. Katzenbach, "Summary of Findings and Recommendations," *Confronting Confinement: A Report of the Commission on Safety and Abuse in America's Prisons* (New York: Vera Institute of Justice) (June 2006), 16.

32. *Ross v. Blake*, 578 U.S. ___ (2016), Docket No. 15-339. This case was decided on June 6, 2016.

33. Schlanger and Shay, "Preserving the Rule of Law."

34. *Brown v. Simmons*, no. 6:03-CV-122, 2007 WL 654920, at *6, S.D. Tex. (Feb. 23, 2007).

35. Schlanger and Shay, "Preserving the Rule of Law," 8.

36. Testimony of Stephen B. Bright regarding the Prison Abuse Remedies Act. To the Subcommittee on Crime, Terrorism, and Homeland Security of the Committee on the Judiciary, U.S. House of Representatives (April 22, 2008), 11. See also Stephen B. Bright, "Counsel for the Poor: The Death Sentence Not for the Worst Crime but for the Worst Lawyer," *Yale Law Journal* 103 (1994), 1835.

37. It was last introduced by Rep. Robert Scott (D-VA) as HB 4335.

38. American Bar Association, Criminal Justice Section, "Report to the House of Delegates, No. 102B," Recommendations Concerning the Prison Litigation Reform Act of 1996 (approved February 2007).

39. See *Hamilton v. Love*, 328 F. Supp. 1182 at 1194, E.D. Ark. (1971); *Gates v. Collier*, 501 F. 2d 1291 1319, CA5 (1974); *Moore v. Morgan*, 922 F. 2d, 1557 n. 4, 11th Cir. (1991); and *Battle v. Anderson*, 564 F. 2d 388, 396, CA10 (1977).

40. 42 U.S.C. §12101(b)(1).

41. U. S. Department of Justice, *Title II Technical Assistance Manual* at II-6.0000 and II-6.3300.

42. *Enforcing the ADA: A Status Report from the Department of Justice*, U.S. Department of Justice, Civil Rights Division, Disability Rights Section (January–March 2007), 2–3.

43. Paul Evans, "The Americans with Disabilities Act and Inmates with Disabilities: The Extent to Which Title II of the Act Provides a Recourse," 22 *Washington University Journal of Law & Policy* 22 (2006), 563.

44. Robert B. Greifinger, "Disabled Prisoners and 'Reasonable Accommodation,'" *Criminal Justice Ethics* (January 1, 2006).

45. U.S. Department of Justice, "Memorandum of Law as Amicus Curiae"; filed in *Buddy Cason v. Jim Seckinger,* 231 F.3d 777 (2000), at 23.

46. ACA, *ACI* (2003) 4-4429 on "Scope of Services," *Standards for Adult Correctional Institutions,* 4th ed. (Lanham, MD: American Correctional Association, 2003) as updated in the *2014 Standards Supplement: Adult Correctional Institutions ACI*, 4th ed. (Alexandria, VA: American Correctional Association, 2014).

47. ACA, *ACI* (2003) 4-4142 on "Housing for the Disabled."

48. ACA, *ACI* (2003) 4-4429-1 on "Scope of Services" as updated in *2014 Standards Supplement.*

49. Deanna Johnson, "The Current State of HIPAA in Corrections," *CorrectCare* (Fall 2013), 14, 25.

50. As seen from judicial decisions such as *Morgan v. Sproat; S.D. v. Parish of Orleans, LA;* and *Gary H. v. Hegstrom.* Citations and further detail about these cases are provided in the next section.

51. Juvenile Justice and Delinquency Prevention Act of 1974, as amended 2002 (42 U.S.C. 5601ff).

52. James Austin, Kelly Dedel Johnson, and Maria Gregoriou, *Juveniles in Adult Prisons and Jails: A National Assessment* (Washington, DC: U.S. Department of Justice, Office of Juvenile Justice and Delinquency Prevention, October 2000), 11.

53. Austin et al., *Juveniles in Adult Prisons.*

54. 42 U.S.C. §1997e *et seq.*

55. *Brock v. Kenton County, KY,* 93 Fed. Appx. 793, 6th Cir. (2004).

56. Feierman, "Testimony of Juvenile Law Center," 3.

57. Feierman, "Testimony of Juvenile Law Center," 2–3.

58. *Schloendorff v. Society of New York Hospital*, 211 N.Y. 125, 105 N.E. 92 (1914).

59. *Spicer v. Williamson*, 191 N.C. 487, 490, 132 S.E. 291, 293 (1926).

60. *Ex parte Hull*, 312 U.S. 546 (1941).

61. *Coffin v. Reichard*, 143 F. 2d 443, 6th Cir. (1944).

62. *Trop v. Dulles*, 356 U.S. 86, 101 (1958).

63. *Monroe v. Pape*, 365 U.S. 167 (1961).

64. *Robinson v. California*, 370 U.S. 660 (1962).

65. *Jackson v. Bishop*, 404 F. 2d 571, 8th Cir. (1968).

66. *Holt v. Sarver*, 442 F. 2d 304 (1971).

67. *Bivens v. Six Unknown Agents of the Federal Bureau of Narcotics*, 403 U.S. 388 (1971).

68. *Procunier v. Martinez*, 416 U.S. 396 (1974).

69. *Wolff v. McDonnell*, 418 U.S. 539 (1974).

70. *Newman v. Alabama*, 349 F. Supp. 278 aff'd. 503 F. 2d 1320, 5th Cir. (1974), cert denied 421 U.S. 948.

71. *Gates v. Collier*, 501 F. 2d 1291 1319. CA5 (1974).

72. *Battle v. Anderson*, 376 F. Supp. 402, E.D. OK (1974) at 26.

73. *Estelle v. Gamble*, 429 U.S. 97 (1976).

74. *Todaro v. Ward*, 565 F. 2d 48 (1977).

75. *Rennie v. Klein,* 462 F. Supp. 1131, D.N.J. (1978).

76. *Rennie v. Klein*, 653 F. 2d 836 at 844–847, 3rd Cir. (1981).

77. *Bell v. Wolfish*, 441 U.S. 520 (1979).

78. *Rogers v. Okin*, 478 F. Supp. 1342, D. Mass. (1979).

79. *Vitek v. Jones*, 445 U.S. 480 (1980).

80. *Carlson v. Green*, 446 U.S. 14 (1980).

81. *Ruiz v. Estelle*, 503 F. Supp 1265, S.D. Texas (1980); rev'd in part 679 F. 2d 1115, 5th Cir. (1982); modified in part, 688 F. 2d 266, 5th Cir. (1982).

82. *Youngberg v. Romeo*, 457 U.S. 307 (1982).

83. *Dean v. Coughlin*, 804 F. 2d 207 (1986).

84. *Turner v. Safley,* 482 U. S. 78 (1987)

85. *West v. Atkins*, 487 U.S. 42 (1988).

86. *Phillips v. Michigan Department of Corrections*, 731 F. Supp. 792, Dist. Court, W.D. Mich. (1990) and affirmed 932 F 2d 969 (1991).

87. *Washington v. Harper*, 494 U.S. 210 (1990).

88. *Wilson v. Seiter*, 501 U.S. 294 (1991).

89. *Helling v. McKinney,* 509 U.S. 25 (1993).

90. *Farmer v. Brennan*, 511 U.S. 825 (1994).

91. *Madrid v. Gómez*, 889 F. Supp. 1146, 1280, N.D. Cal. (1995), 190 F.3d 990 (1999).

92. *Sandin v. Conner*, 515 U.S. 472 (1995).

93. *Lewis v. Casey*, 518 U.S. 343 (1996).

94. *Pennsylvania Department of Corrections v. Yeskey,* 524 U.S. 206 (1998).

95. *Sell v. United States*, 539 U.S. 166 (2003), 123 S. Ct. 2174 (2003).

96. *Stouffer v. Reid*, 413 Md. 491, 993 A2d 104 (2010).

97. *Minneci v. Pollard*, 132 S. Ct. 617 (2012), 565 U.S. ____ (2012)

98. *Coleman v. Brown*, 912 F. Supp. 1282 (1995).

99. *Plata v. Brown*, Docket no. 3:01-cn-01351-TEH, N.D. Cal.

100. *Brown v. Plata*, 131 S. Ct. 1910 (2011), 563 U.S. 493 (2011), 134 S. Ct. 436 (2013).

101. *Ross v. Blake*, 578 U.S. ____ (2016). This case was decided June 6, 2016.

102. *Lollis v. New York State Department of Social Services*, S.D.N.Y., 1970, 322 F. Supp. 473 (1970).

103. *Nelson v. Heyne*, 491 F. 2d 352 (January 31, 1974).

104. *Morgan v. Sproat*, 432 F. Supp. 1130, S.D. Miss. (1977).

105. CRIPA Investigation of Oakley and Columbia Training Schools in Raymond and Columbia, Mississippi (June 19, 2003). Letter from U.S. Assistant Attorney General Ralph F. Boyd Jr. to Ronnie Musgrove, governor of Mississippi, on June 19, 2003.

106. *D.B. v. Tewksbury*, 545 F. Supp. 896, D. Or. (1982).

107. *Morales v. Turman,* 820 F.2d 728, 56 USLW 2045 and 430 U.S. 322 (1977).

108. Texas Youth Commission, "A Brief History of the Texas Youth Commission."

109. *Gary H. v. Hegstrom*, 831 F. 2d 1439 (1987).

110. *Alexander S. v. Boyd*, 876 F. Supp. 773, 778, D.S.C. (1995).

111. *S.D. v. Parish of Orleans, LA* (2001).

112. *United States v. Louisiana et al.*, Civil Action No. 98-947-B-1, M.D. La. (1998).

113. Petitioner's Brief in Support of Motion to Modify (November 27, 2001).

114. Letter and Report from U.S. Department of Justice to Governor Mike Foster.

115. *Jackson v. Ft. Stanton* and *Jackson v. Los Lunas State Hospital and Training School,* 757 F.Supp. 1243 (D.N.M. 1990); 964 F2d 980 (1992).

116. The detailed monitoring reports are available to the public at http://www .jacksoncommunityreview.org. Retrieved May 7, 2016.

117. *A.M. v. Luzerne County Juvenile Detention Center,* 372 F. 3d 572, 3d Cir. (2004).

118. *K.L.W. v. James*, 204-CV-149BN (2005).

119. *Minix v. Pazera*, 3:06-CV-398, 2007 WL 4233455, N.D. Ind. (2007).

120. *J.A. et al. v. Barbour et al.*, 3:07-CV-00394 (2007).

121. Robert B. Greifinger, "The Acid Bath of Cynicism," *CorrectCare* (Spring 2015), 4.

122. Vincent P. Nathan, "Guest Editorial," *Journal of Prison Health Care*, 1 (1985), 3–12.

123. Vincent P. Nathan, "Have the Courts Made a Difference in the Quality of Prison Conditions? What Have We Accomplished to Date?" *Pace Law Review* 24 (December 13, 2004), 420.

124. *Sandin v. Conner*, 515 U.S. 472 (1995).

125. *Lewis v. Casey*, 518 U.S. 343 (1996).

126. For example, *Watts v. Ramos*, 948 F. Supp. 739, N.D. IL. (1996).

127. Vincent P. Nathan, "Have the Courts Made a Difference?" 425.

128. American Correctional Association, "Public Correctional Policy on Term 'Correctional Officer.' " Adopted 1999 and last reviewed and amended January 14, 2009.

129. William C. Collins, "A History of Recent Corrections Is a History of Court Involvement," *Corrections Today* (August 1995), 114, 116, 150.

130. *Madrid v. Gómez,* 889 F. Supp. 1146, 1280, N.D. Cal. (1995). These concerns are discussed in this chapter under "A New Challenge—The Impact of Mass Incarceration" and also in Chapter 3, "Other Challenging Topics in Ethics," under "Housing Mentally Ill in Isolation or Supermax Settings."

131. William C. Collins, "A History of Recent Corrections."

132. Decimus Junius Juvenalis, *Satire No. 6*: 347–348 (circa 120 CE).

133. A full audio transcript of the hearing is available at http://www.oyez.org.

134. 18 U.S.C. § 3626(a)(3) (2006).

135. "Constitutional Law—Eighth Amendment—Eastern District of California Holds that Prisoner Release Is Necessary to Remedy Unconstitutional California Prison Conditions.—*Coleman v. Schwarzenegger*," *Harvard Law Review* 123 (2010), 754, footnote 33.

136. David R. Shaw, *Summary and Analysis of the First 17 Medical Inspections of California Prisons*, Bureau of Audits and Investigations, Office of Inspector General, State of California (August 2010): 2, 3.

137. "*Brown v. Plata*," Legal Information Institute.

138. Rob Kuznia, "An Unprecedented Experiment in Mass Forgiveness," *Washington Post*, February 8, 2016.

139. A comprehensive review of the *Plata v. Brown* saga, its history and implications, and the extreme consequences of mass incarceration, can be found in Jonathan Simon, *Mass Incarceration on Trial: A Remarkable Court Decision and the Future of Prisons in America* (New York: New Press, 2014). Another excellent analysis is available in Keramet Reiter and Natalie Pifer, *"Brown v. Plata,"* Oxford Handbooks Online. Oxford, UK: Oxford University Press, 2014. http://www.oxfordhandbooks.com/view/10.1093/oxfordhb/978019 9935383.001.0001/oxfordhb-9780199935383-e-113.

140. Joseph N. Parsons, "A Constitutional and Political High Wire Act," *University of Pittsburgh Law Review* 75 (Fall 2013) 109.

141. ACA, "Public Correctional Policy on Conditions of Confinement," as amended in August 2006 and reviewed and reaffirmed without amendment July 21012, *ACA Public Correctional Policies* (Alexandria, VA: American Correctional Association, 2012).

142. "Equal Protection—Application to Incarcerated Persons—Inmate Racial Segregation: *Johnson v. California,"* *Harvard Law Review* 119(1) (November 2005), 233, 235, 238.

143. Bradley Schwartz, "Pres. Obama: 80 Billion Dollars for Prisons Hurts USA," prisonpath, April 25, 2016.

CHAPTER 5

1. Robert B. Greifinger, "Inmates As Public Health Sentinels," *Washington University Journal of Law & Policy* 22 (2006), 253.

2. Available at "Health Management Resources," Federal Bureau of Prisons.

3. U.S. Preventive Services Task Force, "Recommendations."

4. NCCHC (2014) P-G-01 (essential) on "Chronic Disease Services," *Standards for Health Services in Prisons, 2014* (Chicago: National Commission on Correctional Health Care, 2014).

5. These principles are also discussed in Chapter 1, "Ethics in the Context of Correctional Health," under "Important Ethical Issues in Corrections."

6. Dean P. Rieger, "When Is a Decision Not to Treat the Right Choice? Distinguishing between Serious and Nonserious Conditions," *Journal of Correctional Health Care* 13(4) (October 2007), 248–249.

7. U.S. Department of Veterans Affairs, Coalition Working Group, *Principles of a Sound Drug Formulary System* (October 2000), 5. The recommendations of the Coalition Working Group were endorsed by the American Medical Association, the Academy of Managed Care Plans, the American Society of Health System Pharmacists, and the U.S. Pharmacopeia.

8. Health through Walls, http://www.healththroughwalls.org.

9. See also Chapter 1, "Ethics in the Context of Correctional Health," under "Organ Transplants."

10. See Chapter 1, "Ethics in the Context of Correctional Health," under "Transgender Issues."

11. Several courts have ruled that lack of funds is neither a defense nor an excuse for failure to provide adequate health care for prisoners. For example, *Anderson v. City of Atlanta*, 778 F. 2d 678 (1985); *Hamilton v. Love,* 328 F. Supp. 1182 at 1194, E.D. Ark. (1971), *Ozecki v. Gaugham,* 459 F. 2d 6, 8, 1st Cir. (1972); *Smith v. Sullivan,* 553 F. 2d 373 (1977). This topic is discussed in Chapter 4, "Legal Issues in Correctional Health Care," under "Adequacy of Funding."

12. John W. Ward and Jonathan H. Mermin, "Simple, Effective, but Out of Reach? Public Health Implications of HCV Drugs," *New England Journal of Medicine* (November 17, 2015).

13. This is discussed earlier in this chapter under "Universal Principles."

14. Barack Obama, "Presidential Proclamation—National Donate Life Month, 2016," April 1, 2016.

15. "Facts and Myths," American Transplant Foundation, Denver, CO.

16. Roderic Gottula, "The Importance of Defining Medical Necessity," *CorrectCare* (Fall 1996), 4.

17. Armond Start, "Physician Recommends Format for Determining Necessity," *CorrectCare* (Fall 1996), 4, 7.

18. Armond Start, MD, MPH, was a highly respected pediatrician who served as statewide medical director for corrections in Oklahoma and Texas during the mid-1970s. He was a passionate champion of professional quality in medical practice and a dedicated advocate for the improvement of health care services of the incarcerated.

19. Armond Start, "Physician Recommends Format for Determining Necessity."

CHAPTER 6

1. The *Diagnostic and Statistical Manual* has been published by the American Psychiatric Association since 1952. The DSM-5 was published in 2013.

2. *Highlights of Changes from DSM-IV-TR to DSM-5*, American Psychiatric Association (2013).

3. Each axis of a multiaxial diagnosis related to a different aspect of a patient's disorder or disability. Axis I: clinical disorders, including major mental disorders and developmental and learning disorders, including depression, anxiety disorders, bipolar disorder, attention deficit hyperactivity disorder, and schizophrenia. Axis II: underlying pervasive or personality conditions, included borderline personality disorder, schizotypal personality disorder, antisocial personality disorder, narcissistic personality disorder, and mild mental retardation, as well as mental retardation. Axis III: acute medical conditions and physical disorders, included drug-related problems. Axis IV: psychosocial and environmental factors contributing to the disorder. Axis V: global assessment of functioning (GAF).

4. Victoria E. Kress et al., *The Removal of the Multiaxial System in the DSM-5: Implications and Practice Suggestions for Counselors The Professional Counselor* 4(3) (2014), 191–201.

5. "Principles for the Protection of Persons with Mental Illness and the Improvement of Mental Health Care." United Nations Resolution 46/119 of 1991.

6. Ahmed Okasha, "Mental Patients in Prisons: Punishment versus Treatment," *World Psychiatry* 3(1) (February 2004), 2.

7. Lisa M. Boesky, *Juvenile Offenders with Mental Health Disorders, Who Are They, and What Do We Do with Them?* 2nd ed. (Alexandria, VA: American Correctional Association, 2010), 10–11.

8. John Howard, *The State of the Prisons in England and Wales* (Warrington, UK: William Eyers, 1777), 16. Digitized by Getty Research Institute (2011).

9. E. Fuller Torrey, *Out of the Shadows: Confronting America's Mental Illness Crisis* (New York: John Wiley & Sons, 1997), 27–28.

10. *Olmstead v. L.C. and E.W.*, 527 U.S. 581 (1999).

11. Mark S. Salzer, Katy Kaplan, and Joanne Atay, "State Psychiatric Hospital Census after the 1999 Olmstead Decision: Evidence of Decelerating Deinstitutionalization," *Psychiatric Services* 57 (October 2006), 1501–1504.

12. U.S. Bureau of the Census.

13. Torrey, *Out of the Shadows*, 10, 100.

14. E. Fuller Torrey et al., *No Room at the Inn: Trends and Consequences of Closing Public Psychiatric Hospitals, 2005–2010*. Arlington, VA: The Treatment Advocacy Center (July 19, 2012).

15. E. Fuller Torrey, "A Dearth of Psychiatric Beds," *Psychiatric Times* (February 25, 2016).

16. "State Mental Health Cuts: A National Crisis," National Alliance on Mental Illness (March 2011). https://www.nami.org/getattachment/About-NAMI/Publications/Reports/NAMIStateBudgetCrisis2011.pdf.

17. Richard M. Austin and Albert S. Duncan, "Handle with Care: Special Inmates, Special Needs," *Corrections Today* (June 1998), 118.

18. Linda A. Teplin, "Policing the Mentally Ill: Styles, Strategies, and Implications," in *Jail Diversion for the Mentally Ill: Breaking through the Barriers,* ed. Henry J. Steadman (Washington, DC: National Institute of Corrections, 1990), 11–13.

19. Ronald Jemelka, "The Mentally Ill in Local Jails: Issues in Admission and Booking," in *Jail Diversion for the Mentally Ill: Breaking through the Barriers,* ed. Henry J. Steadman (Washington, DC: National Institute of Corrections, 1990), 39.

20. Terry A. Kupers, "Testimony before the Commission on Safety and Abuse in America's Prisons" (Newark, NJ, July 28, 2006).

21. Doris J. James and Lauren F. Glaze, "Mental Health Problems of Prison and Jail Inmates," *Bureau of Justice Statistics Special Report,* NCJ 213600 (September 2006), 1.

22. Mark Hornbeck, "Mentally Ill Flood Prisons," *The Detroit News* (December 4, 1997), 13A.

23. James and Glaze, "Mental Health Problems," Table 1. *See also* Andrew F. Angelino, Jeffrey L. Metzner, and Henry C. Weinstein, *Caring for Individuals with Schizophrenia in Correctional Settings* (Chicago: NCCHC, 2009).

24. Jane E. Haddad, "Management of the Chronically Mentally Ill within a Correctional Environment" *CorrectCare* 5(1) (January 1991), 5.

25. Bonita M. Veysey and Gisela Bichler-Robertson, "Prevalence Estimates of Psychiatric Disorders in Correctional Settings," in *Health Status of Soon-To-Be-Released Inmates*, Vol. 2, National Commission on Correctional Health Care (April 2002), 57–80.

26. Miles B. Santamour, *The Mentally Retarded Offender and Corrections* (Lanham, MD: American Correctional Association, 1989).

27. Torrey, *Out of the Shadows*, 31.

28. *Tillery v. Owens*, 719 F. Supp 1256, 1286, W.D. Pa. (1989), aff'd 907 F. 2d 418, 3rd Cir. (1990).

29. Loren H. Roth, "Correctional Psychiatry," in *Forensic Psychiatry and Psychology,* ed. William J. Curran, A. Louis McGarry, and Saleem A. Shah (Philadelphia: F.A. Davis Company, 1986), 434.

30. Leona L. Bachrach, "An Overview of Deinstitutionalization," *New Directions for Mental Health Services* 17 (1983), 5–14.

31. Saundra Maass-Robinson and Pamela Everett Thompson, "Mood Disorders in Incarcerated Women," in *Health Issues among Incarcerated Women,* ed. Ronald L. Braithwaite, Kimberly Jacob Arriola, and Cassandra Newkirk (New Brunswick, NJ: Rutgers University Press, 2006), 104–105.

32. Dean Aufderheide, "Mental Illness in Administrative Segregation: How to Bulletproof Your Program Against Litigation," *CorrectCare* (Spring 2013), 15.

33. Centers for Disease Control and Prevention, "Traumatic Brain Injury in Prisons and Jails: An Unrecognized Problem" (undated).

34. Barbara Burchell Curtis, "Traumatic Brain Injury: How to Assess and Manage an Often-Hidden Condition," *CorrectCare* (Spring 2012), 10, 11.

35. This phenomenon is discussed more thoroughly in Chapter 3, "Other Challenging Topics in Ethics," under "Housing the Mentally Ill in Isolation or Supermax Settings."

CHAPTER 7

1. Tom L. Beauchamp and James F. Childress, *Principles of Biomedical Ethics*, 4th ed. (New York: Oxford University Press, 1994), 189.

2. Cf. Chapter 9, "Corrections and Health Care Working Together," under "Recognizing Differences."

3. Margaret D. Wishart and Nancy N. Dubler, *Health Care in Prisons, Jails and Detention Centers: Some Legal and Ethical Dilemmas* (Bronx, NY: Montefiore Medical Center, 1983).

4. Michelle Staples-Horne, "Sugar and Spice: Understanding the Health of Incarcerated Girls," in *Health Issues among Incarcerated Women,* ed. Ronald L. Braithwaite, Kimberly Jacob Arriola, and Cassandra Newkirk (New Brunswick, NJ: Rutgers University Press, 2006), 73.

5. Jamie S. Brodie, "Caring—The Essence of Correctional Nursing," *CorrectCare* 14(4) (Fall 2000), 15.

6. Judith A. Stanley, "Standing Up to Medication Practice Challenges (Part 2)," *CorrectCare* (Spring 2007), 19.

7. One sometimes views the managed care scene in corrections as only applying to those systems that contract with a "managed care firm" to set up a formal mechanism for approval or denial of costly medical procedures. Some of these approaches make use of highly sophisticated algorithms and formulae, but in a broader sense all correctional health care programs are managed care because the party paying for the care ultimately influences the care to be provided.

CHAPTER 8

1. ACA, *ACI* (2003) 4-4380 (mandatory) on "Health Authority," *Standards for Adult Correctional Institutions,* 4th ed. (Lanham, MD: American Correctional Association, 2003) as updated in the *2014 Standards Supplement: Adult Correctional Institutions ACI,* 4th ed. (Alexandria, VA: American Correctional Association, 2014).

2. NCCHC (2014) P-A-02 (essential) on "Responsible Health Authority," *Standards for Health Services in Prisons 2014* (Chicago: National Commission on Correctional Health Care, 2014).

3. *Estelle v. Gamble*, 429 U.S. at 104–105 (1976), 97 S. Ct. at 291.

4. ACA, *ACI* (2003) 4-4381 (mandatory) on "Provision of Treatment" as updated in *2014 Standards Supplement.*

5. NCCHC 2014 P-A-03 (essential) on Medical Autonomy.

6. APHA, *Standards for Health Services in Correctional Institutions*, 3rd ed. (Washington, DC: American Public Health Association, 2003), 5.

7. ACA *ACI* (2003) 4-4380 (mandatory) on "Health Authority."

8. NCCHC (2014) P-A-02 (essential) on "Responsible Health Authority."

9. B. Jaye Anno, *Prison Health Care: Guidelines for the Management of an Adequate Delivery System* (Chicago: National Commission on Correctional Health Care, 1991), 72.

10. B. Jaye Anno, *Correctional Health Care: Guidelines for the Management of an Adequate Delivery System* (Chicago: National Commission on Correctional Health Care, 2001), 101.

11. Edward M. Brecher and Richard D. Della Penna, *Health Care in Correctional Institutions* (Washington, DC: U.S. Government Printing Office, 1975), 45, 46.

12. Kenneth L. Faiver (research director and principal author), *Key to Health for a Padlocked Society: Design for Health Care in Michigan Prisons* (Lansing, MI: Office of Health and Medical Affairs (March 1975), v, vi, 5, 301. Due credit must be given to members of the Governor's Advisory Committee for State Correctional Health Care and to three talented staff members who contributed to the research and the writing of the report: T. Richard Currier, Joseph A. Droste, and Peter L. Grenier.

13. "Report of the Medical Advisory Committee on State Prisons," Commonwealth of Massachusetts (December, 1971), in *Medical and Health Care in Jails, Prisons, and Other Correctional Facilities: A Compilation of Standards and Materials* (Washington, DC: American Bar Association, August 1974), 97.

14. "The Captive Patient: Prison Health Care: A Report of the Kentucky Public Health Association," (January, 1974), in: *Medical and Health Care in Jails, Prisons, and* Other *Correctional Facilities*, 142.

15. Anno, *Correctional Health Care: Guidelines,* 3rd ed., 98.

16. Anita Cardwell and Maeghan Gilmore, *County Jails and the Affordable Care Act: Enrolling Eligible Individuals in Health Coverage*, National Association of Counties (March 2012), 6.

17. Anno, *Correctional Health Care: Guidelines,* 3rd ed., 107.

18. Anno, *Correctional Health Care: Guidelines,* 3rd ed., 106–107.

CHAPTER 9

1. Armand Start, "Interaction between Correctional Staff and Health Care Providers in the Delivery of Medical Care," in *Clinical Practice in Correctional Medicine*, ed. Michael Puisis (St. Louis: Mosby, 1998), 28.

2. ACA, "Public Correctional Policy on Use of Appropriate Sanctions and Controls," last amended 2008, *ACA Public Correctional Policies* (Alexandria, VA: American Correctional Association 2012).

3. ACA, "Public Correctional Policy on Use of Force" (last amended 2010).

4. Lisa Leone, "Corrections and Health Care Professionals Learn Side by Side," *On the Line* 30(2) (March 2007).

5. Erik N. Schlosser, "A Framework for Correctional/Mental Health Partnership," *CorrectCare* (Winter 2006), 13.

6. Schlosser, "A Framework."

7. Bruce Mendelsohn, "The Right Stuff: An Interview with Dr. Kenneth Moritsugu," *Corrections ALERT Special Report* (Gaithersburg, MD: Aspen Publications, Feb. 26, 1996), 4.

8. ACA, "Public Correctional Policy on Correctional Health Care" (last amended 2011).

9. ACA, *ACI* 4-4381 (mandatory) on "Provision of Treatment," *Standards for Adult Correctional Institutions*, 4th ed. (Lanham, MD: American Correctional Association, 2003) as updated in the *2014 Standards Supplement: Adult Correctional institutions* (ACI), 4th ed. (Alexandria, VA: American Correctional Association, 2014).

10. NCCHC (2014) P-A-03 (essential) on "Medical Autonomy," National Commission on Correctional Health Care, *Standards for Health Services in Prisons* (Chicago: NCCHC, 2014).

11. Joel A. Dvoskin, "Confessions of an Incrementalist," *Public Service Psychology.* American Psychological Association (Spring 1999).

12. ACA, *ACI* (2003) 4-4084 on "Correctional Officers" as updated in *2014 Standards Supplement*; and ACA, *ACI* (2003) 4-4082 on "Orientation."

13. ACA, *ACI* (2003) 4-4389 (mandatory) on "Emergency Response" as updated in 2014 *Standards Supplement.*

14. NCCHC *Standard* (2014) P-C-04 (essential) on "Health Training for Correctional Officers."

15. NCCHC *Standard* (2014) P-C-05 (essential) on "Medication Administration Training."

16. See further discussion on this topic in Chapter 2, "Areas of Significant Ethical Role Conflict," under "Writing Tickets."

17. Gandhi's statement before C. N. Broomfield, I.C.S., District and Sessions Judge, Ahmedabad (March 18, 1922).

18. An excellent presentation on this subject was delivered by Joyce Rackauskis-Anderson titled "Exercise-Induced Rhabdomyolysis in a Correctional Setting" at the Updates in Correctional Health Care Conference (NCCHC) in Orlando, Florida, on May 8, 2007.

19. "Sickle Cell Anemia: Risk Factors," Mayo Clinic.com.

20. "Diseases and Conditions Index: Sickle Cell Anemia," National Heart Lung and Blood Institute.

21. Scott Savage, "After the Zap: Taser Injuries and How to Treat Them," *CorrectCare* (Summer 2005).

Also see J. M. Sanford et al., "Two Patients Subdued with a Taser Device: Cases and Review of Complications," *Journal of Emergency Medicine* (April 23, 2008).

22. The real life heroes in this true story were Dr. Kenneth L. Cole, DO, and Warden Dale E. Foltz of the State Prison of Southern Michigan.

23. ACA, *ACI* (2003) 4-4190-1 on "Use of Restraints" as revised in *2014 Standards Supplement.*

24. ACA "Public Correctional Policy on Use of Restraints with Pregnant Offenders" (ratified 2012).

25. NCCHC (2014) P-G-09 (essential) on "Counseling and Care of the Pregnant Inmate."

EPILOGUE

1. *High Flight,* a sonnet by John Gillespie Magee, an American pilot serving in the Royal Canadian Air Force who was killed in December 1941 during a training flight in Britain at age 19. Arlington National Cemetery Web site: http://arlingtoncemetery.net/highflig.htm.

Bibliography

GENERAL BIBLIOGRAPHY

Abramsky, Sasha. "Return of the Madhouse." *The American Prospect* (February 11, 2002).

Advisory Committee on Human Radiation Experiments (ACHRE). "Chapter 9. Prisoners: A Captive Research Population." *Final Report of the Advisory Committee on Human Radiation Experiments*. Advisory Committee on Human Radiation Experiments. Washington, DC: National Archives and Records Administration, 1995. https://ia80 0209.us.archive.org/2/items/advisorycommitte00unit/advisorycommitte00unit.pdf. Accessed July 6, 2016.

Allen, Scott A., Robert L. Cohen, and William J. Rold. "Dual Loyalties: Our Role in Preventing Inmate Abuse." *CorrectCare* 20(3), Summer 2006.

Alving, Alf S., Branch Craige, Jr., Theodore N. Pullman, C. Merrill Whorton, Ralph Jones, Jr., and Lillian Eichelberger. "Procedures Used at Stateville Penitentiary for the Testing of Potential Antimalarial Agents." *Journal of Clinical Investigation* 27(3) (May 1948), Pt. 2, 2–5.

American Academy of Psychiatry and the Law. *Ethical Guidelines for the Practice of Forensic Psychiatry*. Section II. (2005). http://www.aapl.org/ethics.htm. Accessed May 27, 2016.

American Bar Association (ABA). "Report to the House of Delegates, No. 102B." ABA, Criminal Justice Section. http://www.abanet.org/leadership/2007/midyear/docs /SUMMARYOFRECOMMENDATIONS/hundredtwob.doc. Accessed April 20, 2016.

American Civil Liberties Union (ACLU). *2015 Legislative Report Card*. https://www .acluofnorthcarolina.org/files/legislative/aclunc_2015_legislative_report_card.pdf. Accessed July 13, 2016.

American Civil Liberties Union (ACLU). "Federal Court Upholds Transgender Peoples' Right to Access Medical Treatment in Prison" (August 5, 2011). https://www.aclu .org/news/federal-court-upholds-transgender-peoples-right-access-medical

-treatment-prison?redirect=lgbt-rights/federal-court-upholds-transgender-peoples
-right-access-medical-treatment-prison. Accessed July 13, 2016.

American College of Correctional Physicians (ACCP). "Restricted Housing of Mentally
Ill Inmates: Position Statement." Adopted by the Society of Correctional Physicians
Board of Directors, July 9, 2013. http://societyofcorrectionalphysicians.org
/resources/position-statements/restricted-housing-of-mentally-ill-inmates. Accessed
July 12, 2016.

American College of Correctional Physicians (ACCP). *Code of Ethics.* http://societyof-
correctionalphysicians.org/resources/code-of-ethics. (2016). Accessed May 14,
2016.

American Correctional Association (ACA). *Code of Ethics.* Adopted by the Board of Governors and Delegates Assembly, August 1994. http://www.aca.org/ACA_Prod_IMIS
/ACA_Member/About_Us/Code_of_Ethics/ACA_Member/AboutUs/Code_of
_Ethics.aspx?hkey=61577ed2-c0c3-4529-bc01-36a248f79eba. Accessed July 13,
2016.

American Correctional Association (ACA). *Standards for Adult Correctional Institutions*
(ACI), 4th ed. (Lanham, MD: American Correctional Association, 2003).

American Correctional Association (ACA). *Standards Supplement: Adult Correctional
Institutions* (ACI), 4th ed. (Alexandria, VA: American Correctional Association,
2014).

American Correctional Association (ACA). *Performance-Based Standards for Juvenile Correctional Facilities* (JCF), 4th ed. (Alexandria, VA: American Correctional Association, 2009).

American Correctional Association (ACA). *Public Correctional Policies, 2012* (Alexandria, VA: American Correctional Association, 2012). http://edpdlaw.com/aca.policies
.pdf. Accessed July 25, 2016.

American Correctional Health Services Association (ACHSA). *Code of Ethics.* (2016).
Accessed May 14, 2016.

American Medical Association (AMA). "Chapter 9: Opinions on Professional Self-
Regulation." *AMA Principles of Medical Ethics.* http://www.ama-assn.org/ama/pub
/physician-resources/medical-ethics/code-medical-ethics.page.

American Medical Association (AMA). *Code of Medical Ethics.* (Chicago: American Medical Association, June 2001) (revised).

American Medical Association (AMA). "Court-Initiated Medical Treatments in Criminal
Cases," CEJA Report 4-A-98 (American Medical Association Council on Ethical and
Judicial Affairs), 1998): 1.

American Nurses Association. Position Statement: "Nurses' Role in Capital Punishment" (January 28, 2010). http://www.nursingworld.org/MainMenuCategories/EthicsStandards
/Ethics-Position-Statements/prtetcptl14447.pdf. Accessed May 14, 2016.

American Pharmacists Association. *Code of Ethics for Pharmacists* (October 27, 1994).
http://www.pharmacist.com/code-ethics. Accessed July 3, 2016.

American Pharmacists Association. "House of Delegates Adopts Policy Discouraging
Pharmacist Participation in Executions," March 30, 2015. https://www.pharmacist
.com/apha-house-delegates-adopts-policy-discouraging-pharmacist-participation
-execution. Accessed December 12, 2016.

American Psychiatric Association (APA). "Position Statement on Segregation of Prisoners
with Mental Illness." Approved by Board of Trustees, December 2012, and approved

by the Assembly, November 2012. http://www.dhcs.ca.gov/services/MH/Documents /2013_04_AC_06c_APA_ps2012_PrizSeg.pdf. Accessed July 12, 2016.

American Psychiatric Association. *Highlights of Changes from DSM-IV-TR to DSM-5* (2013). http://www.dsm5.org/documents/changes%20from%20dsm-iv-tr%20to%20 dsm-5.pdf. Accessed June 7, 2016.

American Transplant Foundation. "Facts and Myths" (Denver: American Transplant Foundation, no date). http://www.americantransplantfoundation.org/about-transplant /facts-and-myths. Accessed July 27, 2016.

Angelino, Andrew F., Jeffrey L. Metzner, and Henry C. Weinstein. *Caring for Individuals with Schizophrenia in Correctional Settings* (Chicago: NCCHC, 2009).

Anno, B. Jaye. *Prison Health Care: Guidelines for the Management of an Adequate Delivery System* (Chicago: NCCHC, 1991).

Anno, B. Jaye. *Correctional Health Care: Guidelines for the Management of an Adequate Delivery System* (Chicago: NCCHC, 2001).

Anno, B. Jaye, Carmelia Graham, James E. Lawrence, and Ronald Shansky, *Correctional Health Care: Addressing the Needs of Elderly, Chronically Ill, and Terminally Ill Inmates* (Washington, DC: National Institute of Corrections, February 2004). http:// static.nicic.gov/Library/018735.pdf. Accessed December 12, 2016.

American Public Health Association (APHA). *Standards for Health Services in Correctional Institutions*, 3rd ed. (Washington, DC: American Public Health Association, 2003).

Appelbaum, Kenneth L. "American Psychiatry Should Join the Call to Abolish Solitary Confinement," *Journal of the American Academy of Psychiatry and Law* (43) (2015), 406–415, 407.

Appelbaum, Kenneth L. "Correctional Mental Health Research: Opportunities and Barriers." *Journal of Correctional Health Care* 14(4) (October 2008), 269–277.

Appelbaum, Paul S. "The Parable of the Forensic Psychiatrist: Ethics and the Problem of Doing Harm." *International Journal of Law and Psychiatry* 13(4) (1990), 249–259.

Aufderheide, Dean. "Mental Illness in Administrative Segregation: How to Bulletproof Your Program Against Litigation." *CorrectCare* (Spring 2013).

Austin, James, Kelly Dedel Johnson, and Maria Gregoriou. *Juveniles in Adult Prisons and Jails: A National Assessment* (Washington, DC: U.S. Department of Justice, Office of Juvenile Justice and Delinquency Prevention, October 2000).

Austin, Richard M., and Albert S. Duncan. "Handle with Care: Special Inmates, Special Needs." *Corrections Today* (June 1998).

Bachrach, Leona L. "An Overview of Deinstitutionalization." *New Directions for Mental Health Services* 17 (1983).

Bay, Rebecca. "Medical Management of Transgender, Transsexual and Gender Dysphoria: Time for Policy Revisions." Paper presented at NCCHC National Conference on Correctional Health Care, Orlando, Florida, October 20, 2009.

Beauchamp, Tom L., and James F. Childress. *Principles of Biomedical Ethics*, 4th ed. (New York: Oxford University Press, 1994).

Bell, Carl C. "An Ethical Conundrum in Correctional Health Care." *CorrectCare* (Spring 2012.

Belmont Report. *See* National Commission for the Protection of Human Subjects of Biomedical and Behavioral Research.

Black, Lee, and Robert M. Sade. "Lethal Injection and Physicians: State Law vs Medical Ethics." *Journal of the American Medical Association* 298(23) (December 19, 2007). http://www.deathpenaltyinfo.org/node/2264. Accessed May 27, 2016.

Blue, Ethan. "The Strange Career of Leo Stanley: Remaking Manhood at San Quentin State Penitentiary, 1913–1951." *Pacific Historical Review* 78(2) (May 2009), 210–241.

Boesky, Lisa M. *Juvenile Offenders with Mental Health Disorders: Who Are They, and What Do We Do with Them?* 2nd ed. (Alexandria, VA: American Correctional Association, 2010).

Boisaubin, Eugene V., Alexander G. Duarte, Patricia Blair, and T. Howard Stone. "'Well Enough to Execute': The Health Professional's Responsibility to the Death Row Inmate." *CorrectCare* (Fall 2004).

Borchelt, Gretchen. "Break Them Down: Systematic Use of Psychological Torture by U.S. Forces." Physicians for Human Rights (May 2005). http://physiciansforhumanrights. org/library/documents/reports/break-them-down-the.pdf. Accessed August 1, 2016.

Boston, John. "Court Rules on Smoking Case." *CorrectCare* 8(2) (May 1994).

Bradford, John M. W., and Anne Pawlak. "Double-Blind Placebo Crossover Study of Cyproterone Acetate in the Treatment of Paraphilias." *Archives of Sexual Behavior* (October 1993).

Bradley, Catherine Megan. "Old Remedies Are New Again: Deliberate Indifference and the Receivership in *Plata v. Schwarzenegger*." http://www.law.nyu.edu/sites/default/files /ecm_pro_064617.pdf. Accessed September 26, 2016.

Brecher, Edward M., and Richard D. Della Penna. *Health Care in Correctional Institutions* (Washington, DC: U.S. Government Printing Office, 1975).

"Brief for the Petitioner." *Baze and Bowling v. Rees.* 128 S. Ct. 1520 (2008). http://www .americanbar.org/content/dam/aba/publishing/preview/publiced_preview_briefs _pdfs_07_08_07_5439_Petitioner.authcheckdam.pdf. Accessed February 10, 2016.

"Brief of Professors and Practitioners of Psychology and Psychiatry as *Amicus Curiae* in Support of Respondent," *Reginald A. Wilkinson v. Charles E. Austin* (March 3, 2005). http://www.clearinghouse.net/chDocs/public/PC-OH-0001-0009.pdf. Acc essed August 23, 2016.

Bright, Stephen B. "Counsel for the Poor: The Death Sentence Not for the Worst Crime but for the Worst Lawyer." *Yale Law Journal* 103 (1994). http://www.soc.umn.edu /~samaha/cases/bright_counsel_poor.html. Accessed September 5, 2016.

Bright, Stephen B. "Testimony of Stephen B. Bright regarding the Prison Abuse Remedies Act." To the Subcommittee on Crime, Terrorism and Homeland Security of the Committee on the Judiciary, U.S. House of Representatives (April 22, 2008).

Brodie, Jamie S. "Caring—The Essence of Correctional Nursing." *CorrectCare* 14(4) (Fall 2000).

Brodie, Jamie S. "Caring, the Essence of Correctional Nursing." *Tennessee Nurse* 64(2) (2001), 10–12.

Brodsky, Stanley L. "Ethical Issues for Psychologists in Corrections." In *Who is the Client? The Ethics of Psychological Intervention in the Criminal Justice System,* ed. John Monahan (Washington, DC: American Psychological Association, 1980), 63–92.

"*Brown v. Plata.*" Legal Information Institute. https://www.law.cornell.edu/supct/pdf/09 -1233P.ZD1. Accessed August 2, 2016.

Brown, George R., and Everett McDuffie. "Health Care Policies Addressing Transgender Inmates in Prison Systems in the United States." *Journal of Correctional Health Care* 15(4) (October 2009), 280–291.

Bulman, Philip. "The Psychological Effects of Solitary Confinement." *Corrections Today* (June–July 2012), 58–59. http://www.co.el-paso.tx.us/pdefender/Documents/The _Psychological_Effect_of_Solitary_Confinement.pdf. Accessed July 24, 2016.

Cardwell, Anita, and Maeghan Gilmore. "County Jails and the Affordable Care Act: Enrolling Eligible Individuals in Health Coverage." National Association of Counties (March 2012). http://www.naco.org/programs/csd/Documents/Health%20Reform%20Implementation/County-Jails-HealthCare_WebVersion.pdf. Accessed August 31, 2016.

Centers for Disease Control and Prevention (CDC). "Traumatic Brain Injury in Prisons and Jails: An Unrecognized Problem." (No date). http://www.cdc.gov/traumaticbrainjury/pdf/Prisoner_TBI_Prof-a.pdf. Accessed August 29, 2016.

Chemerinsky, Erwin. *Federal Jurisdiction* (New York: Aspen Publishers, 2003).

Clarke, Margaret E., and W. Benton Gibbard. "Overview of Fetal Alcohol Spectrum Disorders for Mental Health Professionals." *Canadian Child and Adolescent Psychiatry Review* 3 (August 12, 2003), 57–63.

Cohen, Fred. "Isolation in Penal Settings." Written statement submitted by Fred Cohen to the Commission on Safety and Abuse in America's Prisons. Newark, NJ. (July 19, 2005). http://www.prisoncommission.org/statements/cohen_fred.pdf. Accessed December 12, 2010, and no longer available. http://archive.vera.org/files/public-hearing-2-day-1-panel-2-isolation.pdf. Accessed July 31, 2016.

Cohen, Robert L. "Statement before the Commission on Safety and Abuse in America's Prisons" (Newark, NJ: July 20, 2005).

Cohn, Felicia G. "The Ethics of End-of-Life Care for Prison Inmates." *Journal of Law, Medicine and Ethics* 27(3) (Fall 1999), 252–259.

Collins, William C. "A History of Recent Corrections Is a History of Court Involvement." *Corrections Today* (August 1995).

Collins, William C. *Correctional Law for the Correctional Officer*, 5th ed. (Alexandria, VA: American Correctional Association, 2010).

"Constitutional Law—Eighth Amendment—Eastern District of California Holds that Prisoner Release Is Necessary to Remedy Unconstitutional California Prison Conditions. *Coleman v. Schwarzenegger.*" *Harvard Law Review* 123 (2010). http://www.harvardlawreview.org/media/pdf/vol123_coleman_v_schwarzenegger.pdf. Accessed August 1, 2016.

Council for International Organizations of Medical Sciences (CIOMS). *International Ethical Guidelines for Biomedical Research Involving Human Subjects*. Prepared in collaboration with the World Health Organization (WHO) Geneva (2002). www.cioms.ch/publications/guidelines/guidelines_nov_2002_blurb.htm. Accessed January 22, 2016.

Curfman, Gregory D., Stephen Morrissey, and Jeffrey M. Drazen. "Physicians and Execution." *New England Journal of Medicine* 358 (January 24, 2008), 403–404.

Curry, Keith R. "Letter to Donna Brorby, Esq." (March 19, 2002), 6, 7. In *Ruiz v. Gary Johnson*. https://www.hrw.org/reports/2003/usa1003/Texas_ExpertCurry_Re_Ruiz V.Johnson.pdf. Accessed April 14, 2016.

Curtis, Barbara Burchell. "Traumatic Brain Injury: How to Assess and Manage an Often-Hidden Condition." *CorrectCare* (Spring 2012), 10–12.

Dale, Michael J. "Lawsuits and Public Policy: The Role of Litigation in Correcting Conditions in Juvenile Detention Centers." *University of San Francisco Law Review* 32 (Summer 1998).

Death Penalty Information Center. "One Year After Botched Execution, Many States Still Haven't Resumed Executions." http://www.deathpenaltyinfo.org/news/past/109/2015. Accessed May 15, 2016.

"Diseases and Conditions Index: Sickle Cell Anemia." National Heart Lung and Blood Institute. http://www.nhlbi.nih.gov/health/dci/Diseases/Sca/SCA_WhoIsAtRisk.html. Accessed December 17, 2010.

Doing Harm: Health Professionals' Central Role in the CIA Torture Program: Medical and Psychological Analysis of the 2014 U.S. Senate Select Committee on Intelligence Report's Executive Summary. Physicians for Human Rights (December 2014). https://s3.amazonaws.com/PHR_Reports/doing-harm-health-professionals-central -role-in-the-cia-torture-program.pdf. Accessed August 7, 2016.

Dole, Pamela. "Spotlight." *Hepp News* 2(6) (Providence, RI: Brown University School of Medicine, June 1999).

Dostoevsky, Fyodor. *The House of the Dead: Prison Life in Siberia, 1861–1862.* (Project Gutenberg). www.gutenberg.org/ebooks/37536?msg-welcome_stranger. Accessed August 15, 2016.

Dougherty, Sarah, and Vincent Iacopino. "CIA Documents Show How Deeply Doctors and Health Professionals Were Involved in Torture." Physicians for Human Rights (July 25, 2016). http://physiciansforhumanrights.org/blog/cia-documents-show-how-deeply-doctors-and-health-professionals-were-involved-in-torture.html. Accessed August 4, 2016.

Dubler, Nancy N., ed. *Standards for Health Services in Correctional Institutions,* 2nd ed. (Washington, DC: American Public Health Association, 1986).

Dvoskin, Joel A. "Confessions of an Incrementalist." *Public Service Psychology* (Spring 1999). www.vachss.com/guest_dispatches/dvoskin3.html. Accessed February 10, 2016.

Dvoskin, Joel A. "What Are the Odds on Predicting Violent Behavior?" *Journal of California AMI* 2(1). http://www.joeldvoskin.com/Dvoskin_1990.pdf. Accessed June 17, 2016.

"Enforcing the ADA: A Status Report from the Department of Justice." U.S. Department of Justice, Civil Rights Division, Disability Rights Section (January–March 2007). http://www.ada.gov/janmar07.pdf. Accessed April 29, 2016.

"Equal Protection—Application to Incarcerated Persons—Inmate Racial Segregation: *Johnson v. California.*" *Harvard Law Review* 119(1) (November 2005).

Evans, Paul. "The Americans with Disabilities Act and Inmates with Disabilities: The Extent to Which Title II of the Act Provides a Recourse." *Washington University Journal of Law & Policy* 22 (2006). http://openscholarship.wustl.edu/law_journal_law _policy/vol22/iss1/26. Accessed August 9, 2016.

Faiver, Kenneth L. (research director and principal author). *Key to Health for a Padlocked Society: Design for Health Care in Michigan Prisons, Volume 1.* Lansing, MI: Office of Health and Medical Affairs, March 1975.

Farber, Neil J., Brian M. Aboff, Joan Weiner, Elizabeth B. Davis, E. Gil Boyer, and Peter A. Ubel. "Physician's Willingness to Participate in the Process of Lethal Injection for Capital Punishment." *Annals of Internal Medicine* (November 2001). http://www .annals.org/content/135/10/884.full.pdf. Accessed June 15, 2016.

Fathi, David C. "The Common Law of Supermax Litigation." *Pace Law Review* (2004). http://digitalcommons.pace.edu/cgi/viewcontent.cgi?article=1209&context=plr. Accessed August 1, 2016.

Feierman, Jessica. "Testimony of Juvenile Law Center, Youth Law Center, National Center for Youth Law, and Center for Children's Law and Policy for the House Judiciary Subcommittees on Crime, Terrorism and Homeland Security and Constitution, Civil Rights and Civil Liberties" (November 8, 2007).

"Forced Psychotropic Medications Reviewed by Courts." *CorrectCare* 8, no. 2 (May, 1994).

Forsythe, Ian D. "A Guide to Civil Rights Liability under 42 U.S.C. §1983: An Overview of Supreme Court and Eleventh Circuit Precedent" (Orlando, FL: The Constitution Society, no date). http://www.constitution.org/brief/forsythe_42-1983.htm. Accessed May 6, 2016.

Friedman, Alfred M., and Abraham L. Halpern. "The Psychiatrists' Dilemma: A Conflict of Roles in Legal Executions." *Australian and New Zealand Journal of Psychiatry* 33 (1999), 620–635. http://www.wpanet.org/uploads/Publications/WPA_Books/Additional_Publications/WPA_Forums_on_Current_Opinion/psychiatrists-death-penalty.pdf. Accessed July 14, 2016.

Fry, Rodney L. "Transsexualism: A Correctional, Medical or Behavioral Health Issue?" *CorrectCare* (Winter 2003).

Gandhi, Mohandas. "Gandhi's statement before C. N. Broomfield, I.C.S., District and Sessions Judge." Ahmedabad (March 18, 1922).

García-Arroyo, José Manuel and María Luisa Domínguez-López (2014). "Subjective Aspects of Burnout Syndrome in the Medical Profession," *Psychology* 5, 2064–2072. http://dx.doi.org/10.4236/psych.2014.518209.Accessed January 4, 2017.

Gawande, Atul. "When Law and Ethics Collide—Why Physicians Participate in Executions." *New England Journal of Medicine* 354(12) (March 23, 2006), 1221–1229.

Gibbons, John J., and Nicholas de B. Katzenbach. "Summary of Findings and Recommendations." *Confronting Confinement: A Report of the Commission on Safety and Abuse in America's Prisons* (New York: Vera Institute of Justice, June 2006). http://archive.vera.org/sites/default/files/resources/downloads/Confronting_Confinement.pdf. Accessed April 27, 2016.

Goliszek, Andrew. *In the Name of Science: A History of Secret Programs, Medical Research, and Human Experimentation* (New York: St. Martin's Press, 2003).

Gostin, Lawrence O. "Biomedical Research Involving Prisoners: Ethical Values and Legal Regulation." *Journal of the American Medical Association* 297 (February 21, 2007), 737–740. http://Scholarship.law.Georgetown.edu/cgi/viewcontent.cgi?article=1478&context=facpub. Accessed January 25, 2016.

Gostin, Lawrence O., Cori Vanchieri, and Andrew Pope, eds. *Ethical Considerations for Research Involving Prisoners* (Washington, DC: Institute of Medicine, National Academies Press, 2006), 1–253. http://www.NAP.edu/catalog/11692.html. Accessed February 24, 2016.

Gottula, Roderic. "The Importance of Defining Medical Necessity," *CorrectCare* (Fall, 1996), 4.

Grassian, Stuart. "Psychiatric Effects of Solitary Confinement." Redacted from a declaration submitted in September 1993 in *Madrid v. Gomez*, 889 F. Supp. 1146, and presented as an attachment to testimony before the Commission on Safety and Abuse in America's Prisons (July 19, 2005).

Grassian, Stuart. "Testimony on Impact of Isolation." Written testimony for the Commission on Safety and Abuse in America's Prisons (July 19, 2005).

Greifinger, Robert B. "Commentary: Is It Politic to Limit Our Compassion?" *Journal of Law, Medicine and Ethics* 27(3) (Fall 1999), 235–236.

Greifinger, Robert B. "Disabled Prisoners and 'Reasonable Accommodation.'" *Criminal Justice Ethics* (January 1, 2006). http://www.thefreelibrary.com/Disabled+prisoners+and+%22reasonable+accommodation%22.-a0202365829. Accessed April 29, 2016.

Greifinger, Robert B. "Five Steps toward an Ethical Practice." *CorrectCare* (Fall 2009).

Greifinger, Robert B. "Inmates As Public Health Sentinels." *Washington University Journal of Law & Policy* 22 (2006), 253–264. http://openscholarship.wustl.edu/law _journal_law_policy/vol22/iss1/21. Accessed August 9, 2016.

Greifinger, Robert B. "The Acid Bath of Cynicism," *CorrectCare* (Spring 2015).

Grunberg, Frederic. "Patients and Society: the Double Allegiance of Psychiatrists." *Bulletin.* Canadian Psychiatric Association (October 2002). https://ww1.cpa-apc.org /Publications/Archives/Bulletin/2002/october/grunberg.pdf. Accessed May 13, 2016.

Haddad. Jane E., "Management of the Chronically Mentally Ill within a Correctional Environment." *CorrectCare* 5(1) (January 1991).

Hale, Janet Fraser, Arthur M. Brewer, and Warren Ferguson. "Correctional Health Primary Care: Research and Educational Opportunities." *Journal of Correctional Health Care* 14(4) (October 2008), 278–289.

Haney, Craig. "Second Report to the Court" (December 2003). In *Osterback v. Moore.* Case no. 97-2806-CIV-HUCK (S.D. Florida, 2001). http://www.clearinghouse.net/chDocs /public/PC-FL-0011-0006.pdf. Accessed July 13, 2016.

Hansen, Chris, and Gordon C. Kanska. "Ethical Problems: Cases and Commentaries." *Journal of Prison Health* 1(2) (Fall–Winter 1981), 97–104.

"Health Care Associations Join to Oppose Participation in Executions." *CorrectCare* 8(2) (May 1994).

"Health Groups Oppose A.G. on Executions." *CorrectCare* 7(1) (January–February 1993).

"Health Management Resources." Federal Bureau of Prisons. https://www.bop.gov /resources/health_care_mngmt.jsp. Accessed August 29, 2016.

Health through Walls. http://www.healththroughwalls.org. Accessed August 29, 2016.

Hilton, Robert. "Crushing Medications." *CorrectCare* 7(4) (November 1993).

Hodges, Robert E., James Hood, John E. Canham, Howerde E. Sauberlich, and Eugene M. Baker. "Clinical Manifestations of Ascorbic Acid Deficiency in Man." *American Journal of Clinical Nutrition* 24 (April 1971), 432–443. http://www.ajcn.org/cgi /content/abstract/24/4/432. Accessed March 19, 2016.

Hornbeck, Mark. "Mentally Ill Flood Prisons." *The Detroit News* (December 4, 1997).

Hornblum, Allen M. *Acres of Skin: Human Experiments at Holmesburg Prison* (New York: Routledge, 1998).

Howard, John. *The State of the Prisons in England and Wales* (Warrington, UK: William Eyers, 1777). Digitized by Getty Research Institute (2011). https://ia800206.us .archive.org/24/items/stateofprisonsin00howa/stateofprisonsin00howa_bw.pdf. Accessed August 29, 2016.

Institute of Medicine. *Crossing the Quality Chasm* (Washington, DC: The National Academies Press, 2001). http://www.iom.edu/~/media/Files/Report%20Files/2001 /Crossing-the-Quality-Chasm/Quality%20Chasm%202001%20%20report%20 brief.pdf. Accessed July 25. 2016.

Isele, William P. "Right to Treatment/Right to Refuse Treatment." *Corrections Today* (June 1983).

James, Doris J., and Lauren F. Glaze. "Mental Health Problems of Prison and Jail Inmates." *Bureau of Justice Statistics Special Report* (September 2006), NCJ 213600.

Jemelka, Ronald. "The Mentally Ill in Local Jails: Issues in Admission and Booking." In *Jail Diversion for the Mentally Ill: Breaking through the Barriers,* ed. Henry J. Steadman. (Washington, DC: National Institute of Corrections, 1990).

Johnson, Deanna. "The Current State of HIPAA in Corrections." *CorrectCare* (Fall 2013).

"Justice, Texas Style." *Newsweek* (October 6, 1986).

Juvenalis, Decimus Junius. *Satire No. 6*, 347–348 (circa 120 CE).

Juvenile Justice and Delinquency Prevention Act of 1974, as amended 2002. 42 U.S.C. 5601ff. http://www.ojjdp.gov/about/jjdpa2002titlev.pdf. Accessed September 5, 2016.

Kaeble, Danielle, Lauren E. Glaze, Anastasios Tsoutis, and Todd D. Minton. "Correctional Populations in the United States, 2014." Bureau of Justice Statistics (December 29, 2015) NCJ 249513. http://www.bjs.gov/index.cfm?ty=pbdetail&iid=5519. Accessed September 10, 2016.

Kagle, Jill Doner, and Sandra Kopels. "Confidentiality after *Tarasoff*." *Health and Social Work* 19(3) (August, 1994).

Kendig, Newton E. "Introduction." *Journal of Correctional Health Care* 14(4) (October 2008), 260–262.

Kress, Victoria E., Casey A. Barrio Minton, Nicole A. Adamson, Matthew J. Paylo, and Verl Pope. *The Removal of the Multiaxial System in the DSM-5: Implications and Practice Suggestions for Counselors.* (2014). http://tpcjournal.nbcc.org/the-removal-of-the-multiaxial-system-in-the-dsm-5-implications-and-practice-suggestions-for-counselors. Accessed June 7, 2016.

Kupers, Terry A. "Testimony before the Commission on Safety and Abuse in America's Prisons." Newark, New Jersey (July 28, 2006).

Kupers, Terry. "No Equal Justice: The Prison Litigation Reform Act in the United States." *Human Rights Watch* (June 16, 2009). Human Rights Watch telephone interview with Terry Kupers on November 14, 2008. https://www.hrw.org/report/2009/06/16/no-equal-justice/prison-litigation-reform-act-united-states#page. Accessed July 24, 2016.

Kurtzman, Josh. "Overcoming the Exhaustion Requirement of the Prison Litigation Reform Act." *Young Advocates E-Newsletter.* American Bar Association (January 7, 2016). apps.americanbar.org/litigation/committees/youngadvocate/articles/winter2016-0116-overcoming-exhaustion-requirement-prisoner-litigation-reform-act.html. Accessed May 5, 2016.

Kuznia, Rob. "An Unprecedented Experiment in Mass Forgiveness." *Washington Post,* February 8, 2016.

Laiño, Rubens. "Ethics in Prison Health Care." Paper presented at Second World Congress on Prison Health Care, Ottawa, Canada (August 31, 1983), and attended by the author. Excerpted from 16-page copy of Dr. Laiño's presentation issued by the Canadian Secretary of State to conference attendees.

LeBaron, Wayne D. *America's Nuclear Legacy* (Commack, NY: Nova Publishers, 1998).

Leone, Lisa. "Corrections and Health Care Professionals Learn Side by Side." *On the Line* 30(2) (March 2007).

Lerman, Daniel N. "Second Opinion: Inconsistent Deference to Medical Ethics in Death Penalty Jurisdictions." *Georgetown Law Journal* (August 2007) 1941–1978, http://georgetownlawjournal.org/files/pdf/95-6/Lerman.PDF.10.

Letter and report from U.S. Department of Justice to Governor Mike Foster (undated, estimated circa 1998). https://www.justice.gov/crt/louisiana-juveniles-findings-letter-1. Accessed August 1, 2016.

Letter from U.S. Assistant Attorney General Ralph F. Boyd, Jr. to Ronnie Musgrove, Governor of Mississippi. "CRIPA Investigation of Oakley and Columbia Training Schools in Raymond and Columbia, Mississippi (June 19, 2003)." U.S. Department of Justice under the Civil Rights for Institutional Persons Act of 1980. http://www

.justice.gov/crt/split/documents/oak_colu_miss_findinglet.pdf. Accessed May 8, 2010, but no longer available. http://nospank.net/msgulag.htm. Accessed September 6, 2016.

Maass-Robinson, Saundra, and Pamela Everett Thompson. "Mood Disorders in Incarcerated Women." In *Health Issues among Incarcerated Women,* ed. Ronald L. Braithwaite, Kimberly Jacob Arriola, and Cassandra Newkirk (New Brunswick, NJ: Rutgers University Press, 2006), 91–111.

"Mass Incarceration: The Whole Pie 2016." *Prison Policy Initiative.* www.prison policy .org/reports/pie2016.html. Accessed September 9, 2016.

McCormick, Brian. "Ethics Panel Spells Out Physician Role in Executions." *American Medical News* (December 28, 1992).

McCullough, Lawrence, and Richard Stubbs. *Ethical Challenges of Physician Executives* (Tampa, FL: The American College of Physician Executives, July 1995).

McDirmid, M. A. U.S. Department of Labor, Occupational Safety and Health Administration. Letter to Jay Bagley, Administrator, Utah Occupational Safety and Health Division (November 1993).

McDonald, Douglas C. *Managing Prison Health Care and Costs* (Washington, DC: National Institute of Justice, 1995).

McKay Robert D. (The McKay Commission). *Attica: the Official Report of the New York State Special Commission on Attica* (New York: Bantam Books, 1972).

Mears, Daniel P. *Evaluating the Effectiveness of Supermax Prisons* (Washington, DC: U.S. Department of Justice, January 2006). https://www.ncjrs.gov/pdffiles1/nij/grants /211971.pdf. Accessed April 14, 2016.

Medici, Lt. Col. John, U.S. Army Chemical Corps (ret.). "Emergency Response to Incidents Involving Chemical and Biological Warfare Agents" (Quincy, MA: National Fire Protection Association, 1997). http://www.disaster-info.net/lideres/english /jamaica/bibliography/ChemicalAccidents/NFPA_Sup14_EmergencyResponsetoI ncidentsInvolvingChemicalandBiologicalWarfareAgents.pdf. Accessed July 13, 2016.

Mendelsohn, Bruce. "The Right Stuff: An Interview with Dr. Kenneth Moritsugu." *Corrections ALERT Special Report* (Gaithersburg, MD: Aspen Publications, Feb. 26, 1996).

Merrill, Jeffrey D. Sr. *Maine State Prison: 1824–2002* (Charleston, SC: Arcadia Publishing, 2009).

Metcalf, Hope, Jamelia Morgan, Samuel Oliker-Friedland, Judith Resnick, Julia Spiegel, Haran Tae, Alyssa Work, and Brian Holbrook. *Administrative Segregation, Degrees of Isolation, and Incarceration: A National Overview of State and Federal Correctional Policies* (New Haven, CT: Yale Law School, Liman Public Interest Program, June 25, 2013), 4.

Metzner, Jeffrey L. "Mental Health Considerations for Segregated Inmates." *CorrectCare* (Fall 2015).

Mill, John Stuart. *On Liberty.* London: Longman, Roberts, & Green, 1859. Library of Economics and Liberty. Accessed July 27, 2016. http://www.econlib.org/library/Mill /mlLbty1.html.

Mitford, Jessica. "Experiments behind Bars: Doctors, Drug Companies, and Prisoners." *Atlantic Monthly* 23 (January 1973): 64–73.

Mitford, Jessica. *Kind and Usual Punishment: The Prison Business* (New York: Alfred A. Knopf, 1973).

Monahan, John. "The Prediction of Violent Behavior." *American Journal of Psychiatry* 141 (1984), 5–8.

Monahan, John. *The Clinical Prediction of Violent Behavior* (Northvale, NJ: Jason Aronson, 1995).

Morreim, E. Haavi. *Balancing Act: The New Medical Ethics of Medicine's New Economics* (Boston: Kluwer Academic, 1991).

Mossman, Douglas. "Is Prosecution 'Medically Appropriate'?" *Mossman Macro* (New England School of Law), 15–80. http://www.nesl.edu/userfiles/file/nejccc/vol31/1/MOSSMAN.pdf. Accessed May 27, 2016.

Munetz, Mark R., Patricia A. Galon, and Frederick J. Frese III. "The Ethics of Mandatory Community Treatment." *Journal of the American Academy of Psychiatry and Law* 31 (2003), 173–183.

Muse, Mary. "Caring: an Integral Aspect of Nursing." Paper presented at the NCCHC National Conference on Correctional Health Care, Orlando, Florida, October 19, 2009, and attended by author.

Muse, Mary. "Examining Correctional Nursing Practice and Moral Distress." Paper presented at the NCCHC National Conference on Correctional Health Care, Orlando, Florida, October 20, 2009, and attended by author.

Nathan, Vincent P. "Guest Editorial," *Journal of Prison Health Care* 1 (1985), 3–12.

Nathan, Vincent P. "Have the Courts Made a Difference in the Quality of Prison Conditions? What Have We Accomplished to Date?" *Pace Law Review* 24 (December 13, 2004).

National Coalition to Abolish the Death Penalty (NCADP). http://www.ncadp.org/blog/entry/apha-votes-to-oppose-participation-in-execution. Accessed December 12, 2016.

National Coalition to Abolish the Death Penalty (NCADP). http://www.ncadp.org/blog/entry/news-drug-maker-akorn-bans-use-of-midazolam-for-executions. Accessed December 20, 2016.

National Commission on Correctional Health Care (NCCHC). *Standards for Health Services in Prisons (1992)* (Chicago: National Commission on Correctional Health Care, 1992).

National Commission on Correctional Health Care (NCCHC). *Standards for Health Services in Juvenile Detention and Confinement Facilities (1995)* (Chicago: National Commission on Correctional Health Care, 1995).

National Commission on Correctional Health Care (NCCHC). *Standards for Health Services in Jails (1996)* (Chicago: National Commission on Correctional Health Care, 1996).

National Commission on Correctional Health Care (NCCHC). *Standards for Health Services in Prisons 2014* (Chicago: National Commission on Correctional Health Care, 2014).

National Commission on Correctional Health Care (NCCHC). "Competency for Execution." Position statement adopted by NCCHC Board of Directors on October 30, 1998, and reaffirmed in October 2012.

National Commission on Correctional Health Care (NCCHC). "Correctional Health Care Professionals' Response to Inmate Abuse." Position statement adopted by NCCHC Board of Directors in October 2012.

National Commission on Correctional Health Care (NCCHC). "Transgender, Transsexual, and Gender Nonconforming Health Care in Correctional Settings." Position statement adopted by the National Commission on Correctional Health Care Board of Directors on October 19, 2009, and reaffirmed with revision April 2015. http://www

.ncchc.org/transgender-transsexual-and-gender-nonconforming-health-care. Accessed April 9, 2016.

National Commission for the Protection of Human Subjects of Biomedical and Behavioral Research. *The Belmont Report: Ethical Principles and Guidelines for the Protection of Human Subjects of Research* (Bethesda, MD: National Institutes of Health, Office of Human Subjects Research, April 18, 1979). http://or.org/pdf/BelmontReport.pdf. Accessed July 6, 2016.

National Commission for the Protection of Human Subjects of Biomedical and Behavioral Research. *Report and Recommendations: Research Involving Prisoners* (1976). https://repository.library.georgetown.edu/bitstream/handle/10822/559374/Research_involving_prisoners.pdf?sequence=1&isAllowed=y. Accessed August 3, 2016.

National Institute on Alcohol Abuse and Alcoholism (NIAAA). www.niaaa.nih.gov/alcohol-health/fetal-alcohol-exposure. Accessed June 20, 2016.

News Briefs. "Force-Feeding of Inmate Deemed Legal." *Corrections Today* (June 2008).

Norman, Silas (Board Certified in Internal Medicine and *olim* Medical Director of the State Prison of Southern Michigan in Jackson, MI). Memorandum to Kenneth L. Faiver on March 4, 1988.

Nuremberg Code. *Trials of War Criminals before the Nuremberg Military Tribunals under Control Council Law No. 10. Volume 2* (Washington, DC: U.S. Government Printing Office, 1949).

O'Keefe, Maureen L., Kelli J. Klebe, Alysha Stucker, Kristin Sturm, and William Leggett. *One Year Longitudinal Study of the Psychological Effects of Administrative Segregation* (Colorado Springs: Colorado Department of Corrections and University of Colorado, 2010). http://www.ncjrs.gov/pdffiles1/nij/grants/232973.pdf. Accessed April 14, 2016.

Obama, Barack. "Presidential Proclamation—National Donate Life Month, 2016" (April 1, 2016). www.whitehouse.gov/the-press-office/2016. Accessed July 26, 2016.

Obasogie, Osagie K. "Prisoners and Clinical Trials: Cruel and Unusual Ethics?" *Genetics and Society* (June 29, 2007). www.geneticsandsociety.org/article.php?id=3203. Accessed July 25, 2016.

Office of Human Research Protections (OHRP). *Institutional Review Board Guidebook: Chapter VIII—Special Classes of Subjects,* Section E—Prisoners. (Washington, DC: U.S. Department of Health and Human Services). Last updated 1993. http://archive.hhs.gov/ohrp/irb/irb_chapter6ii.htm. Accessed June 21, 2016.

Office of Human Research Protections (OHRP). "Guidance: Special Subject Populations: Prisoners." UCLA. Office of the Human Research Protection Program. Last updated October 24, 2011. http://ora.research.ucla.edu/OHRPP/Documents/Policy/9/Prisoners.pdf. Accessed July 12, 2016.

OHSRP, "Standard Operating Procedure/Policy Approval & Implementation." February 25, 2016. http://ohsr.od.nih.gov/ohsr/public/SOP_10_v3_2-24-2016_508.pdf

Office of Human Research Protections (OHRP). "Standard Operating Procedure/Policy—14C" (Bethesda, MD: Office of Human Research Protections, Department of Health and Human Services, National Institutes of Health). ohsr.od.nih.gov/ohsr/public/SOP_14C_v4_2-25-2016_508.pdf. Accessed May 23, 2016.

Okasha, Ahmed. "Mental Patients in Prisons: Punishment versus Treatment." *World Psychiatry* 3(1) (February 2004). http://www.ncbi.nlm.nih.gov/pmc/articles/PMC1414650. Accessed June 9, 2016.

Paar, David, Carol Bova, Jacques Baillargeon, William Mazur, and Larry Boly. "Infectious Disease in Correctional Health Care: Pursuing a Research Agenda." *Journal of Correctional Health Care* 14(4) (October 2008), 263–268.

Parker, Jr., Frederick R., and Charles J. Paine. "Informed Consent and the Refusal of Medical Treatment in the Correctional Setting" *Journal of Law, Medicine and Ethics* 27(3) (Fall 1999), 240–251.

Parsons, Joseph N. "A Constitutional and Political High Wire Act." *University of Pittsburgh Law Review* 75 (Fall 2013).

Petitioner's Brief in Support of Motion to Modify (November 27, 2001). *S.D. v. State of Louisiana.* http://www.clearinghouse.net/chDocs/public/JI-LA-0009-0001.pdf. Accessed June 25, 2016.

Pinel, Philippe. See "Pinel, Philippe" in *Complete Dictionary of Scientific Biography* (2008). www.encyclopedia.com/topic/Philippe_Pinel.aspx. Accessed July 12, 2016.

Plato. Book 1, line 352d, *Republic* (circa 390 BCE). Translated from the original Greek by the author.

Protecting Inmate Rights: Prison Reform or Prison Replacement? A Report of the Ohio Advisory Committee to the United States Commission on Civil Rights, February 1976.

Rackauskis-Anderson, Joyce. "Exercise-Induced Rhabdomyolysis in a Correctional Setting." Paper presented at the Updates in Correctional Health Care Conference (NCCHC) in Orlando, Florida, and attended by author on May 8, 2007.

Rantz, Liz. "Ask ACHSA: A Regular Column Responding to YOUR Questions." *CorHealth Newsletter* (Spring 2008), 3.

Rawls, John. *A Theory of Justice* (Cambridge, MA: Harvard University Press, 1971).

Reams, Patricia N., Martha Neff Smith, John Fletcher, and Edward Spencer. "Making a Case for Bioethics in Corrections." *Corrections Compendium* 24(12) (November 1997).

Reiter, Keramet A. "Experimentation on Prisoners: Persistent Dilemmas in Rights and Regulations." *California Law Review* 97(2) (April 9, 2009). http://www.californialawreview.org/7experimentation-on-prisoners-persistent-dilemmas-in-rights-and-regulations. Accessed July 7, 2016.

Reiter, Keramet A. "Statement of Keramet A. Reiter before the U.S. Senate Committee on the Judiciary, Subcommittee on the Constitution, Civil Rights and Human Rights, February 21, 2014." https://www.prisonlegalnews.org/media/publications/Reassessing%20Solitary%20Confinement%20II%20Keramet%20Reiter%20Congressional%20Testimony%202014.pdf. Accessed May 23, 2016.

Reiter, Keramet, and Natalie Pifer. *"Brown v. Plata."* Oxford Handbooks Online (Oxford, UK: Oxford University Press, 2014). http://www.oxfordhandbooks.com/view/10.1093/oxfordhb/9780199935383.001.0001/oxfordhb-9780199935383-e-113. Accessed May 6, 2016.

"Report of the Medical Advisory Committee on State Prisons." Commonwealth of Massachusetts (December 1971). In *Medical and Health Care in Jails, Prisons, and Other Correctional Facilities: A Compilation of Standards and Materials* (Washington, DC: American Bar Association, August 1974).

"Report of the Survey Team of the Washington State Medical Association" (December 15, 1971). In *Medical and Health Care in Jails, Prisons, and Other Correctional Facilities: A Compilation of Standards and Materials* (Washington, DC: American Bar Association and American Medical Association, August 1974).

"Review of Burnout: Stages of Disillusionment in the Helping Professions; Burnout and Health Professionals: Manifestations and Management; and Stress, Health and Psychological Problems in the Major Professions." *Family Systems Medicine*, 2(4) (1984), 444–448. http://dx.doi.org/10.1037/h0091836. Accessed January 3, 2017.

Rice, Marnie E., and Grant T. Harris. "Treatment for Prisoners with Mental Disorders." In *Successful Community Sanctions and Services for Special Offenders: Proceedings of the 1994 Conference of the International Community Corrections Association*, ed. Barbara J. Auerbach and Thomas C. Castellano (Lanham, MD: American Correctional Association and International Community Corrections Association, April 1998).

Rieger, Dean P. "When Is a Decision Not to Treat the Right Choice? Distinguishing between Serious and Nonserious Conditions." *Journal of Correctional Health Care* 13(4) (October 2007), 248–249.

Roth, Loren H. "Correctional Psychiatry." In *Forensic Psychiatry and Psychology*, ed. William J. Curran, A. Louis McGarry, and Saleem A. Shah (Philadelphia: F. A. Davis, 1986).

Salzer, Mark S., Katy Kaplan, and Joanne Atay. "State Psychiatric Hospital Census after the 1999 Olmstead Decision: Evidence of Decelerating Deinstitutionalization." *Psychiatric Services* 57 (October 2006), 1501–1504.

Sanford, J.M., G.J. Jacobs, E.J. Roe, and T.E. Terndrup. "Two Patients Subdued with a Taser(R) Device: Cases and Review of Complications." *Journal of Emergency Medicine* (April 23, 2008). Accessed December 17, 2010. http://www.ncbi.nlm.nih.gov/pubmed/18439781.

Santamour, Miles B. *The Mentally Retarded Offender and Corrections*. Lanham, MD: American Correctional Association, 1989).

Sargent, D. A. "Treating the Condemned to Death." *Hastings Center Report* 16(6) (December 1986).

Savage, Scott. "After the Zap: Taser Injuries and How to Treat Them." *CorrectCare* (Summer 2005).

Schlanger, Margo, and Giovanna Shay. "Preserving the Rule of Law in America's Prisons: The Case for Amending the Prison Litigation Reform Act." *American Constitution Society for Law and Policy* (March 2007). http://www.acslaw.org/files/Schlanger%20Shay%20PLRA%20Paper%203-28-07.pdf. Accessed April 7, 2016.

Schlosser, Erik N. "A Framework for Correctional/Mental Health Partnership." *CorrectCare* (Winter 2006).

Schoenly, Lorry. "Chapter 2. Ethical Principles for Correctional Nursing." In *Essentials of Correctional Nursing*, ed. Lorry Schoenly and Catherine M. Knox (New York: Springer, 2013).

Schoenly, Lorry. "Moral Distress and Correctional Nursing," CorrectionalNurse.net.http://correctionalnurse.net/moral-distress-and-correctional-nursing/. Accessed January 6, 2017.

Schwartz, Bradley. "Pres. Obama: 80 Billion Dollars for Prisons Hurts USA." *Prison Path* (April 25, 2016). http://www.prisonpath.com/pres-obama-80-billion-dollars-for-prisons-hurts-usa. Accessed May 7, 2016.

Shaw, David R. *Summary and Analysis of the First 17 Medical Inspections of California Prisons* (Sacramento: Bureau of Audits and Investigations, Office of Inspector General, State of California, August 2010). http://www.oig.ca.gov/media/reports/MIU/SUMMARY/Summary%20and%20Analysis%20of%20the%20First%20

17%20Medical%20Inspections%20of%20California%20Prisons.pdf. Accessed May 5, 2016.

"Sickle Cell Anemia: Risk Factors." Mayo Clinic.com. http://www.mayoclinic.com/health/sickle-cell-anemia/DS00324/DSECTION=prevention. Accessed December 15, 2010.

Simon, Jonathan. *Mass Incarceration on Trial: A Remarkable Court Decision and the Future of Prisons in America* (New York: New Press, 2014).

Smith, C. Gregory, and Woodhall Stopford. "Health Hazards of Pepper Spray." *North Carolina Medical Journal* 60(5) (September–October 1999). http://duketox.mc.duke.edu/pepper%20spray.pdf. Accessed July 13, 2016.

Smith, Sue. "Stepping through the Looking-Glass: Professional Autonomy in Correctional Nursing." *Corrections Today* (February 2005).

Somnier, F. E., and I. K. Genefke. "Psychotherapy for Victims of Torture." *British Journal of Psychiatry* 149 (1986), 323–329.

Southwick, Arthur F. *The Law of Hospital and Health Care Administration* (Ann Arbor, MI: Health Administration Press, 1978).

Spinaris, Caterina, Michael Denhof, and Gregory Morton. *Impact of Traumatic Exposure on Corrections Professionals*, White paper, NIC Cooperative Agreement 12CS14GKM7. December 21, 2013, 17–18. http://static.nicic.gov/UserShared/2015-02-03_nic12cs14gkm7white_paper_122113(1).pdf. Accessed January 6, 2017.

Stanley, Judith A. "Standing Up to Medication Practice Challenges (Part 2)." *CorrectCare* (Spring 2007).

Staples-Horne, Michelle. "Sugar and Spice: Understanding the Health of Incarcerated Girls." In *Health Issues among Incarcerated Women,* ed. Ronald L. Braithwaite, Kimberly Jacob Arriola, and Cassandra Newkirk (New Brunswick, NJ: Rutgers University Press, 2006), 67–87.

Start, Armond. "Interaction between Correctional Staff and Health Care Providers in the Delivery of Medical Care." In *Clinical Practice in Correctional Medicine,* ed. Michael Puisis (St. Louis: Mosby, 1998), 26–31.

Start, Armond. "Physician Recommends Format for Determining Necessity." *CorrectCare* (Fall, 1996).

"State Mental Health Cuts: A National Crisis." National Alliance on Mental Illness (March 2011). http://www.nami.org/getattachment/about-nami/publications/reports/namistatebudgetcrisis2011.pdf. Accessed June 8, 2016.

Steadman, Henry J. "The Right Not to Be a False Positive: Problems in the Application of the Dangerousness Standard." *Psychiatric Quarterly* 52(2) (Summer 1980), 84–99.

Stern, Marc F. "Force-Feeding for Hunger Strikers." *CorrectCare* (Spring 2009).

Stinneford, John F. "Incapacitation through Maiming: Chemical Castration, the Eighth Amendment, and the Denial of Human Dignity." *University of St. Thomas Law Journal* (2006). http://scholarship.law.ufl.edu/cgi/viewcontent.cgi?article=1175&context=facultypub. Accessed July 7, 2016.

Sultan, Bonnie. "Working Behind the Wall: Mental Health of Correctional-Based Staff." PsychAlive. Accessed January 6, 2017. http://www.psychalive.org/working-behind-the-wall-mental-health-of-correctional-based-staff/.

Teplin, Linda A. "Policing the Mentally Ill: Styles, Strategies, and Implications." In *Jail Diversion for the Mentally Ill: Breaking through the Barriers,* ed. Henry J. Steadman (Washington, DC: National Institute of Corrections, 1990).

Texas Youth Commission. "A Brief History of the Texas Youth Commission." http://www
.tyc.state.tx.us/about/history.html. Accessed November 29, 2010 and no longer available. https://tshaonline.org/handbook/online/articles/mdt35. Accessed September 5, 2016.

"The Captive Patient: Prison Health Care: A Report of the Kentucky Public Health Asso-
ciation." In *Medical and Health Care in Jails, Prisons, and Other Correctional
Facilities: A Compilation of Standards and Materials* (January 1974) (Washington,
DC: American Bar Association, August, 1974).

Thomas, David L., and Nicholas Thomas. "Bioethics in Corrections." *Correctional Health
Today* 1(1) (2009).

Toch, Hans. *Men in Crisis: Human Breakdowns in Prisons* (Chicago: Aldine, 1975).

Torrey, E. Fuller, Doris A. Fuller, Jeffrey Geller, Carla Jacobs, and Kristina Ragosta. *No
Room at the Inn: Trends and Consequences of Closing Public Psychiatric Hospitals, 2005–2010* (Arlington, VA: The Treatment Advocacy Center, July 19, 2012).
http://www.tacreports.org/storage/documents/no_room_at_the_inn-2012.pdf.
Accessed June 8, 2016.

Torrey, E. Fuller. "A Dearth of Psychiatric Beds," *Psychiatric Times* (February 25, 2016).
http://www.psychiatrictimes.com/psychiatric-emergencies/dearth-psychiatric
-beds. Accessed June 8, 2016.

Torrey, E. Fuller. *Out of the Shadows: Confronting America's Mental Illness Crisis* (New
York, Wiley & Sons, 1997).

United Nations. "Principles for the Protection of Persons with Mental Illness and the
Improvement of Mental Health Care." United Nations Resolution 46/119 of 1991.
http://www.un.org/documents/ga/res/46/a46r119.htm. Accessed June 9, 2016.

United Nations. "Principles of Medical Ethics Relevant to the Role of Health Personnel,
Particularly Physicians, in the Protection of Prisoners and Detainees against Torture and Other Cruel, Inhuman or Degrading Treatment or Punishment." Adopted
by United Nations General Assembly resolution 37/194 of 18 December 1982.
http://www.ohchr.org/EN/ProfessionalInterest/Pages/MedicalEthics.aspx.
Accessed May 23, 2016.

United Nations. Office of the United Nations High Commissioner for Human Rights.
"International Covenant on Civil and Political Rights." Article 7. (Adopted Decem-
ber 16, 1966). http://www.ohchr.org/en/professionalinterest/pages/ccpr.aspx. Accessed
August 2, 2016.

Urbina, Ian. "Panel Suggests Using Inmates in Drug Trials." *The New York Times* (August 13,
2006). http://www.nytimes.com/2006/08/13/us/13inmates.html?pagewanted=print
. Accessed June 6, 2016.

U.S. Central Intelligence Agency. "Death Investigation—Gul Rahman." https://www
.thetorturedatabase.org/files/foia_subsite/pdfs/cia_production_c06555318_death
_investigation-_gul_rahman_0.pdf. Accessed August 4, 2016.

U.S. Central Intelligence Agency. *OMS Guidelines on Medical and Psychological Support
to Detainee Rendition, Interrogation, and Detention (December 2004)*. Approved
for Release 6-10-2016. https://www.cia.gov/library/readingroom/docs/0006541536
.pdf. Accessed July 30, 2016.

U.S. Department of Justice. "Memorandum of Law as *Amicus Curiae*." Filed in *Buddy
Cason v. Jim Seckinger*, 231 F. 3d 777 (2000), at 23. http://www.ada.gov/briefs
/casonbr.doc. Accessed April 28, 2016.

U.S. Department of Justice. *Title II Technical Assistance Manual* at II-6.0000 and II-6.3300. http://www.ada.gov/taman2.html. Accessed August 28, 2016.

U.S. Department of Veterans Affairs, Coalition Working Group. *Principles of a Sound Drug Formulary System* (October 2000), 5. http://www.pbm.va.gov/linksotherresources /docs/FormularyPrinciplesCoalition.pdf. Accessed July 27, 2016.

U.S. Preventive Services Task Force. "Recommendations." http://www.uspreventiveser-vicestaskforce.org/BrowseRec/Index. Accessed August 28, 2016.

"U.S. Supreme Court Redefines 'Deliberate Indifference.' " *CorrectCare* 5(3) (July 1991).

Veysey, Bonita M., and Gisela Bichler-Robertson. "Prevalence Estimates of Psychiatric Disorders in Correctional Settings." In *Health Status of Soon-To-Be-Released Inmates*. Vol. 2 (Chicago: National Commission on Correctional Health Care, April 2002). http://www.ncchc.org/health-status-of-soon-to-be-released-inmates.   Accessed August 29, 2016.

Vogt, Robert P. "When an Inmate Refuses Care." *CorrectCare* (Summer 2005).

Vulcano, David. "Research Involving Prisoners in Non-Prison Settings: FDA and OHRP Regulations." *Journal of Clinical Research Best Practices* 6, no. 1 (January 2010). Accessed January 25, 2016. http://firstclinical.com/journal/2010/1001_Prisoners .pdf.

Ward, John W., and Jonathan H. Mermin. "Simple, Effective, but Out of Reach? Public Health Implications of HCV Drugs." *New England Journal of Medicine* (November 17, 2015).

Watson, Jean. *Human Caring Science: A Theory of Nursing*, 2nd ed. (Boston: Jones & Bartlett, 2012).

Weiner, Janet, Kim Thorburn, Ron Shansky, Steve Spencer, Armond Start, Gregg Bloche, Henry Schwarzchild, Lee Tucker, Jim Welsh, David Rothman, et al. *Breach of Trust: Physician Participation in Executions in the United States* (American College of Physicians, Human Rights Watch, National Coalition to Abolish the Death Penalty, and Physicians for Human Rights, 1994). http://www.hrw.org/legacy/reports/1994 /usdp/index.htm. Accessed July 1, 2016.

Weiskopf, S. J. "Nurses' Experience of Caring for Inmate Patients." *Journal of Advanced Nursing* 49(4) (2005), 336–343.

Williams, Peter C., and Joan Hirsch Holtzman. "Ethical Problems: Cases and Commentaries." *Journal of Prison Health* 1(1) (Spring–Summer, 1981), 44–54.

Winner, Ellen J. "An Introduction to the Constitutional Law of Prison Medical Care." *Journal of Prison Health* 1(1) (Spring–Summer 1981), 67–84.

Wishart, Margaret D., and Nancy N. Dubler. *Health Care in Prisons, Jails and Detention Centers: Some Legal and Ethical Dilemmas* (Bronx, NY: Montefiore Medical Center, 1983).

Wolf, Richard and Jayne O'Donnell, "Pfizer Rules on Lethal Injection Drugs May Limit Death Penalty Executions," USA Today (May 13, 2016). http://www.usatoday.com /story/news/2016/05/13/pfizer-lethal-injection-drugs-supreme-court-executions -death/84344628/.

World Medical Association (WMA). "WMA Statement on Body Searches of Prisoners," Adopted by 45th World Medical Assembly at Budapest, Hungary, October 1993; editorially revised by 170th WMA Council Session at Divonne-les-Bains, France, May 2005. http://www.wma.net/en/30publications/10policies/b5/index.html. Accessed August 5, 2016.

World Medical Association (WMA). *"Declaration of Malta* on Hunger Strikers." Adopted by 43rd World Medical Assembly at Malta, November 1991, and last revised by 57th WMA General Assembly at Pilanesberg, South Africa, October 2006. http://www.wma.net/en/30publications/10policies/h31/index.html. Accessed August 8, 2016.

World Medical Association (WMA). "International Code of Medical Ethics." Adopted in October 1949 and last amended at 57th WMA General Assembly at Pilanesberg, South Africa, October 2006. *World Medical Association Bulletin* 1(3) (1949), 109, 111. www.wma.net/en/30publications/10policies/c8. Accessed August 5, 2016.

World Medical Association (WMA). "World Medical Association Supports Doctors Refusing to Participate in Torture." 49th WMA General Assembly at Hamburg, Germany, November 17, 1997, Universidad de Navarra. www.unav.es/cdb/ammhamburgo5.html. Accessed July 4, 2016.

World Medical Association (WMA). *Declaration of Helsinki.* "Ethical Principles for Medical Research Involving Human Subjects." Adopted at Helsinki, Finland, in June 1964 and amended at Fortaleza, Brazil, in October 2013. http://www.wma.net/en/30publications/10policies/b3/17c.pdf. Accessed July 3, 2016.

World Medical Association (WMA). *Declaration of Tokyo.* "Guidelines for Physicians Concerning Torture and other Cruel, Inhuman or Degrading Treatment or Punishment in Relation to Detention and Imprisonment." Adopted by the 29th World Medical Assembly, Tokyo, Japan, October 1975 and last revised at the 173rd WMA Council Session, Divonne-les-Bains, France, May 2006. www.wma.net/en/30publications/10policies/c18/index.html. Accessed July 14, 2016.

World Psychiatric Association (WPA). *Declaration of Madrid.* Approved by the General Assembly of the World Psychiatric Association on August 25, 1996. http://www.wpanet.org/detail.php?section_id=5&content_id=48. Accessed July 14, 2016.

Index

Page numbers followed by *t* indicate tables

Abuse—physical or sexual
and biomedical experiments, 87–90.
See also Biomedical research and
experimentation
and body cavity searches, 34–35.
See also Body cavity searches
legal redress of limited by PLRA,
140
by mace spray, 58–59
of mentally ill, 206, 219, 220
numbers of sex-abused incarcerated
women, 39
reporting of, 15, 35, 39, 58, 78–81,
161, 278, 288–289
and strip search, 36, 38, 39. *See also*
Strip searches
of transgender persons, 29, 30
of women and girls, 38–39
zero tolerance for, 161
Abuse of drugs, 42–43, 101, 121
ACA. *See* American Correctional
Association (ACA)
Academy of Correctional Health
Professionals (ACHP), 164
ACCP. *See* American College of
Correctional Physicians (ACCP)

Accreditation, 94, 102, 161, 164–167,
245, 292. *See also* American
Correctional Association (ACA);
National Commission on
Correctional Health Care
(NCCHC)
limitations of, 165, 167
and prison research—American
Correctional Association, 94–95,
102
ACHP. *See* Academy of Correctional
Health Professionals (ACHP)
ACHRE. *See* Advisory Committee on
Human Radiation Experiments
(ACHRE)
ACHSA. *See* American Correctional
Health Services Association
(ACHSA)
Acute psychiatric facility, 41, 220–221
ADA. *See* Americans with Disabilities
Act (ADA)
Addictive behavior—learning of and
acquiring, 121
Adequate health care, xxiii, xxiv,
137, 143, 167, 173, 178, 182,
284

Administrative remedies—exhaustion of
  under PLRA. *See* Prison Litigation
  Reform Act (PLRA)
Administrative segregation. *See also*
  Isolation in penal settings;
  Security housing units (SHUs);
  Segregation
  health care services difficult in,
    106–107, 283
  NIC study, 108–109
  Yale Law School study, 106
Adverse side effects, 44, 57, 187, 194,
  196, 199, 275
  and court ordered medical treatment,
    116–117
  of mace, 58–59
Advisory Committee on Human Radiation
  Experiments (ACHRE), 90–91,
  94–95
Advocacy, 7, 13, 49, 84, 120, 122, 162,
  182, 224, 232, 236, 238, 243, 244,
  247, 252, 254, 256, 269, 283, 288,
  289. *See also* Patient advocacy
AJA. *See* American Jail Association
  (AJA)
Alternative treatment intervention, 194,
  195, 197, 273
AMA. *See* American Medical Association
  (AMA)
Ambience, part of treatment, 223, 257
American Academy of Psychiatry and
  Law, 72
American College of Correctional
  Physicians (ACCP)
  code of ethics of, 74
  medicine only for diagnosed illness, 61
  mental health input of in disciplinary
    system, 114–115
  and physician involvement in execution,
    74
  professionalism in correctional health
    care, 164
  restricted housing of mentally ill
    inmates, 114, 115
  treatment after informed consent, 61
  witnessing use of force, 63
American Correctional Association
  (ACA), 15, 34, 35, 45, 49, 56, 62,

94–96, 101, 148, 153, 169, 243,
  244, 245, 264, 266, 270, 275, 286
  accreditation and prison research, 102
  accreditation programs of, 164–165, 167
American Correctional Association
  (ACA)—public policies
  Code of Ethics (reporting unethical
    behavior; officers, not guards), 80,
    164
  Conditions of Confinement (safe
    population limit), 169
  Correctional Health Care (officer
    involvement), 270
  Correctional Mental Health Care
    (segregation access), 107
  Research and evaluation (no
    experimental subjects), 96
  Use of Appropriate Sanctions and
    Controls (least restrictive), 264
  Use of Force (stabilize and deescalate),
    266
  Use of Restraints with Pregnant
    Offenders (prohibits), 286
American Correctional Association
  (ACA)—standards, xiii–xiv
  4-JCF-4C-63 (2009) on Contraband
    Control (body cavity searches), 34
  ACI (2003) 4-4084 on Correctional
    Officers (officer training
    requirements), 275
  ACI (2003) 4-4142 on Housing for the
    Disabled (access to services and
    programs), 148
  ACI (2003) 4-4190 on Use of Restraints
    (not used as punishment), 62
  ACI (2003) 4-4190-1 on Use of
    Restraints (on pregnant women),
    286
  ACI (2003) 4-4191 on Use of Restraints
    (notify health care of four-point),
    62
  ACI (2003) 4-4193 on Control of
    Contraband (body cavity searches),
    34, 35
  ACI (2003) 4-4256 on Admission and
    Review of Status (segregation), 45
  ACI (2003) 4-4258 on Supervision
    (segregation), 45

ACI (2003) 4-4264 on General Conditions of Confinement (food loaf), 49

ACI (2003) 4-4320 on Therapeutic Diets (food loaf), 49

ACI (2003) 4-4365 on Health Appraisal (classification), 56

ACI (2003) 4-4380 on Health Authority (defines role of), 243, 245

ACI (2003) 4-4381 on Provision of Treatment (medical autonomy), 244, 271

ACI (2003) 4-4389 on Emergency Response (officers' health training), 275

ACI (2003) 4-4396 on Confidentiality (medical records), 15

ACI (2003) 4-4400 on Segregation (transfer to), 56

ACI (2003) 4-4402 on Research (prohibition of), 96, 102

ACI (2003) 4-4414 on Transfers (health record confidentiality), 15

ACI (2003) 4-4429 on Scope of Services (no disability discrimination), 148

ACI (2003) 4-4429-1 on Scope of Services (disability advisor), 148

4-JCF-4C-63 (2009) on Contraband Control (body cavity searches), 34

American Correctional Association Health Professional Interest Section (ACA–HPIS), 164

American Correctional Health Services Association (ACHSA)
code of ethics of, 61–63, 74, 164
medicine only for diagnosed illness, 61
physician involvement in executions, 74
witnessing use of force, 61–62

American Jail Association(AJA), 164

American Medical Association (AMA)
code of ethics, 118
ethical directives of, 66, 73, 77, 118
on interrogation by physicians, 77
on organ donation by condemned prisoners, 66
on physician participation in execution, 63, 66–67

physicians not following AMA ethical codes, 73
precursor to correctional health standards of ACA and NCCHC, xiii–xiv
on torture, 77

American Nurses Association—nurse participation in executions, 63

American Pharmacists Association (APhA), 68, 69, 70

American Psychiatric Association
on extended segregation of mentally ill, 105–106
and lack of opposition to deinstitutionalization, 207

American Public Health Association (APHA)
body cavity searches standards of, 33–34
confidentiality, 15
duty to report mental, physical, or sexual abuse, 80
medical autonomy of health care providers, 244
and participation in executions, 63
and witnessing use of force, 62

American Society of Anesthesiologists
and opposition to participation in execution, 67

Americans with Disabilities Act (ADA) of 1990. *See also* Disability lawsuits
as applied to inmates, 145–146, 155
PLRA impact on, 146–147

Anno, B. Jaye
and prison health care in 1970s, 4
and recommendation for organizing correctional health care, 251, 254–255
and tensions between care and custody in prisons, xxvii

Antipsychotic medications, 21–22, 70–72, 152, 155, 207, 218. *See* Psychotropic medications

Anxiety
from correctional environment, 108–109, 113
disabling, 218

Anxiety (*cont.*)
  from disruption of circadian rhythm,
    105
  in supermax settings, 105, 108, 109,
    113
  during torture, 76, 77, 113
  of transgender patient, 29
  over trial, 214, 219
Anxiety disorder in jails and prisons,
    211–212
APhA. *See* American Pharmacists
    Association (APhA)
APHA. *See* American Public Health
    Association (APHA)
Appelbaum, Dr. Kenneth, 106
Appelbaum, Dr. Paul, 72
Asthma, 58, 177, 183, 195, 275
Attica riot, 127
Aufderheide, Dean H. 107, 217
Autonomy, 18, 19, 92, 99, 178, 179.
    See also Medical autonomy;
    Patient autonomy
Awareness of facts and risks. *See Farmer v.
    Brennan,* 134–135

Basic human rights, 8–9, 88, 99, 101,
    205
Behavior
  control of by drugs, 60–61, 85, 121
  and influence on decision to treat in
    prison, 190
Belief in patient, importance of, 23
Belief systems, corrections and health
    care compared, 261*t*, 266–267
Bell, Dr. Carl C., 120–121
Belmont Report, 91, 101
Beneficence, 14, 20, 71
  biomedical research principle of, 91
  definition of, 14
  and hunger strikers, 52
  and physician participation in chemical
    castration, 117
  and psychiatrists, 72, 74
  and punitive denial of medical care,
    190
  and standards of professional practice,
    178–179
  and tissue specimen collection, 31

Benefit, 186–187
Bioethics committee, 13, 14
Biomedical research and experimentation,
    88–104
  and Advisory Committee on Human
    Radiation Experiments, 90–91,
    94–95
  and Belmont Report, 91, 101
  and biomedical research principles, 91
  and history of experiments on prisoners,
    88–90
  and National Commission for
    Protection of Human Subjects,
    90–93
  and Office of Human Research
    Protection, 94, 98, 99
  and regulation of in U.S. prisons,
    90–101
BJC. *See* Bureau of Justice Statistics
Bleach to disinfect needles, 48
Blood and tissue specimen
  drawing of through bars, 45–46
  ethical concerns on use of, 31
Body cavity searches, 33–36
  alternatives to, 35
  and imaging. *See* Imaging
    technologies
  physician involvement through CIA,
    76
  of pretrial detainees—*Bell v. Wolfish,*
    153
  probable cause for, 35
  standards on, 33–35
  warden's authorization for, 35–36
  who conducts, 34
  World Medical Association on, 36
Boesky, Dr. Lisa, 205
Boot camps, 260
Boundary issues and caring, 22–23,
    26–27, 235. *See also* Corrections
    and health care
Brain function in chronic mentally ill,
    216
Breach of trust, 34
Brecher, Edward, 249–250
Brodie, Jamie S., 231
Budgetary limitations, 187
Burnout, 81–84, 256

Califano, Joseph, 94–95
Capital punishment, 62–70, 72–75
    and ACCP, ACHSA, AMA, ANA,
        APHA, NCCHC, and WMA on
        participation in, 62–63
Cardozo, Justice Benjamin, 18, 151
Castration,
    and sterilization of mentally defectives,
        116
    See also Chemical castration
Celebrity status and decision to treat, 191
Cell door, 17, 44–45, 106, 110, 111, 132,
    284, 287
Central health authority, 250, 254, 255
Central Intelligence Agency (CIA)
    and release of documents on torture,
        76–77
Certification of professionals, 164–165
Chemical castration
    by court order, 115–120
    effects and side effects of, 117
    ethics of physician involvement in,
        116–121
    legality of, 115–116
Chemoprophylaxis, 41, 198
Chemotherapy, 196
Chief medical officer, 243
Chronic mental illness, 215
Chronicity of care, 198
Circadian rhythm, 105
Civil death, 124, 125, 169
Civil disobedience, 6, 126
Civil Rights Act of 1871, 126, 129–130,
    133–137, 142, 144
Civil Rights Act of 1964, 30
Civil rights movement of the 1960s, 126
Civil Rights of Institutionalized Persons
    Act of 1980 (CRIPA), 135–136
Civil rights suit, 131, 135
Classification
    and communication between health care
        and corrections, 56–57
    by health status and need, 285–286
    of transgender inmates, 28
Clinic areas
    design of with health care staff input, 272
    encounters and privacy in, 284–285
    safety and security in, 282–283

Clinical guidelines, 176–178
Clinical judgment
    and competing loyalties, 80
    and final authority of responsible
        physician, 245
    of forensic psychiatrist, 72
    and medical autonomy, 14
    and patient advocacy, 252
    and physician discretion, 265
    practitioner guidelines, 177
Clinical responsibility, line of, 256
Closed head injuries, 218–219
CN spray, 58
Codes of professional ethical conduct, 8,
    63, 164. *See also* Ethical codes
Coercive measures
    and IOM recommendations on research,
        100
    as treatment, 118–120
Cognitive behavioral therapy (CBT), 23,
    109, 114
Cognitive impairment
    from solitary confinement, 113
Cognitive skills
    impairment of, 211
Cohen, Fred, 105–106
Cohen, Dr. Robert, 81
Cohn, Felicia
    ethical rationale for prisoner entitlement
        to basic rights, 8–10
    on organ transplants and ethics, 43
Collins, William, 166
Comforting environment, 187, 213–214,
    221–224, 229
Command-control approach, 265
Commission on Safety and Abuse in
    America's Prisons, 81, 105–106,
    111–112, 140, 210
Common Rule, 95
Community norms and standards, 7,
    18, 28, 29, 41, 124, 137, 165,
    178–180, 183, 192, 196, 220,
    238
Community practice, 18, 81, 160, 182,
    185, 189, 228, 232
Comorbidity
    and reduce treatment outcomes, 199
Compassion fatigue, 83. *See* Burnout

Competence evaluation
    for execution, 72–75
    by other than treating psychiatrist or
        psychologist, 39, 40
    for trial, 70–72
    and use of treatment record, 39, 40
Compounding pharmacies and lethal
    injection drugs, 67
Computerized management information
    system 272
Conditions of confinement, 84, 111, 112,
        127, 129, 152, 153, 157, 162, 165,
        169, 248, 252, 254
    ACA Public Policy on, 169
    in federal court, 129
    Holt v. Sarver and, 127–128, 152
Condoms, 48
Confidentiality, 11–17, 159. *See also*
        Privacy
    breach of, 13, 17, 44
    of custody staff, 16–17
    in ethical codes, 15
    of health professionals, 11, 12, 40
    and HIPAA, 149
    limits on, 16–17
    and medical records, 15, 179, 253,
        368
    priority of corrections and health care,
        259
    of private and sensitive information, 31,
        241
Conflict avoidance with correctional staff,
        278
Conflict of interest, 74, 278
Conklin, Dr. Thomas, 112
Conscience, 8, 10, 69, 127, 151, 292
Consent to treatment
    and requirement of signed form, 18
Conspiracy of silence on inmate abuse,
        79–80
Constitutional protection of prisoners, 9
Contagious disease prevention, 17, 48,
        101, 275, 276
    and fellow prisoners, 188
    and role of medical staff, 257
Contemporary standards of community
        practice, 178, 182–183. *See also*
        Community norms and standards

Contemporary standards of health in free
        world, 178–180
Continuous quality improvement (CQI),
        272
Contraband, 31, 34–38, 48, 235, 278
Contractor liability, 153–154
Contributory negligence, 131
Co-payment programs, 30, 161
Correctional agencies
    mission fulfilment of, 262
Correctional environment. *See also*
        Corrections and health care
    bad for mentally ill, 213–214,
        219–220
    coercive measures in, 263–264
Correctional fatigue, 83. *See also*
        Burnout
Correctional health care
    contrast with noncorrectional health
        care, 260–267
    historical perspective of, 2–6
    and professionals' responses to inmate
        abuse (NCCHC), 78–79
    under single responsible health
        authority, 253–254
Correctional officers
    difference from guards, 164
    training in medical care and mental
        health care, 161, 274–277
Correctional systems
    restoring health to entering condition,
        176
    rule violation in, 264
    segregation policies of, 106
Corrections and health care, 2, 242,
        260–267, 268–269, 270–271
    bridging gap between cultures and,
        270
    clear and consistent policies of, 242
    comparison between cultures, 261*t*
    comparison of, 2, 242, 260–262,
        263–264
    crossed lines between, 235–236
    and dialogue with respectful
        deliberation, 272–274
    and how custody depends on health
        care, 269–270
    interdependence of, 268–278

means used to fulfill missions of, 262–263
and the mentally ill, 219–220
purposes of, 260–262
and relationship between custody and institutional services, 268–269
shared priorities of, 259
solid ethical and professional foundation for, 242
staff training styles for, 265–266
system of beliefs of, 266–267
working together, 270–27
Cosmetic experiments, 96–97, 102
Cosmetic treatment
facelifts and surgery, 181, 185, 196
Cost of health care, 185–189, 194–195, 198–199
cost–benefit equation in, 186
cost-effectiveness of, 249, 259
perspectives on, 187–189
Counseling, 10, 262, 264, 288
Counter-therapeutic environment, 104, 212–215
Court-imposed medical procedures and informed consent, 117–120
Courts
hands-off policy in, 124–136
impact of, xxiv, 163–169
pulling in the reins of, 136–143.
See also Prison Litigation Reform Act (PLRA)
role of, 123–124
CQI. See Continuous quality improvement
Criminal justice reform, 10, 171
Criminalization of the mentally ill
Hinkley effect on, 209–212
CRIPA. See Civil Rights of Institutionalized Persons Act (CRIPA)
Crisis intervention, 221–223
Cross training. See Training
Crossed lines
health care and corrections, 235–236
Crowding
amelioration of, 163
in California prisons, 168–169, 171
and court orders, 113

and exacerbated stress, 215
from mass incarceration, 217
and the mentally ill, 219
Cruel and unusual punishment. See also Conditions of confinement; Eighth Amendment
and capital punishment, 67, 72, 115
and chemical castration, 115, 117
clause applies to states—Robinson v. California, 151
and evolving standards of decency. See Decency, evolving standards of
and execution of the insane, 72
future court rulings on, 137
mentally ill in supermax or solitary confinement, 113, 114, 224
and reasonable access to medical care, 132–133
and totality of a prison's conditions, 127
CS spray, 58
Cultural factors and sensibilities, xxvi, 178
Curry, Keith
on segregating the mentally ill, 108, 114
Curtis, Barbara
on TBIs and behavior problems, 219
Custody and health care, 269–270
and mutual cooperation, 2. See also Mutual respect
and primacy of custody, 238
recognizing differences between, 2
relationship between, 227
Cynicism, 54–55, 84

Danger to self or others
limits of confidentiality, 17
DBT. See Dialectical behavioral treatment (DBT)
Death penalty states, 63–64
Decency, xxvi, 8, 37, 85, 87, 117, 131, 147, 151, 157, 291, 292
and ADA application of to prisons and jails, 147
and biomedical research in prisons, 87. See also Biomedical research and experimentation
and Eighth amendment, 117, 131. See also Eighth Amendment

Decency (*cont.*)
  evolving standards of, 8, 37, 117, 131,
    151, 291. *See also Trop v. Dulles*
  and human dignity of sex offenders, 117
  and transsexual surgery, 185
  and use of strap, 151
Decision analysis
  conceptual framework, 180–182
Decision-making model, 183–200
Decision to treat, 189–200
  and factors considered in making
    decision, 193*t*
Declaration of Helsinki
  and medical research, 96–97
  and risk–benefit analysis for research,
    96, 99, 103
Declaration of Madrid
  and prohibition of psychiatrists in
    executions, 74, 205
  and treatment by least-restrictive, 205
Declaration of Malta
  and forced feeding, 52
Declaration of Tokyo
  and denunciation of torture and role in
    executions, 63, 78
  and prohibition on forced feeding,
    51–52
Decompensation of mentally ill in jails and
    prisons, 104, 212
Deference to professional judgment
  Youngberg v. Romeo, 153
Deflect and deescalate tense situations,
    278
Dehumanizing terms
  offenders versus patients, xx, 82, 148,
    227–240, 283
Deinstitutionalization, 205–212, 215, 217
  history of, 206–209
  position of American Psychiatric
    Association on, 207
Deliberate indifference, 30, 37, 129,
    131–137, 141, 147, 152–154, 175,
    181, 212, 243
  definition of, 131–133
  Estelle v. Gamble, 126, 128–132, 137,
    152, 180, 243–244
  Farmer v. Brennan, 134–135, 154
  to mental health needs, 212–213

  reckless disregard of known risk,
    131–133
  to serious medical needs, 128–134
  serious mental illness defined—*Tillery
    v. Owens*, 212
  violates Eighth Amendment, 152.
    See also Eighth Amendment
Delinquent, xx, 228
Della Penna, Richard, 249–250
Denial of access to medical care
  Todaro v. Ward, 152
Department of Health, Education and
    Welfare (DHEW), 91–92
Department of Health and Human Services
    (DHHS)
  on biomedical research, 121, 126
  on HIPAA, 94
Depo-Provera, 116–117
Depression, 26, 29, 117, 215, 212
  prevalence of, 208, 211–212
  and segregation, 105, 106, 107, 108, 113
Designated mental health clinician, 243
Detainee; 37, 70, 74, 76–77, 158
  as term, xiv, 228–230
Determination of competence to be
    executed, 66, 72–75
Devices and prosthetics, 17, 184, 263
DHHS. *See* Department of Health and
    Human Services (DHHS)
Diabetes, 58, 117, 183, 195
  clinical guidelines for, 177, 179–180
  transport of patients with, 286
Diagnosis under less-than-satisfactory
    conditions, 43–48
*Diagnostic and Statistical Manual of
    Mental Disorders* (DSM-5),
    203–204
Dialectical behavioral treatment (DBT)
Diet, 22, 49–50, 268, 269, 282
Dignity of humans, 1, 2, 6, 8–10, 27, 28,
    36, 37, 42, 53, 96, 114, 115, 117,
    118, 131, 151, 169, 171, 174, 179,
    180, 205, 229, 230, 232, 234, 241,
    242, 256, 259, 262, 270, 288, 291.
    See also Decency
Dimensions of necessity, 192–194
Dioxin, 89
Direct orders, 261*t*, 266

Directly observed therapy (DOT), 41–42
Disability issues in correctional facilities, 143–148. *See also* Americans with Disabilities (ADA)
  ACA standards and discrimination against, 148
  exclusion from programs, 147
  "reasonable accommodation," 147–148
Disability law suits, 145–146
Disciplinary measures
  communication between corrections and health care staff over, 56–57
Disciplinary segregation, 55–58, 163 *See also* Segregation
Discipline and punishment of mentally ill, 104, 107, 108, 115, 163, 223–224
Disparities between corrections and medicine, 82, 260–268
Disproportionate minority representation, 170–171
Dissonance, 55, 90, 230
Distress, 27, 113. *See also* Moral distress; Psychological distress
Distributive and corrective justice, 10
Dix, Dorothea, 205–206
DNA testing, 32–33
Doctors
  as advocates for patients, 288
  use best clinical judgment, 265
Doctors without Borders, 183
Documentation of patient information, 24, 80, 148, 159, 160, 236. *See also* Health records
Dole, Dr. Pamela, 39
Door design and patient assessment, 44. *See also* Cell door
Dostoyevsky, Fyodor, xi, 171
DOT. *See* Directly observed therapy (DOT)
Drug companies and non-prisoner research, 94
Drug formulary, 149, 182, 287
DSM. *See Diagnostic and Statistical Manual of Mental Disorders* (DSM-5)
Due process, 19–21, 37, 74, 114, 126, 138, 149–158, 176, 179, 180, 260, 264
  in *Lewis v. Casey*, 155, 163

relaxation of protections for, 163
  rights of, 152
  in *Sandin v. Conner*, 154–155
  in *Wolff v. McDonnell*, 152
Duration of stay in facility, 194
Duty to warn, 17, 57
Dvoskin, Joel, 40, 84–85, 274
Dwight, Louis, 205–206

Economic factors and standards, 178
  Education programs in corrections, 10
  Efficient resource use, 2, 242, 282
Eighth Amendment
  and ADA, 147. *See* Americans with Disabilities Act (ADA)
  and denial of care, 152
  on discomfort and humiliation, 134
  and inhumane conditions, 135
  and juveniles, 149–150
  and prohibition on cruel and unusual punishment, 124. *See also* Cruel and unusual punishment
  and transgender inmate, 154
Elderly prisoners, 196, 200, 277, 278, 280
Elective procedures
  defined, 184–185
Eleventh Amendment (ADA and state's rights), 145–146
Emergency and disaster preparedness
  emergency scenario in, 273
  as health care training topic, 278
  importance of to both corrections and health care, 1, 241, 259
Emergency room trips
  other options for, 284
Emergency medical treatment
  and consent—*Schloendorff v. Society of New York Hospital,* 151
  and surrogate consent, 18–19
Emergency medical technicians and executions, 69
Employee burnout, 256–257
Enforced feeding, 50–53. *See also* Hunger strikes
Enforced medical treatment, 18–22. *See also* Patient autonomy; Informed consent

Enhanced interrogation techniques, 77
  See also Torture
Entitlement, 7, 8, 127
Environment favorable to treatment of
    mental health, 213
Environmental safety and sanitation, 256
Equipment, 47–48, 255
Equitable care, 24
Erosion, 81, 82, 256
Escape plan
  limits of confidentiality about, 17
Ethical challenges in correctional health
    care, 120–121, 224–225
Ethical codes, 10–14, 61, 62, 63, 64
Ethical conflicts
  facing health professionals, xxvi
Ethical decisions, 53–54. *See also*
    Beneficence; Confidentiality;
    Decency—evolving standards of;
    Nonmaleficence; Patient
    autonomy; and Privacy
Ethical delivery of humane health care,
    122
Ethical issues, 55–79
  abuse of inmates. *See* Abuse—physical
    or sexual
  acceptability, 15–16
  application of ethical principles, 7
  beneficence. *See* Beneficence
  body cavity searches. *See* Body cavity
    searches
  burnout, 26, 81–84, 256
  caring approach. *See* Caring
  certifying competency for execution, 73
  competence evaluation. *See* Competence
    evaluation
  confidentiality. *See* Confidentiality
  crushing medication, 42–43
  defective or inadequate equipment,
    47–48
  determination of competence for
    execution, 66, 72–75
  diagnosing under unsatisfactory
    conditions, 43–48
  directly observed therapy (DOT), 41–42
  dissonance, 55, 230
  DNA testing, 32–33
  drawing blood through bars, 45–46

fetal alcohol syndrome disorder,
    120–121
forensic use of medical information and,
    30–40
harm-reduction strategies and, 48, 49,
    101
and housing the mentally ill in extended
    isolation, 104–115, 161
and hunger strikes, 50–53
and informed consent. *See* Informed
    consent
and involvement in torture, 75–79
and medical autonomy. *See* Medical
    autonomy
and medical clearance for punishment,
    56–58
and medical neutrality, 14
and medical parole, 40
and medical restraints, 41, 261*t*, 264
and medication for behavior control, 56,
    60–61, 85
and organ donations by condemned
    prisoners, 66
and organ transplants. *See* Organ
    transplants
and participation in court-imposed
    treatment, 117–120
participation in executions, 62–75
and patient assessment through closed
    doors, 44–45
and patient autonomy. *See* Patient
    autonomy
and prediction of danger, 40
and preventing blood-borne
    transmission, 17, 48, 101, 276
and privacy. *See* Privacy
and reporting staff abuse of patients,
    79–81
research on prisoners. *See* Biomedical
    research and experimentation
and role conflicts, 55–85
and shakedowns by health professionals,
    61
and strip searches, 36–39
and transgender issues. *See* Transgender
    inmates
and treatment to render competence for
    execution, 72–75

and treatment to render competence for trial, 70–72
and treatment under unsatisfactory conditions, 45–48
and unnecessary risks to health care staff, 46–47
and use of force, 61–62
use of torture and, 75–79
writing tickets and, 59–60
Ethical reasoning, 87–88
Ethical role conflicts, 55–121
Ethical values erosion and employee burnout, 26, 81–84, 256
Ethicists from outside the agency, 13–14
Ethics
and certifying competency for execution, 72–74
codes of. See Ethical codes
definition of, 6–8
and dignity of the human person, 8–10. See also Decency
and law, 7–8
study of as framework for defining right and wrong behavior, 6
Ethnicity
as factor in decisions, 8, 14, 24, 189–190, 280
Evaluation for Approval of Major Medical Procedure. Start, 200–201
Evaluation of competency. See Competence evaluation
Evidence gathering, 34
Evidence-based treatment—Dr. Robert Greifinger, 176–177
Evolving community standards, 182, 185, 187, 189. See also Decency
Examination room, 17, 288
Excessive exercise and rhabdomyolysis, 280–281
Excessive sanctions versus least-restrictive environment, 264
Executions
and health professionals, 62–75
of insane persons as violation of Eighth Amendment, 72
See also Competence evaluation
Executive functions of brain, 216
Expected practices, xx

Expertise,
and clinical guidelines, 176
professional obligation to use for wellness of patients, 63, 170
of university-based state health care providers, 252
Extend life, 176, 186–187
Extreme segregation
vicious cycle of, 107–115
Eye problems and mace-type sprays, 58

Facility, xix, 17
Facility presence by responsible health care authority, 246–248
Faith traditions and medical ethics, xxv–xxvi
Fears of inmates
of female inmates, 37–39
of mentally ill inmates, 108–109, 113, 212, 214–219
Federal Bureau of Prisons clinical guidelines, 177
Feierman, Jessica, 139
Fetal alcohol spectrum disorder (FASD), 120–121
Filing fees, 143, 146
Firearms proficiency, 235
Food as disciplinary measure, 49
Food loaf (Nutraloaf), 49–50
Food slot, 44–45, 106, 110, 284
Forced feeding, 51
Forced medication for mental health, 20–21, 153–154
Forensic psychiatrist not acting qua physician
American Academy of Psychiatry and Law, 72
Forensic use of medically obtained information, 30–40
Formulary, pharmaceutical, 149, 182, 287
Forsythe, Ian, 133
Fourth Amendment rights, 37, 136, 153
Francis, Pope, 171
Fry, Rodney, 30
Function, restoration of, 175, 176, 183, 192, 193t, 194, 196, 199, 200, 228, 261t

Funding
    limited budget does not justify
        insufficient care, 143
    and politics, 262
Fuzzy reasoning or faux defenses, 88

Gandhi, Mohandas
    on noncooperation with evil, 289
Gawande, Dr. Atul, 63, 66, 67
Gender, 37, 39, 211
    not relevant to certain decisions, 8, 14,
        189, 190, 280
    sensitivity to, 16, 24, 101, 277
Gender incongruence treatment, 28–30,
    181, 185
Golden rule and ethics, 7
Gostin, Lawrence O., 101
Government
    and delegation of liability to private
        vendors, 242
    and duty to protect prisoners from harm,
        124
    and enforcement of regulations, 165
Grassian, Dr. Stuart, 111–112
Greifinger, Dr. Robert
    and cynicism among correctional health
        care staff, 162
    and disabled prisoners needing
        reasonable accommodation, 147
    and evidence-based treatment
        guidelines, 177
    and harm-reduction approaches, 49
Grievances, 24–26. See also Prison
        Litigation Reform Act (PLRA)
    dismissal of on technicalities, 24–26,
        231
    and implementation of effective
        grievance system, 157, 159, 162,
        278
Guardian ad litem, 139, 150
Guilty but mentally ill, 209–210

Handcuffs during transport, 286
Handicapped, 144. See also Disability
        issues in correctional facilities
Hands-off policy, 124–136
Haney, Craig, 59, 108, 113
Harm prevention, 1, 241, 259

Harm to third party and privacy issue
        limits, 16–17
Harm-reduction strategies, 48–49, 101
Healing profession, xiv, 55, 69, 75. See
        also Health care staff and burnout,
        82
    and torture, 90. See Torture
Health aspects of officers' training,
        274–277
Health care
    comparison of with corrections, 2, 242,
        260–262, 263–264
    costs of, 185–189, 194–195, 198–199
    defining appropriate and necessary, 137,
        173–201
    funding adequacy for, 143
    objectives of—preventive and
        therapeutic, 262
    for prisoners pre-1970, 2–6, 123
    rationing of and human dignity, 43,
        174–175, 188
    See also Corrections and health care
Health Care Management Issues in
        Corrections, xii
Health care program, 1, 2, 159, 165, 177,
        232, 235, 241, 242, 250, 251, 255,
        271, 274
Health care staff
    and boundaries with patients, 22–23,
        26–27, 235, 283
    as fully qualified by community
        standards, 159
    in-service training for, 159
    as patient advocates, 162. See also
        Patient advocacy; Advocacy
    and prohibitions on witnessing use of
        force, 62–63
    safety concerns of, 46–47
    and special accommodations, 203, 263
Health care staff training, 265–266
    on security and institutional aspects,
        277–279
    See also Training
Health care treatment
    comparison of jails, prisons, juvenile
        facilities, 176
Health care unit furnishings and design
        reinforce therapeutic function, 235

Health care workers
    inurement of to violence and needs of
        prisoners, 81
Health certification or approval for
    punishment, 34
Health classification. *See* Classification
Health Insurance Portability and
    Accountability Act (HIPAA), 149,
    159
Health records, 15, 18, 41, 149, 159, 177,
    212, 213, 238, 246. *See also*
    Medical records
Health records and forms
    use of term *patient* and not *inmate*,
        232–233
Health screening area privacy, 284–285
Health services in New York City jails,
    251
Health status
    monitoring of, 268–269
Health through Walls, 183
Heart problems
    and use of mace, 58
Hemodialysis, 155, 195, 197, 199
Hepatitis C (HCV), 42, 101, 184, 188–189,
    195, 198
Hinkley effect, 209
HIPAA, and correctional compliance with,
    149
Hippocratic oath, xxvi, 7, 12, 14, 56, 60,
    65, 80, 91, 119, 179, 233, 228
History of patient
    and compliance with treatment, 199
    documentation of, 148
    and mental health problems, 210, 212,
        215, 219, 222*t*
HIV-positive individuals, 17, 48–49
HIV treatment, 42, 184, 198
Holmesburg Prison, 89
Homosexual activity, 48
Hormonal therapy, 28, 29, 30, 185
Hospitalization, 19, 40, 160, 195, 281
    psychiatric, 206, 207, 208, 212, 215
Housing mentally ill. *See* Isolation;
    Segregation; Supermax prisons;
    Intermediate care unit for mentally
    ill
Housing of transgender inmates, 28

Howard, John, 205
Human dignity. *See Trop v. Dulles,* 151
Human Rights Watch, 64, 138
Humane treatment, 270
    of confined children, 150, 157
    of mental health patients, 206, 215,
        224
    of youth in adult facilities, 150
Hunger strikes, 50–53, 168
Hygiene, 1, 2, 28, 30, 182, 241, 242, 257,
    259, 262, 269, 276, 277
Hyphenated labels, 234
Hypoglycemic patient transport, 286

Illegal or excessive use of force
Imaging technologies
    and body cavity searches, 35, 37–38
    and brain of mentally ill, 216
    for medical use, 184, 196
Imminent risk of danger to patient, 12, 17,
    20, 70, 88
Impact of the courts, xxiv, 163–169
Impaired cognitive skills, 97, 109, 112,
    113, 138, 204, 205, 211, 221
Important events in patient's life, 213
Improvement in function, 192, 196
Improvement of health-treatment goal,
    192, 196
Incarceration rate, 171
Independent contractor physician
    no qualified immunity for, 134
    West v. Atkins, 134, 153
Individual accommodations sought by
    health care staff, 263
Individual responsibility, 263
Individualized treatment plan
    good health care practice and, 263
    Infectious diseases and privacy issue
        limits, 17
Infirmary, 41, 53, 235, 264
Inflict no harm. *See* Hippocratic oath
Informed consent, 18–22, 75, 151, 160,
    263. *See also* Autonomy; Patient
    Autonomy
    bioethicists advise on, 14
    and chemical castration, 118–120
    and court-initiated medical procedure,
        118

Informed consent (*cont.*)
 and death row prisoners, 57
 and experimentation on prisoners,
  91–98, 100
 and enforced treatment, 18–22
 and medication for behavior control,
  60–61
 in mental health unit, 234
 and privacy and autonomy, 18–19
 requirements of, 18
 of tissue-specimen collection, 31, 32
Informed refusal, 22
Inmates
 abuse by staff, 79–80
 behavior, 190–191
 and handling health care, 3–4
 misbehavior in medical care, 59–60
 "nurses" in 1970s, 3
 or prisoner versus patient, 227–228. *See*
  Dehumanizing terms
Inpatient unit
 for the mentally ill, 220–224
 and restraints, 41
Insanity defense, 209
Institute of Medicine (IOM) , 98–104
Institution Review Board (IRB)
 Guidebook, 93–94
Intake health care screening, 176
Intellectual disability, 109, 204
Interdependence of corrections and health
 care, 268–279
Interference with prescribed treatment,
 128, 152
Intermediate care unit for the mentally ill,
 104, 105, 109, 114, 220, 264
International Association of Compounding
 Pharmacists
 opposition to participation in
  executions, 70
International ethical guidelines for
 biomedical research using human
 subjects, 97–98
Interrogation
 AMA prohibition for doctors, 73, 77
 NCCHC opposes for correctional health
  care staff, 78–79
 physician role in CIA interrogations,
  76–77

Intervention by medical staff, 12, 14, 18,
 179
 and beneficence. *See* Beneficence
 and contributing behavior, 190–191
 and forced feeding, 50, 52
 and influencing factors, 189–201
 and medical research, 97
 not for forensic purposes, 32
 practitioner guidelines for, 176–178
 for reducing risk of violence, 40
 in suicide. *See* Suicide intervention
Involuntary administration of antipsychotic
 medication, 21, 70, 154
Involuntary treatment, 70, 152, 153, 154,
 179, 264
 court order needed for prolonged
  treatment, 20
 in mental health unit, 19
 and restraints, 62, 264
 for trial readiness, 21
IOM, *See* Institute of Medicine (IOM)
IRB Guidebook, 93–101
Isolation in penal settings. 104–106.
  See also Supermax

Jails
 countertherapeutic environment in, 122,
  212–215, 230
 definition of, xix
 health care treatment in, 176, 198
 as major intake centers for health,
  welfare, social problems,
  209–211
 as poor persons' mental health facility,
  210
JJDPA. *See* Juvenile Justice and
  Delinquency Prevention Act
  (JJDPA)
Johnson, Perry, xi, 250, 272
Judicial oversight for improvement,
 165–167
Junker, Gary N., 267
Just deserts, 10
Justice, 10, 91, 101
Juvenal, 167
Juvenile correctional facilities
 definition of, xix
 health care treatment in, 176

impact of PLRA on, 139, 149, 150, 143, 166
protecting detainees from harm, 156
Juvenile Justice and Delinquency Prevention Act (JJDPA), 150
Juveniles
and Eighth Amendment, 149–150
and Fourteenth Amendment on due process, 149
and informed consent of parent or guardian, 18

Keep-on-person (KOP) drugs, 42, 160, 244, 287
Kendig, Dr. Newton, 102–103
Kupers, Dr. Terry, 138, 210
Kurtzman, Josh, 138

Language influence on actions, 229–235
Law and order, 165, 171, 262
Law versus ethics, 7–8
Lawsuits
and plan of correction, 162–163
LEAA 1975 study of health care in U.S. prisons and jails, 249–250
Legal issues in correctional health care, 123–171
Legal liability, 17, 18, 22, 129, 130, 133, 134, 135, 139, 140, 148, 154, 192, 242, 245, 265
Legal services programs, 142
Legible documentation, 148, 159
Legitimate medical requirements, 33, 44, 81, 162, 239, 266, 273
Lethal force, 65, 264
Lethal injection, 64–70
and compounding pharmacies, 67
Leukemia, 196
Level of care, 104, 114, 180–182, 222t
Life-skills training, 144, 191, 262
Lighting, 44, 46, 110
and circadian rhythms, 105
importance of, 47, 48
or Linan Public Interest Program, 106
Line of responsibilitycareful delineation of, 254–257
Litigation-reduction strategies, 159–163
Lockdown, 262, 264, 273

Loss of control, 113, 214, 218, 265
Lottery approach, 195

Mace
and COPD patients, 58
use and effects of, 58–59
Maiming
federal statute and, 115
Maintain and improve program quality, 2, 24, 161, 167, 177, 242, 248
adherence to ethical and professional standards, 164, 231, 241
principle of corrections and health care, 175, 181, 235, 241, 272
Malingering, 223–224
Malpractice suits, 44, 120, 129, 130, 131, 180, 242
Managed care system, 178, 236–237
Manic disorders of inmates compared to general population, 208, 210
Mann, Horace, 205–206
Marshall, Justice Thurgood, 129
Mass incarceration, 167. *See also* Crowding
May, Dr. John, 183
McKay Commission, 127
Medicaid coverage, 196
Medical and mental health staff
participation in punitive measures, 55, 79, 161, 260–264
Medical appointments, 109, 244, 268, 288
Medical authority, 244–245, 248
Medical autonomy, 14, 46, 61, 162, 243–245, 263–264, 271
for clinical decisions, 244, 271
definition of, 14
Estelle v. Gamble, 243–244
with security restrictions, 244
Medical care
and contemporary standards in free world, 179–180, 182–183
to meet routine and emergency needs of patients, 152
of prisoners, 128
Medical clearance, 56–58
Medical confidentiality limits, 16–17, 276

Medical director, 243, 247–248
Medical equipment, 47, 246
Medical ethics
  and faith traditions, xxvi
Medical malpractice, 44
  and contemporary standards of
    community, 180
  Gamble, 129, 132
  success factors for suit on, 131
  tort of negligence, 130
Medical necessity, 183–187, 192–194,
    196–197
Medical neutrality defined, 14
Medical parole, 40
Medical records, 3, 82, 123, 168, 177–179,
    253. *See* also Documentation of
    patient information; Health records
  computerized, 148
  confidentiality in, 15. *See also*
    Confidentiality
  disclosure and privacy rights of, 149
  filing and retention of, 148
  and HIPAA, 149, 159
  legible documentation in, 148, 159
Medical restraints or seclusion, 41, 62,
    261*t*, 262, 264
Medication
  administration of, 160
  for behavior control, 60–61, 85, 121,
    161.
  crushing of, 42–43
  DOT, 41–42
  and high cost of, 188–189
  keep on person (KOP), 42, 160, 244,
    287
  mood-altering drugs, 60–61
  prompt refills, 24, 160
  psychotropic. *See* Psychotropic
    medications; Antipsychotic
    medications
  in transit, 286
  used in lethal injection, 67–70
Mental disorders
  among inmates, 120–121
  rooted in biological causes, 204. *See
    also Diagnostic and Statistical
    Manual of Mental Disorders*
    (DSM-5)

Mental health levels of care, 105, 221,
    222*t*, 223
  beds for, 104–105, 220
  procedural protections for, 19, 153
  state guidance for, 41
Mental health professionals
  and belief in patients, 266
  as correctional resources, 266
  encouraging compliance by persuasion,
    266
  and inmate potential for change, 267
  and staff training in conflict resolution,
    266
Mental health unit
  discharge to general population, 217,
    220
  special features of, 234
Mental illness
  as chronic condition, 203–205, 216,
    221–224
  consequences of failing to recognize
    chronicity of, 221–224
  and correctional environment. *See*
    Correctional environment
  and deinstitutionalization, 205–212
  and lighting, 105
  prevalence of in correctional
    populations, 210–211
  and remission, 217
  treated not punished, 225
  waxes and wanes, 215–219
Mental retardation, 120–121, 135, 204, 208
  intellectual disability in DSM-5,
    203–204
Mentally ill in corrections
  advocacy about, 122. *See also* Advocacy
  levels of care, 220–223
  and closed-head injured, 218–219
  and correctional officer escort versus
    trained worker, 287
  discharge into general population of jail
    or prison, 217
  discrimination against, 144
  and disruptiveness in general prison
    population, 220
  follow-up frequency for, 221
  and housing in correctional facilities,
    204–205

in inpatient units and intermediate care settings, 220
involuntary treatment of. *See* Involuntary treatment
in isolation or supermax setting, 104–115
and *Madrid Declaration*, 205
management problems of, 104
medication as primary treatment for, 216
in prison longer than nonmentally ill, 210
and segregated housing for, 104–114, 161
in sheltered living units, 219–220
staff training for dealing with, 220
therapeutic environment as effective treatment for, 216
in therapeutic settings, 114
transition out of long-term segregation, 109
World Psychiatric Association on, 204–205
Methamphetamine abuse, 101, 121
Metzner, Dr. Jeffrey, 105
Mill, John Stuart, on harm principle, 15
Mitford, Jessica, 90
Models of organization, 248–254
Moral distress
of caregivers, 26
ethics committee as remedy to, 26
as psychological imbalance—Lorry Schoenly, 83
Morality, 6, 9
Mortisugu, Dr. Kenneth P., 269–270
Mossman, Dr. Douglas, 70–72
Muse, Mary, 26
Mutual respect and trust, xxvii, 2, 255, 270, 271, 272, 274, 281–282

Name tags, 283
Names, derogatory, 228
Nathan, Vincent, 163–164
National bioethics forum for corrections, 14
National Commission for Protection of Human Subjects of Biomedical and Behavioral Research, 90–93, 95
National Commission on Correctional Health Care (NCCHC), xvi, 15, 29, 33, 34, 45, 56, 63, 73, 78, 80, 96, 102, 153, 232, 243, 244, 245, 246, 271, 275, 286
beneficial impact of accreditation and other programs, 164–165, 167
National Commission on Correctional Health Care—position statements
Competency for Execution, 73, 74
Correctional Health Care Professionals' Response to Inmate Abuse, 78–79, 80
Transgender, Transsexual, and Gender Nonconforming Health Care in Correctional Settings, 29
National Commission on Correctional Health Care—standards, xiii–xiv, xx–xxi
P-A-02 on Responsible Health Authority, 243, 246
P-A-03 on Medical Autonomy, 244, 271
P-A-08 on Communication on Patients' Health Needs, 56
P-C-04 on Health Training for Correctional Officers, 275
P-C-05 on Medication Administration Training, 275
P-E-09 on Segregated Inmates, 45
P-G-01 on Chronic Disease Services, 178
P-G-09 on Counseling and Care of the Pregnant Inmate, 286
P-H-02 on Confidentiality of Health Records, 15
P-I-03 on Forensic Information, 33, 34
P-I-06 on Medical and Other Research, 96
P-I-07 on Executions, 63, 73
National Institute of Corrections (NIC) study on administrative segregation, 108–109
National Institute on Alcohol Abuse and Alcoholism, 120
Nationality and human worth or dignity, 8
Nature of crime and decision to treat, 190
Nazi death camps, 75

NCCHC. *See* National Commission on Correctional Health Care (NCCHC)
Necessary care, 181–182, 187, 192–194
Necessity
    of custody procedures, 35, 37, 39, 58
    of medical procedures, 183–186, 192–200, 244
Negative aspects of correctional environment, 214
Negligence, 131
Net benefit, 179, 186
New employee orientation. *See* Training
Noise, 44, 46, 212, 219, 223
Nomenclature, 283
Nonmaleficence principle, 14, 179.
    See also Beneficence
Not guilty by reason of insanity, 209
Notoriety, 191
Number of incarcerated people, xxv
Number of prisons and jails, xxv
Nuremberg Code, 92–93
Nurses
    and moral distress versus custody staff, 83
    and protocols to prevent litigation, 160
Nursing care and contemporary standards, 179–180
Nurturing, 213, 214

Obama, President Barack, 171
Obasogie, Osagie K., 99
OC spray. *See* Mace, use and effects of
Off-site appointments, 268–269, 273, 284
"Offender"
    implications of word, 228–229
Office of Human Research Protection (OHRP), 94, 98, 99
Ohio State Advisory Committee
    and medical decision making in 1970s, 4–5
OHRP. *See* Office of Human Research Protection (OHRP)
Okasha, Dr. Ahmed, 204–205
Orderly management of institution
    common mission of corrections and health care, 241
    part of properly managed health care program, 2

shared priority of corrections and health care, 259
Organ donation by condemned prisoners
    American Medical Association position on, 66
Organ transplants, 194–195
    allocation of, 195
    bioethicist advice on, 14
    Felicia Cohn on, 43
    and medical considerations, 43
Organizing correctional health care, 241–257
Outpatient care, 20, 40, 104, 114
    psychiatric, 104, 114, 220, 221
Outside public health authorities, 251–254
Overcrowding. *See* Crowding
Overuse of incarceration, 170

Pain control inadequacy, 192, 196, 232
Paradox of the Commons, 188
Paramilitary staff training for corrections, 265
Parole, medical, 40
Pat-down searches, 39
Patient
    acceptability of medical and psychiatric procedures, 15–16
    autonomy of, 14–15, 178–179
    as beneficiary of health care services, 228
    best interest of, 70–72, 75
    definition of, xix, 82, 227–239
    and dignity and standards of professional practice, 179
    education of, 101, 161
    liberty of, 179
    privacy of, 187, 284–285
    rights of, 80
    safety of, 182
Patient advocacy, 236–237, 252. *See also* Advocacy
Patient autonomy, 14, 52, 53, 71, 88, 91, 92, 97, 99, 101, 117, 178, 179.
    See also Informed consent
Patient Protection and Affordable Care Act (PPACA) of 2010, 173–174, 178, 192
Patient-centered care components, 24

Patient–provider
    relationship and forensic evidence
        collection, 32–34, 179, 266
Pattern of neglect, 132
Peer pressure, 52, 53, 55
Peer review and role of medical director,
    248
Pelvic exams, 39
Penal servitude, 124, 164, 169
Pepper spray. *See* Mace, use of
Personal dignity, 8–10, 270, 288. *See also*
    Decency
Personal liability, 135
Personality-disordered patients' treatment,
    23
"Persons" and qualified immunity,
    133–134
Persons' value and religious belief
    systems, 8–9
Persons with disabilities—Section 504 of
    Rehabilitation Act, 143–148
Pharmaceutical companies, 94
Pharmaceutical formulary, 149, 182, 287
Pharmacists and executions, 68–71
Phlebotomists, 66, 69
Physical restraints. *See* Restraints
Physician practice clinical guidelines,
    160
Physician roles
    in correctional facilities in 1970s, 3
    in determining competence for
        execution, 72
    and help with capital punishment, 75
    and help in torture, 76
Physician–nurse on-call arrangements,
    159
Physicians
    adherence to ethical practices, 7, 73
    as agents of state in corrections, 90
    duty of, 96
    ethics of involvement in chemical
        castration, 116–121
    on-call arrangements of, 159, 284
    participation in executions, 62–68, 72
    as patient advocate, 13
    providers of treatment and not agents of
        social control, 120
Pill lines for directly observed therapy, 42

Pinel, Philippe, 105
PLRA, Prison Litigation Reform Act,
    137–143
    applicability to juveniles, 139, 150
    attorney compensation limited under,
        140, 147
    exhaust all administrative remedies,
        138, 146
    filing fee, 146
    and grievance-system problems, 139,
        140, 142, 150, 158, 166
    impact of, 146–147, 166
    limits appointment of special masters,
        139
    objectives—limiting number of
        frivolous cases, 141–142
    precludes claims that do not show a
        physical injury, 142, 138, 146
    prospective/injunctive relief
        prohibited, 146
    reform is needed, 140–143
    special masters versus monitors and
        receivers under, 140
    termination of existing settlements
        and consent decrees, 136–137
    unreasonably limits access to the
        courts, 164
Policies and practices of good correctional
    system, 1, 2, 241
Politics and prison expenditures for health
    care, 136–137, 165
Posttraumatic stress disorder, 83, 212,
    218
Practitioner guidelines, 176–178
Predicted dangerousness, 40
Preexisting conditions, 189–190, 191–192
Pregnant women, 286
Pretrial detainees' body searches—*Bell v.
    Wolfish*, 153
Prevalence of mental illness and disorders,
    210–211, 219
Preventive and therapeutic health care
    objectives, 262
Primary client, 264
Primun non nocere (above all do no harm),
    12, 60, 228, 230
Principles common to corrections and
    health care, 1, 241

Prison health care in 1970s, 4
Prison Litigation Reform Act of 1996
        (PLRA). *See* PLRA Prison
        Litigation Reform Act
Prison overcrowding. *See* Crowding
Prison versus free community choice of
        health care, 6–7
Prisoners
        and consent—protection from
                exploitation, 93
        definition of in IOM
                recommendations, 102
        experimentation on, 93–94
        have constitutionally guaranteed right
                to health care, 6–7
        privacy of. *See* Privacy
        rehabilitation of, 10, 262
        rights of, 8–10, 151, 180
        as slaves of the state—*Ruffin v.*
                Commonwealth, 124
        well-being of as priority of
                corrections and health care, 259
Prisons and jails and the mentally ill, 76,
        204, 212, 215
Privacy, 284–285. *See also* Confidentiality
        auditory or visual, 285
        as basis for patient autonomy, 14
        in booking and health screening areas,
                285
        limits on, 16–17
        rights of patients and HIPAA
                applicability, 149
Private prisons
        personnel of shielded from Bivens
                action, 155
Privatization, 251
Probability of successful outcomes, 43,
        196–197
Profession of patients and decision to treat,
        191
Professional and medical ethics
        compromising of, 274
Professional certification programs,
        164–165.
Professional code of ethics, 10–14, 164.
        See also Ethical codes
Professional judgment
        and correctional health care, 265

Professional standards, 178. *See also*
        Standards of correctional
        organizations
Professionalism. 164. *See also*
        Responsible health authority
        and mutual respect. *See* Mutual respect
        and trust
Pronouncing death, 63–66, 68–69, 75
Protecting from harm, 17, 35, 56, 62, 74,
        80, 124–126
        of employees who report abuse,
                79–80
        of juveniles, 149–150
        of offenders with disabilities, 148.
                See also Americans with
                Disabilities Act (ADA)
        of public health, 265. *See also*
                Quarantine
        of society, 1, 11, 12, 260, 261*t*
        of therapeutic relationship, 33. *See also*
                Therapeutic alliance
        of vulnerable inmates, 28–29, 38–39,
                59, 97, 111, 114, 212, 268
Psychiatric care and contemporary
        standards, 179–180
Psychiatric hospitals, 208
Psychiatric procedures, 15–16
Psychiatric treatment
        hospitalization for, 19
        involuntary, 19, 20
        mandatory outpatient, 19–21
        Vitek v. Jones, 19, 153
Psychiatrist
        concern for conditions of confinement,
                247–248
        involvement in treatment planning,
                248
Psychiatrists' role in execution or
        punishment, 74. *See also*
        Declaration of Madrid
Psychological distress
        of patients, 27, 113, 220, 222, 232, 268
Psychologists, 265
Psychosis, 108, 112, 195, 210, 218.
        See also Posttraumatic stress
        disorder
Psychosocial treatment interventions, 215,
        217

Psychotropic medications, 58, 114, 152–154, 160, 198, 210, 247, 280. *See also* Antipsychotic medications
  and heat sensitivity, 57
  involuntarily administered in medical setting only, 41
  and patients' liberty interest, 21
  Washington v. Harper, 21
PTSD. *See* Posttraumatic stress disorder (PTSD)
Public health
  advocacy. *See* Advocacy; Patient advocacy
  and balance of individual and public goods, 265
  and fetal alcohol issues, 120–121
  and methods of risk reduction, 49
  and outside public health authority, 251–252
  and role of medical staff, 257
  role of responsible physician in, 247–248
Public opinion on overuse of incarceration, 170–171
Public safety as priority of corrections and health care, 259
Punishment
  and Eighth Amendment, 151
  environment of, 230
  health care involvement in, 56–58, 79
  and *Jackson v. Bishop*, 151
  of mentally ill, 280, 283
Punitive dealings with patients
  and burnout, 81
  and comparison of corrections and health care, 264
  as sanctions, 260–262, 264

Qualified immunity, 133–134
Qualified staff, 159
Quality improvement
  monitoring of, 24, 161
  priority of corrections and health care in, 259
  role of medical director in, 248
Quality of life, 176, 186, 187, 199, 200
Quality of medical care required
  Battle v. Anderson, 152

Quality-control program, xxiv, 81, 164, 242
Quarantine
  TB testing and medications, 21

Race
  and decision to treat, 189–190
  discrimination, 152, 170
  and human worth or dignity, 8
Radiation experiments on prisoners, 89–91
Reasonable modifications, 147
Receivership, 140
Receiving screening, 282
Recipient rights, 41
Referral to specialist, 195
Refusal to take psychotropic drugs, 152–153
Regimentation, 262
Rehabilitation
  as goal of criminal justice system, 10, 288
  and justice through programs in corrections, 10
  mission of correctional agencies in, 262, 288
  programs for, 262
Rehabilitation Act of 1973, Section 504. *See* Americans with Disabilities Act (ADA)
Reiter, Keramet, 99–100, 102
Relief of pain, 192, 196
Remedy for deprivation of federally protected rights, 151
Reporting abusive behavior by staff, 79–80
Research
  and ethical protections, 98–104
  on prisoners, 93–94
  topics suggested for prisons, 101
Residential care, 220–222
Respect
  for dignity and rights of inmates, 241, 242, 259
  for shared mutual responsibility, 28, 270, 272
  and teamwork, 255
Respectful deliberation, 272–274

Respondeat superior (vicarious liability), 135

Responsible health authority, 242–248
    duties of, 246–247
    and ethical orientation of responsible physician, 256
    and improving recruitment, 245
    legal liability issues of, 245
    person and not agency, 243
    rationale for designating, 245–246
    standards on, 243–246
Responsible physician , 243. *See also* Medical director
Restoration of function, 199
Restrained inmates
    monitoring of, 269
Restraint and good health care practice, 264
Restraints, 62. *See also* Medical restraints
    ambulatory, 41
    four-point, 62
    monitoring inmates in, 62
    on pregnant women, 286
    reduction in use, 282
    restraining chair, 41
Restrictive measures, 262
Retribution and restraint versus rehabilitation, 10
Rhabdomyolysis, 280–281
Rieger, Dr. Dean P.
    and determining serious medical needs, 181
Right of access to courts, 125, 145 151
Right to refuse treatment, 19, 51, 52, 151, 197, 263
Rights of prisoners versus state's interest, 37
Rights retention, 152
Risk–benefit analysis
    and Declaration of Helsinki, 103
Risk-prone areas, 159–162
Role conflicts, 55–85, 213
    and writing tickets, 59–60
Rudimentary medical practice in Third World Countries, 182

Safe and secure environment, 1, 241, 259
Safety
    in clinic, 282
    community standards of, 179

and good order, 237, 284
    in health care and corrections, 241, 282
    and security, 46–47, 234–235, 241
Sanitation
    in health care and corrections, 282
    as part of properly managed health care program, 1
Sanity of defendant, 39, 73
Sargent, D. A., 73
Satellite facilities, 247
Scarcity of resources, 2, 9, 10, 13, 83, 176, 180
Schizophrenia, 20, 217
Schlanger, Margo, and Giovanna Shay, 141–142
Schlosser, Erik, 267
Schoenly, Lorry, 26
Seasonal affective disorder (SAD)
Seclusion, medical, 41, 262, 264
Secondary gain, 112, 187
Section 1983 suits, 126, 129–130. *See also* Civil Rights Act of 1871; Deliberate indifference
Secure therapeutic environment, 283
Security
    constraints impairing cost-effective health care, 287–288
    criteria for hires as domain of correctional authority, 244
    as issue in health care staff training, 277–279
    as necessary for good treatment, 234
    problems with, 234, 266–267
Security housing units (SHUs). *See* Segregation
    and exercise time, 283
    removal of mentally ill from, 283
    visits by nurse or psychologist through food slot, 44–45, 106, 110, 284
Segregation. *See also* Isolation in prison settings; Supermax prisons
    of mentally ill persons, 107–109
    outpatient care of, 114
    proper rounding inessential, 45, 161
    reduction in use of, 282
Segregation cells, 41
Segregation units, 110–111, 224

Self-harm, 190–191
Self-monitoring, 165–167
Sense of self-worth, 232, 262, 288
Sensitivity to heat, 57
Sensory deprivation of mentally ill in
    segregation, 108, 111, 224–225
Serious medical conditions defined, 153
Severe isolation. *See* Security housing
    units (SHUs)
Sex-reassignment surgery, 28–30
Sexual abuse and duty to report, 80
Sexual orientation and preference
    and decision to treat, 189–190
    and human worth or dignity, 8
Sexually traumatized women—Dr. Pamela
    Dole on, 39
Shackling pregnant women during labor,
    286
Shakedowns by health professional staff,
    61, 278
Shared priorities of health care and
    corrections, 259–260, 270
Short-term facilities, xix, 176, 198. *See
    also* Detention centers; Jails
Should I quit my job? 84–85
SHU. *See* Security housing units (SHUs)
Sick call, 3, 4, 5, 6, 22, 48, 81, 106, 128,
    157, 159, 161, 244, 268, 272
Skin test for TB, 46
Slaves of the state, 124, 164, 169
Sleep deprivation and CIA physicians
    and psychologists, 76. *See also*
    Torture
Social and family skills for rehabilitation
    programs, 10, 262
Social and psychological problems of
    prisoners as research topics, 93
Social class, 191
Social contract theory and ethical basis of
    prisoners' rights, 9
Social standing and decision to treat, 191
Social worker's professional standards,
    153
Social worth, 174, 195
Societal perspective on extent of health
    care, 188
Sociopaths and societal benefits from
    treatment of, 23

Socrates, 7
Solitary confinement, 51, 111–112
    and cognitive impairment, 113
Speaking out, 36, 58, 79–81, 161, 278,
    288–289. *See also* Advocacy;
    Patient advocacy
Special masters versus monitors—PLRA
    rules, 139–140
Specialty care on site, 284
Spectrum of care model, 183–189
Staff training
    on conflict resolution, 266
    paramilitary for corrections, 265
    styles of, 265–266
Standards of correctional organizations.
    See ACA standards; NCCHC
    standards
Standards of decency
    evolution of, 291
Stanley, Judith, 232
Staples-Horne, Dr. Michelle, 229
Start, Dr. Armond H., 200–201
State and federal jurisdiction over
    Section 1983 suits, 133–134
State Prison of Southern Michigan, 94–95
Sterilization of mentally defective inmates,
    116
Stevens, Justice John, 132–133
Stinneford, John, 115
Strategic planning, 282
Stress
    and chronic nature of mental illness,
        221, 223–224
    from crowding, 215
    and factors affecting patients, 213
    and housing, 217, 219–220
    and medication, 217
    of mentally ill in prisons and jails, 216
    from overly restrictive environment, 280
    of prisons and jails, 212, 214, 215, 217
    and public health role of staff in
        reduction of, 257
Stress management and burnout treatment,
    82
Stress reduction and role of medical staff,
    257
Stressful influences in general population,
    223

Strip searches, 36–39
    constitutional issues involved with, 36
    cross-gender searches, 36
    imaging technology as possible
        substitute, 36
    mental health implications of, 36
    and PTSD, 38
Subacute care, 222
Subjective awareness, 132, 134
Substance abuse, 10, 248
    new disorders of in DSM-5, 204
    tests for not done by health care staff,
        31–32
    treatment of outside health services
        division, 248
Suicidal ideation, 113, 212, 268, 276
Suicidal tendencies
    recognizing and responding to, 278
Suicide prevention training standards,
    275
Suicide risk surveillance, 268
Sultan, Bonnie, 83
Supermax prisons. See also Isolation in
        penal settings; Segregation
    characteristics of, 110
    costs, goals, and impacts in Urban
        Institute DOJ study of, 112
    cruel and unusual punishment and,
        113–115
    and high rates of psychological trauma
        Craig Haney, 113
    and isolation, 109–115
    and mental health care in Texas, 112
    sensory deprivation and social isolation
        in, 110–115
    and unconstitutional confinement of
        seriously mentally ill persons, 114
System of beliefs, 242, 266–267
Systemwide health authority, 243

Taser and rhabdomyolysis, 280–281
TB, medication for tuberculosis, 41–42
TBI. See Traumatic brain injury
Tear gas. See Mace, use and effects of
Technological advances, 8, 35–39, 174,
        178, 181–182, 185, 189
Tension between care and custody in
        prisons, xxvii

Teplin, Linda, 209–210
Terms for patients in juvenile facilities,
    228
Testicular transplant experiment on
        prisoners, 90
Therapeutic activities , 264
Therapeutic alliance, 23, 31, 34, 161, 201
Therapeutic environment for mentally ill,
        225. See also Intermediate care
        unit
Therapeutic response rather than
        punishment by health care staff,
        264
Therapeutic seclusion or restraint ordered
        by medical staff, 262–263
Third-party payers, 13, 173, 178, 192, 196,
        244
Thorazine, 207
Tickets and ticketing, 21, 55, 59–60, 218,
        234, 260, 278
Tissue and blood collection by outside
        health professionals, 31
Tissue specimen collection, 31
Title 42 U.S.C. Section 1983. See Civil
        Rights Act of 1871; Deliberate
        indifference
Title II of ADA. See Americans with
        Disabilities Act (ADA)
Toch, Hans, 113
Torrey, E. Fuller
    plight of incarcerated mentally
        disordered persons, 212
    state psychiatric bed decline, 208
Tort liability, 18, 130–131
Torture, 30, 55, 72, 75–79, 80, 87, 90, 98,
        113, 115, 121, 152
Total quality management (TQM), 285
    Touching, appropriate, 26
Tours by responsible health authority, 246
Toxic sprays
    decontamination from, 59
    not as punishment, 59
    not ethical to clear prisoners for, 59
Training
    cooperation in crossover areas, 161,
        274–275, 277–278
    curriculum for, 256
    methodology of, 268, 278–279

and new employee orientation, 80, 84,
227, 231, 233, 236, 238–239, 274,
279
and staff training style, 265–266
style compared, 265–266
Tranquilizing drugs, misuse of, 156
Transfer of patients to medical facilities,
41, 275
Transgender inmates, 27–30. *See also*
Transsexual patient treatment
assault potential on, 28, 29
bioethicist advice on managing, 14
Farmer v. Brennan, 154
housing of, 28
Obergefell v. Hodges on, 30
treatment start in prison, 28–29
Wisconsin law on, 29–30
Transition of mentally ill out of long-term
segregation, 109
Transport, 272, 286
delay of medical, 244
and medications en route, 286
of patients, 286
Transsexual inmate—*Phillips v. Michigan
Department of Corrections*, 154
Transsexual patient treatment, 30, 154,
184, 185
Traumatic brain injury (TBI), 218–219
Treatment
and celebrity status, notoriety, social
class, and profession, 191
and contributory behavior, 131
delays and outcome of, 199
goals for, 192–194
and refusal and informed refusal form
and nurse, 22
to render person competent for
execution, 74–75
through bars, 45–46
for trial competency, 70–72
under less-than-satisfactory conditions,
45–48
Treatment Advocacy Center
report on decline in psychiatric beds,
208
Trust
breach of, 34
Tuberculosis, 41, 42

Unethical behavior—reasons for engaging
in, 122
United Nations
and International Covenant on Civil and
Political Rights on
experimentation, 98
and physician certification of persons
for punishment, 74
United States
Department of Justice, 249
Department of Labor, 58
Preventive Services Task Force,
177–178
Universal health insurance, 183
Universal precautions, 17, 275
University research on correctional
populations, 103–104
Unnecessary risk, 46–47
Unnecessary suffering and , 92
Urban Institute DOJ study of supermax
prisons, 112
Urgency, 194, 197–198
Urine collection for forensic drug testing,
31–32
Use of force, 58, 61–62, 65, 107, 264.
See also Capital punishment;
Executions; Forced feeding
Utilitarian calculus, 10, 71
Utilization review, 173, 181–182, 200

Vaccine trials and research on prisoners,
93–94
Value of persons
in different religious belief systems, 8–9
Venipuncture, 46
Vicarious liability, 135
Vietnam War protests, 126
Violent behavior prediction, 40
Violent crimes, 32, 210
Vital signs, 44, 64, 66
Vodka
and effective cooperation between
physician and warden to save lives,
281–282
as treatment for toxic alcohol poisoning,
281–282
Voluntary compliance, 266
Voluntary consent of subjects, 92

War on Poverty, 127

Warden (superintendent, supervisor, jail administrator), xix

Warder is responsible for well-being of ward, 180

Washington State Medical Association, 5

Waste avoidance in health care programs, 2

Waterboarding, 76

Weapons training of health care staff, 278

Well-being of prisoners as shared priority, 259, 270

Well-being of society as shared priority, 270

WHO. See World Health Organization

Window coverings and safety, 17

Wisconsin law on transgender inmates, 29–30

Wishart, Margaret, and Nancy Dubler, 126, 229

Witnessing use of force. See Use of force

Women and girls, 38
    impact of strip searches on, 38
    and sexual abuse, pelvic exams, and personal body searches, 39

Women and minorities
    integration by courts into ranks of line and professional staff, 163

Women's correctional facilities
    and advocacy about alcohol and FASD, 120–121

Words and language
    impact on attitudes and behaviors, 227–240

Work restrictions and special accommodations, 263

Workplace violence as stressor, 83

World Health Organization (WHO), xi, 14, 97

World Medical Association (WMA), xiv, 12
    on body cavity searches, 36
    and Declaration of Helsinki on medical research, 96–97
    and Declaration of Tokyo denunciation of torture, 78
    and Declaration of Tokyo prohibition of participation in capital punishment, 63
    and Declaration of Tokyo prohibition on forced feeding, 51–52
    and International Code of Medical ethics on patient rights to confidentiality, 12–13

World Psychiatric Association
    and, Declaration of Madrid, 74, 204–205

Writing tickets
    and role conflict, 59–60

Wrong but legal actions, 6

Yale Law School
    study on administrative segregation, 106

Youth detained in adult facilities, 150. See also Juveniles; Students

Index of Legal Cases

A.M. v. Luzerne County Juvenile Detention Center, 372 F. 3d 572, 3d Cir. (2004), 158

Alexander S. v. Boyd, 876 F. Supp. 773, 778, D.S.C. (1995), 157

Anderson v. City of Atlanta, 778 F. 2d 678 (1985), 143

Babcock v. White, 102 F.3rd 267, 7th Cir. (1996), 133

Battle v. Anderson, 376 F. Supp. 402, E. Dist. OK (1974), 5–6, 152

Battle v. Anderson, 564 F. 2d 388, 396, CA10 (1977), 143

Baugh v. Woodard, 808 F. 2d 333, 335 n. 2, 4th Cir. (1987), 19

Baze v. Rees, 553 U.S. 35, 128 S. Ct. 1520 (2008), 68–69

Bell v. Wolfish, 441 U.S. 520 (1979), 37, 153

Bivens v. Six Unknown Agents of the Federal Bureau of Narcotics, 403 U.S. 388 (1971), 136, 152, 153, 155

Booth v. Churner, 532 U.S. 731 (2001), 307n.30

Brock v. Kenton County, KY, 93 Fed. Appx. 793, 6th Cir. (2004), 150

Brown v. Plata, 131 S. Ct. 1910 (2011), 563 U.S. 493 (2011), 134 S. Ct. 436 (2013), 155, 167–169, 171

Brown v. Simmons, no. 6:03-CV-122, 2007 WL 654920, at *6, S.D. Tex. (Feb. 23, 2007), 142

Buck v. Bell, 274 U.S. 200 (1927), 116

Buddy Cason v. Jim Seckinger, 231 F. 3d 777 (2000), 308n.45

Carlson v. Green, 446 U.S. 14 (1980), 153

Cody v. Hillard, 304 F. 3d 767, 776, 8th Cir. (2002), 307n.30

Coffin v. Reichard, 143 F. 2d 443, 6th Cir. (1944), 124, 125, 151

Coleman v. Brown, 912 F. Supp. 1282 (1995), 155, 167

Coleman v. Schwarzenegger, 912 F. Supp. 1282 (1995), 155, 167

Cruzan v. Missouri Department of Health, 497 U.S. 261 (1990), 47

D.B. v. Tewksbury, 545 F. Supp. 896, D. Or. (1982), 156

Dean v. Coughlin, 804 F. 2d 207 (1986), 153

Estelle v. Gamble, 429 U.S. 97 (1976), 126, 128–132, 137, 152, 180, 243–244

Ex parte Hull, 312 U.S. 546 (1941), 125, 151

Fante et al. v. Department of Health and Human Services et al., U.S. District Court, E.D. Mich., S. Div., Civil Action No. 80-72778 (1981), 94

Farmer v. Brennan, 511 U.S. 825, 837 (1994), 134–135, 154

Fields v. Smith (previously *Sundstrom v. Frank*). 2010 Westlaw 1929819, E.D, 30

Ford v. Wainwright, 477 U.S. 399, 409–10 (1986), 72

Fulwood v. Clemmer, 295 F. 2d 171 (1961), 126

Gary H. v. Hegstrom, 831 F.2d 1439 (1987), 157

Gates v. Collier, 501 F. 2d 1291 1319, CA5 (1974), 143, 152

Goodman v. Georgia (*United States v. Georgia et al.*), 126 S. Ct. 877, 882 (2006), 145–146

Hamilton v. Love, 328 F. Supp. 1182 at 1194, E.D. Ark. (1971), 143

Hancock v. Payne, 2006 WL 21751 at *3, S.D. Miss. (2006), 138

Hays v. Jefferson County, Ky., 668 F. 2d 869, 874, 6th Cir. (1982), 135

Haywood v. Drown, 556 U.S., 129 S. Ct. 2108 (2009),133–134

Helling v. McKinney, 509 U.S. 25 (1993), 137, 154

Holt v. Sarver, 442 F. 2d 304 (1971), 127–128, 152

Hope v. Pelzer, 536 U.S. 730 (2002), 134

Inmates of Suffolk County Jail v. Rouse et al., 129 F. 3d 649, 654, 1st Cir. (1997), 307n.30

J.A. et al. v. Barbour et al., 3:07-CV-00394 (2007), 158–159

Jackson v. Bishop, 404 F. 2d 572, 8th Cir. (1968), 143, 151

Jackson v. Ft. Stanton and Jackson v. Los Lunas State Hospital and Training School, 757 F.Supp. 1243 (D.N.M. 1990); 964 F2d 980 (1992), 158

John Does 1-100 v. Boyd. 613 F. Supp. 1514, 1522, D.C. Minn. (1985), 37

Johnson v. California, 543 U.S. 499 (2005), 170

Jones v. Bock, 127 S. Ct. 910 (2007), 140–141

Jones 'El et al. v. Berge et al., 164 F. Supp. 2d 1096 (2001), 111, 113–114

Jordan v. Gardner 986 F. 2d 1521, 9th Cir. en banc (1993), 37

Justice v. City of Peachtree City, 961 F. 2d 188, 192, 11 Cir. (1992), 37

K.L.W. v. James, 204-CV-149BN (2005), 158

Knecht v. Gillman, 488 F. 2d 1136 (1973), 161

Lewis v. Casey, 518 U.S. 343 (1996), 155, 163

Lollis v. New York State Department of Social Services, 322 F. Supp. 473 (1970), 156

Madrid v. Gómez, 889 F. Supp. 1146, 1280, N.D. Cal. (1995), 190 F. 3d 990 (1999), 113–114, 154, 166

Martin v. Hadix, 527 U.S. 343 (1999), 307n.30

Mary Beth G. v. City of Chicago. 7th Cir. 1983, 723 F. 2d at 1272, 37

McNabb v. Department of Corrections, 180 P. 3d 1257, Washington (2008), 51

Miller v. French, 530 U.S. 327 (2000), 307n.30

Minix v. Pazera, 3:06-CV-398, 2007 WL 4233455, N.D. Ind. (2007), 139, 158

Minix v. Pazera, 2005 WL 1799538, N.D. Ind. (2005), 139, 158

Minneci v. Pollard, 132 S. Ct. 617 (2012), 565 U.S. ___ (2012), 136, 155

Monroe v. Pape, 365 U.S. 167 (1961), 126, 151

Moore v. Morgan, 922 F. 2d, 1557 n. 4, 11th Cir. (1991), 143

Morales v. Turman, 820 F. 2d 728, 56 USLW 2045 and 430 U.S. 322 (1977), 156–157

Morgan v. Sproat, 432 F. Supp. 1130, S.D. Miss. (1977), 156

Nelson v. Heyne, 491 F. 2d 352 (1974), 156

Newman v. Alabama, 349 F. Supp. 284 (October 4, 1972), 503 F.2d 1320 (1974), 522 F.2d 71 (1975), 5, 128, 152

Obergefell v. Hodges. 135 S. Ct. 2584 (2015), 30

Olmstead v. L.C. and E.W., 527 U.S. 581 (1999), 206–207

Olmstead v. U.S. 277 U.S. 438 (1928), 14

Osterback v. Moore, Case No. 97-2806-CIV-HUCK, S.D. Florida (2001), 298n.10, 304n.61

Ozecki v. Gaugham, 459 F. 2d 6, 8, 1st Cir. (1972), 143

Pennsylvania Department of Corrections v. Yeskey, 524 U.S. 206 (1998), 145, 155

Phillips v. Michigan Department of Corrections, 731 F. Supp. 792, Dist. Court, W.D. Mich. (1990) and affirmed 932 F. 2d 969 (1991), 30, 154

Plata v. Brown, Docket no. 3:01-cn-01351-THE, N.D. Cal, 155, 167

Plata v. Schwarzenegger, Docket no. 3:01-cn-01351-THE, N.D. Cal, 155, 167

Porter v. Nussle, 534 U.S. 516 (2002), 307n.30

Procunier v. Martinez, 416 U.S. 396 (1974), 152

Rennie v. Klein, 462 F. Supp. 1131, D.N.J., (1978), 653 F.2d 836 at 844–847, 3rd Cir. (1981), 720 F.2d 266 (1983), 152, 153

Rhodes v. Chapman, 452 U.S. 146, 131

Robinson v. California, 370 U.S. 660 (1962), 126, 151

Rogers v. Okin, 478 F. Supp. 1342, D. Mass. (1979), 153

Ross v. Blake. 578 U.S. ___ (2016), Docket No. 15-339, 141, 155–156

Ruffin v. Commonwealth of Virginia, 62 Va. (21 Gratt.) 790, 796 (1871), 124

Ruiz et al. v. Gary Johnson, et al., 304n.62

Ruiz v. Estelle, 503 F. Supp. 1265, S.D. Texas (1980); rev'd in part 679 F. 2d 1115, 5th Cir. (1992); modified in part, 688 F. 2d 266, 5th Cir. (1982), 153

Sandin v. Conner, 515 U.S. 472 (1995), 154–155, 163

Schloendorff v. Society of New York Hospital, 211 N.Y. 125, 105 N.E. 92 (1914), 18, 151

S.D. v. Parish of Orleans, LA (2001), 157

Sell v. United States. 539 U.S. 166 (2003), 123 S. Ct. 2174 (2003), 21, 70, 155

Shelton v. Tucker 364 U.S. 479 (1960), 15

Singletary v. Costello. 665 So. 2d. 1099, Fla. App. 4th Dist. (1996), 51

Smith v. Sullivan, 553 F. 2d 373 (1977), 143

Spencer v. Earley, 278 Fed. Appx. 254, 261, 4th Cir. (2008), 146

Spicer v. Williamson, 191 N.C. 487, 490, 132 S.E. 291, 293 (1926), 124–125

Stouffer v. Reid, 413 Md. 491, 993 A2d 104 (2010), 155

Sundstrom v. Frank. See *Fields v. Smith*, 296n.59

Tarasoff v. Board of Regents of the University of California, 551 P. 2d 334 (1976), 295n.29

Tennessee v. Lane, 541 U.S. 509 (2004), 145

Thor v. Superior Court of Solano County (Howard Andrews, Real Party in Interest), 855 P. 2d 375—1993—Cal. Supreme Court, 264

Tillery v. Owens, 719 F. Supp 1256, 1286, W.D. Pa. (1989), aff'd, 907 F. 2d 418, 3rd Cir. (1990), 212

Todaro v. Ward, 565 F. 2d 48 (1977), 132, 152

Torcasio v. Murray, 57 F. 3d. 1340, 4th Cir. (1995), 145

Trop v. Dulles, 356 U.S. 86, 101 (1958), 37, 117, 131, 151

Turner v. Safley, 482 U.S. 78 (1987), 153

United States v. Louisiana et al., Civil Action No. 98-947-B-1, M.D. La. (1998), 157

Vitek v. Jones, 445 U.S. 480, 494–96, 100 S. Ct. 1254 (1980), 153

Walker v. Montana, 68 P. 3d 872 and 885, Mont. (2003), 114

Washington v. Harper, 494 U.S. 210 (1990), 21, 70, 154

Watts v. Ramos, 948 F. Supp. 739, N.D. IL. (1996), 164

West v. Atkins, 487 U.S. 42 (1988),
    153–154

Wilkinson v. Austin, 544 U.S. 74 (2005)
    372 F. 3d 346, affirmed in part,
    reversed in part, and remanded,
    114

Wilson v. Seiter, 501 U.S. 294 (1991), 137,
    154

Witzke v. Johnson. 656 F. Supp. 294,
    297–98, W.D. Mich. (1987), 19–20

Wolff v. McDonnell, 418 U.S. 539 (1974),
    152

Woodford v. Ngo, 126 S. Ct. 2378 (2006),
    307n.30

Youngberg v. Romeo, 457 U.S. 307 (1982),
    153

About the Author

KENNETH FAIVER's educational background includes a bachelor of arts (AB) in psychology and Latin, licentiate (master's) in sacred theology (STL) from Catholic University, master's in labor and industrial relations (MLIR) from Michigan State University, master's of public health (MPH) in medical care organization from the University of Michigan, and doctorate of public health (ABD) in Health Care Administration from the University of Michigan.

Faiver served for 11 years as a priest of the Diocese of Lansing, six of them as pastor of Cristo Rey parish and codirector of the Cristo Rey Community Center in Lansing, Michigan. During and after this time, he was also active in the civil rights movement in Michigan and elsewhere.

For three years, Faiver was associate director of the Inner City Development Project, a large antipoverty program in Milwaukee. He then spent a year researching the process and outcomes of deinstitutionalization and community placement of the mentally ill and developmentally disabled in Michigan. In 1974, he was introduced to the world of correctional health when he was drafted to direct a year-long study of the Michigan prison health care system. After a brief stint as research director for the Bureau of Manpower in the Michigan Department of Labor, the prison health study led to 16 years of service as the associate director of the Michigan Department of Corrections health care program followed by three years as chief medical coordinator for the Puerto Rican prison system. Since then, his interest and passion to contribute to the improvement of the practice of correctional health care have found expression in various ways.

In 1994, Faiver became actively involved in the accreditation of correctional institutions and has visited well over 100 correctional facilities either as lead surveyor for the National Commission on Correctional Health Care or as a health care auditor for the American Correctional Association. In 1995, he formed a small company to recruit and supply qualified health professionals for work in state prison facilities; he managed the company for 20 years. For some of this time, he also directed a program to provide cognitive behavioral therapy drug rehabilitation services in some Michigan jails. Since 1980, he has remained active as a consultant or expert witness in cases regarding correctional health care and has done some writing—papers at national conferences, articles in journals, and now three books.

He is happily married to Rosemary. They have five children and eight engaging grandchildren, all delightful and creative, yet each a unique and truly awesome individual. On any good weather day, you may also find him wearing a broad smile when flying high in his aircraft "just to get a better view of things."